Research and Innovation on the Road to Modern Child Psychiatry

Volume 1

Festschrift for

Professor Sir Michael Rutter

Research and Innovation on the Road to Modern Child Psychiatry

Volume 1

Festschrift for

Professor Sir Michael Rutter

Edited by Jonathan Green and William Yule

GASKELL & The Association of Child Psychology and Psychiatry

Queries concerning copyright should be addressed to The Royal College of Psychiatrists

Cover images:
Front: photographers Anita and John O'Grady, © The British Council 1989
Back: © The Wellcome Trust Medical Library 1996

Gaskell is an imprint of the Royal College of Psychiatrists
17 Belgrave Square, London SW1X 8PG

British Library Cataloguing-in-Publication Data
A catalogue record for this book is available from the British Library.
ISBN 1-901242-62-5

Distributed in North America by American Psychiatric Press, Inc.

Printed by Bell & Bain Limited, Glasgow, UK.

Contents

A series of 12 plates begins opposite p. 80

	List of contributors	vi
	Foreword	vii
1	Prospect and retrospect Lessons from longitudinal research *Barbara Maughan*	1
2	The significance of genetic variation for abnormal behavioural development *Jim Stevenson*	20
3	Reflections on the past and future of developmental psychopathology *Dante Cicchetti*	37
4	Autism Two-way interplay between research and clinical work *Michael Rutter*	54
5	Developmental neuropsychiatry The foundations of neuropsychiatry in childhood *Eric Taylor*	81
6	Five decades of research on autism Progress and promise *Fred R. Volkmar*	93
7	Classification and categorisation revisited *David Shaffer*	104
8	Making sense of the increasing prevalence of conduct disorder *Lee N. Robins*	115
9	Psychosocial adversity and child psychopathology *Michael Rutter*	129
10	Appreciation of Professor Sir Michael Rutter *Ann Le Couteur*	153
	Index	163

Contributors

Dante Cicchetti   Director, Mount Hope Family Center, University of Rochester, 187 Edinburgh Street, Rochester, NY 14608, USA

Ann Le Couteur   Professor of Child and Adolescent Psychiatry, Fleming Nuffield Unit, University of Newcastle, Burdon Terrace, Jesmond, Newcastle upon Tyne NE2 3AE, UK

Jonathan Green   Senior Lecturer and Honorary Consultant in Child and Adolescent Psychiatry, University of Manchester, Academic Department of Child and Adolescent Psychiatry, Booth Hall Children's Hospital, Blackley, Manchester M9 7AA, UK

Barbara Maughan   External Scientific Staff, Medical Research Council Social, Genetic and Developmental Psychiatry Research Centre, Institute of Psychiatry, De Crespigny Park, London SE5 8AF, UK

Lee N. Robins   4501 Lindell Boulevard, Apt 16b, St Louis, MI 63108-2039, USA

Michael Rutter   Professor of Developmental Psychopathology, Medical Research Centre Child Psychiatry Unit and Social, Genetic and Developmental Psychiatry Research Centre, Institute of Psychiatry, De Crespigny Park, London SE5 8AF, UK

David Shaffer   Irving Philips Professor of Child Psychiatry, Columbia University College of Physicians and Surgeons, New York State Psychiatric Institute, 1051 Riverside Drive, New York, NY 10032, USA

Jim Stevenson   Professor of Psychology, Centre for Research into Psychological Development, Department of Psychology, University of Southampton, Highfields, Southampton SO17 1BJ, UK

Eric Taylor   Professor of Child and Adolescent Psychiatry, Institute of Psychiatry, De Crespigny Park, London SE5 8AF, UK

Fred R. Volkmar   Professor of Child Psychiatry, Pediatrics and Psychology, Child Study Center, Yale University, PO Box 207900, New Haven, CT 06520, USA

William Yule   Professor of Applied Child Psychology, Institute of Psychiatry, De Crespigny Park, London SE5 8AF, UK

Foreword

Jonathan Green and William Yule

The retirement of Professor Sir Michael Rutter from the MRC Child Psychiatry Unit in 1998 was a landmark event for child mental health research and practice, both in the UK and around the world. Not that any of his colleagues expected this formal transition to affect his ongoing research work and productivity. Indeed, his retirement coincided with the opening of the Social, Genetic and Developmental Psychiatry Research Centre at the Institute of Psychiatry, of which he was prime mover and initial director. However, the formal retirement did lead the Child and Adolescent Faculty of the Royal College of Psychiatrists and the Association for Child Psychology and Psychiatry independently to plan events to celebrate his life and work until that point. When we realised each other's plans, the decision was made to combine forces and to publish the contents of the separate events as a single Festschrift volume in honour of Michael Rutter's achievement and contribution. In addition, a second, companion, volume was planned which would reproduce some of Mike's classic papers: this would act both a celebratory compilation and as source material for much of what is referred to in the Festschrift.

It is appropriate that the Festschrift should have originated as it did. Michael Rutter is very much a child and adolescent psychiatrist, but cross-disciplinary association with academic psychologists, educationalists and developmentalists of all kinds has distinguished his work. Many of the contributors to this volume make clear that the evolution of developmental psychopathology as a theoretical model and basis for research strategies has been greatly influenced by his efforts in linking across specialisms and bringing a rigorous developmental perspective to the field.

The Association for Child Psychology and Psychiatry held their event in London in June 1998 and the Royal College of Psychiatrists held theirs in Bristol in September 1998. Each meeting was the occasion for a major presentation from Mike himself, both subsequently published and reproduced here. These two presentations appropriately represent twin pillars of his research activity and achievement. The first was a broad review of the development of scientific research into autism: a progress that has established the genetic basis of the disorder and made it amenable to emerging molecular genetic research strategies. Mike reminded us in this lecture what huge conceptual advances there had been since he first entered this field and how the early genetic studies required an imaginative challenge to many dominant assumptions of the day. His own work over 30 years has been seminal to this progress. The other lecture, delivered to the Child and Adolescent Faculty of the Royal College of Psychiatrists as the inaugural Michael Rutter lecture, represented the other pole of Mike's achievement. Entitled 'Psychosocial adversity and child psychopathology' it was a review of a broad sweep of psychosocial research, refining over the years the areas in which psychosocial adversity and risk factors affect the development of child mental health. Again Mike could point to his own work at the forefront of many of these developments.

Just the mention of these two titles of course illustrates the massive range of Mike's achievement. The newly established Social, Genetic and Developmental Psychiatry Research Centre pulls the two threads together into a new generation of research: modelling complex interactions between genetic vulnerability and psychosocial experience. Between these two poles Mike has been greatly influential in defining the boundaries of modern child mental health thinking. A number of the contributors to this volume enlarge on these influences. Fred Volkmar amplifies the work on autism and Jim Stevenson gives further coverage of genetic advances. On the other side, Lee Robins and Barbara Maughan amplify the work in psychosocial development and make reference to joint work that they have both done with Mike in the field.

However, there has been activity in even more areas. Mike has been at the forefront of the evolution of classification systems and of bringing US-based and European-based systems rather closer together in recent years. The history of this work is described in this volume by David Shaffer, with whom he collaborated on much of it. Mike's early work, stemming from the Isle of Wight studies on the consequences of brain disorder for psychopathology, are illustrated in Eric Taylor's chapter. Dante Cicchetti pays tribute to Mike's work at the forefront of advances in developmental psychopathology. As a number of these contributors point out, Mike has also been a great ambassador for child mental health in wider areas of scientific endeavor (particularly as a Fellow of the Royal Society), and in policy-making (witness his reassessment of maternal deprivation and the impact of school on children's development). Through all this he has played a leading role in a transformation of the way that clinical child mental health work has been practiced over four decades.

Ann Le Couteur's more personal appreciation addresses a number of other aspects of Mike's career, as family man, colleague, teacher and boss. She touches on a question that must have entered the minds of all Mike's audiences worldwide and over time: what is the secret of this man's astonishing breadth and productivity? As a friend, Ann both suggests the question and resists a simplistic answer. We are left at the end of this volume – as we were in the warm atmosphere of both meetings – celebrating and enjoying Mike's productivity and the benefits that it has reaped for the field of child and adolescent mental health and, through this, for children and families worldwide. Neither meeting was marked by overblown tributes or exaggerated hyperbole: this is not his style. As a committed scientist Mike lets the facts speak for themselves without excessive gloss. What is illustrated in this and the companion volume is a sober, imaginative and sophisticated elaboration of research practice across the whole field over four decades – and that is his real legacy.

1 Prospect and retrospect

Lessons from longitudinal research

Barbara Maughan

Throughout his career, Michael Rutter has been a strong advocate of the value of longitudinal research in advancing our understanding of both normal and abnormal development (Rutter, 1977, 1981, 1988, 1989, 1991, 1993, 1994). Longitudinal studies play a central role in charting the stability of personality traits and psychiatric symptoms throughout development, in identifying early predictors of later adverse outcomes and in highlighting the processes that reinforce poor functioning in some individuals but allow more positive developmental trajectories in others. Knowledge about patterns of later outcome can cast important light back on our models of child psychopathology and forward on our understanding of both intra- and intergenerational continuities in disorder and distress. If we are serious in our commitment to a developmental perspective on psychopathology, longitudinal research must form part of our scientific armoury.

Rutter's own concern with longitudinal methods has been far from purely theoretical. The Isle of Wight studies (Rutter *et al*, 1976) were among the first to introduce a longitudinal element into epidemiological investigations of childhood, and he has since directed and collaborated on a wide range of longer-term follow-ups, stretching from childhood to adult life (e.g., Quinton & Rutter, 1988; Harrington *et al*, 1990; Quinton *et al*, 1990; Rutter & Mawhood, 1991; Maughan *et al*, 1996). It is this long-term perspective on psychopathology, spanning distinct developmental periods, that forms the main focus of this chapter. In addition to its theoretical significance, long-term longitudinal research of this kind is in a unique position to build bridges to clinical practice. For practitioners, the almost universal separation of child and adult services inevitably constrains perspectives: workers in children's services often remain unaware of the long-term outlook for the children they treat, while those in adult settings have few chances to observe the early roots of their patients' difficulties. The life-span perspective offered by longitudinal research provides one key means of bridging that divide.

Over a decade ago, Rutter took the theme of pathways from childhood to adulthood for his Jack Tizard Memorial Lecture to the Association for Child Psychology and Psychiatry (Rutter, 1989). He began by highlighting some central principles that have emerged from longitudinal research on both normal and abnormal development: the need to see each phase of development within a full life-span perspective; the need to pay attention to key transitions in development and to the social contexts in which they occur; the need to focus on both continuities and discontinuities in poor functioning, and the processes that contribute to each; and the variety of mechanisms – genetic, biological and experiential – that contribute to development over time. In the late 1980s, when he set out those issues, the number of empirical studies of psychopathology spanning the childhood to adult years was still quite limited. Over the intervening years the research base has expanded markedly. Increasing numbers of well-researched childhood cohorts have matured to adulthood, and a widening range of adult studies have included retrospective reports of childhood disorder and experiences. Methodological investigations have clarified both the limitations and the utility of retrospective reports (Rutter *et al*, 1997*a*), and advances in statistical methodology have made possible increasingly sophisticated modelling of developmental processes (e.g., Fergusson, 1997; Willett *et al*, 1998). Developments in each of these areas have served to confirm and elaborate on the propositions Rutter set forth. Below I highlight just a few key themes emerging from this more recent work.

Developmental trends in disorders

A first need has been to delineate age trends and continuities in disorder across the childhood and early adult years. Although a large number of studies have now examined segments of this age span, detailed data on the same samples, and covering the full age period, are still limited. The most comprehensive evidence to date comes from the Dunedin Multidisciplinary Study of Health and Development (Silva, 1990). This study assessed a representative, community sample of about 1000 young people at 2- to 3-yearly intervals from age 3 years, and included formal assessments of psychiatric disorder between the ages of 11 and 21 years.

A rich longitudinal data-set of this kind provides a variety of perspectives on the development of disorder. The first, focusing on age trends in disorder, comes from cross-sectional estimates of prevalence at different ages. Figure 1.1 shows 1-year prevalence rates of any psychiatric disorder in the Dunedin cohort over five consecutive study contacts, beginning at age 11. Rates remained relatively stable between ages 11 and 13, and showed just a slight rise at age 15. Between ages 15 and 18, however, there was a dramatic increase, followed by a levelling out in the early 20s (Newman *et al*, 1996). Over the course of adolescence, overall rates of disorder increased two-fold, from 18% at age 11 to a high point of 41% at age 18. In addition to disorders arising for the first time in childhood, the transitional years from middle to late adolescence appear to mark a major increase in risk for psychopathology.

These cross-sectional findings reflect aggregate trends. The power of longitudinal data, however, lies in their capacity to reveal continuity and change at the individual level. Two different perspectives are available here: one, as it were, looking backwards from early adulthood, the second forwards from middle adolescence. Each tells a slightly different story. Looking backwards, the picture seems one of strong continuity in vulnerability to disorder between childhood and early adult life. Figure 1.2 illustrates this, showing the proportions of young adults identified as suffering from a disorder at age 21 who had shown difficulties at earlier ages. In each of the main diagnostic categories, at least 70% of young people who met DSM–III–R criteria for disorder (American Psychiatric Association, 1987) at age 21 had already been identified as showing disorder at one or more of the previous study contacts (Newman *et al*, 1996). Rates of new adult onset were highest for mood and substance disorders, lowest for dysthymia and antisocial personality. By comparison with new-onset cases, young adults with histories of prior disorder were

2 ∎

Fig. 1.1 Age trends in psychiatric disorder, ages 11–21 years. (Dunedin, NZ; from Newman et al, 1996.)

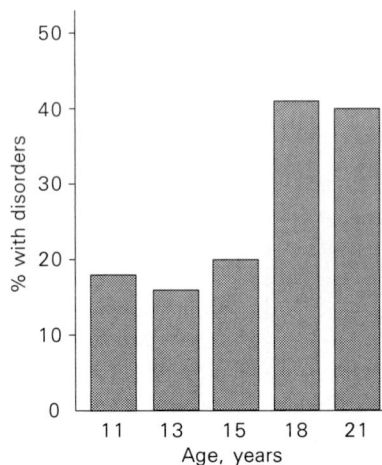

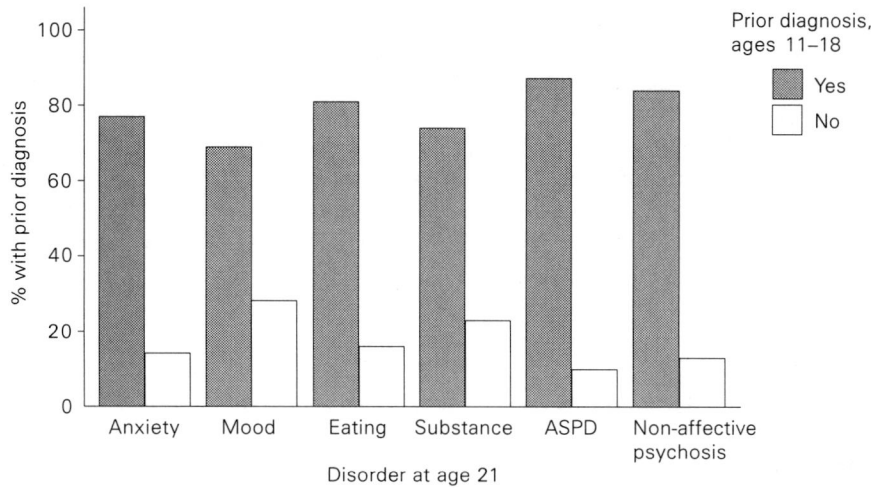

Fig. 1.2 Looking backwards: disorder at age 21, prior diagnosis at ages 11–18. ASPD, antisocial personality disorder. (Dunedin, NZ; from Newman et al, 1996.)

more severely affected at age 21, more likely to have comorbid diagnoses and showed more indicators of clinical impairment. Retrospective studies in adulthood (e.g., Christie *et al*, 1988) and the few other prospective studies to have presented 'follow-back' analyses of this kind (e.g., Pine *et al*, 1998) support a similar view. Much adult disorder has ITS roots in childhood problems; many young adults with psychiatric problems are likely to show difficulties that are chronic, or episodically remitting at best.

Viewed prospectively, the data highlight somewhat different features. Figure 1.3 illustrates this, focusing on developments in the Dunedin cohort between ages 15 and 18. It divides the sample into three broad groups according to their status at age 15: those with no disorder in the mid-teens; those with predominantly emotional difficulties; and those with antisocial/disruptive disorders (Feehan *et al*, 1993). As we might anticipate from the steep overall rise in rates of disorder in late adolescence, about a third of the young people without marked problems at age 15 showed a new onset of disorder later in their teens. Emotional difficulties were most prominent among these 'new' disorders, but, in addition, some 18-year-olds began to show 'adolescence-limited' problems in the domains of antisocial behaviour and substance use, and a small group showed a mixed pattern of difficulties. Identifying the biological, psychological and social factors that contribute to this steep rise in vulnerability to disorder in the late teens is an urgent priority for future longitudinal research projects.

For young people already showing disorder at age 15, three main features are of note. First, although risks of disorder later in adolescence were markedly higher than for groups without disorders, continuities were far from complete. About a third of these young people showed no marked problems later in their teens. Although continuities in disorder seemed strong looking backwards, looking forwards the picture seemed much less deterministic. This same contrast has been highlighted in other long-term studies. Probably the best-known example comes from Robins' (1966) classic follow-up of child

■ 3

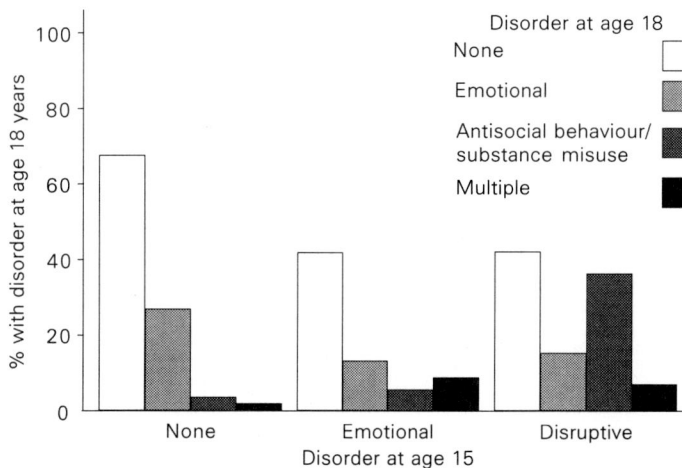

Fig. 1.3 Looking forwards: continuities in disorder, ages 15–18 years. (Dunedin, NZ; from Feehan et al, 1993.)

guidance patients. Looking backwards from adulthood, an early history of antisocial behaviour seemed almost a prerequisite for severe antisocial problems in adult life. Looking forwards from childhood, only about a third of severely antisocial children went on to be antisocial adults. A similar picture appears to hold in relation to anxiety disorders (Pine *et al*, 1998). As Rutter argued (1989), our models of development need to account for both continuity and change.

Two other key features of outcomes for young people with disorder in mid-adolescence are highlighted in Fig. 1.3. First, overall risks of persistence were closely similar for 15-year-olds with either emotional or behavioural problems. But second, the nature of those continuities varied in important ways. For adolescents who had had emotional problems in their mid-teens, anxiety and depression continued to constitute much the most likely pattern of problems 3 years later. Continuities were predominantly homotypic to phenotypically similar disorders later in the teens. For those with antisocial disorders, later outcomes were more varied. Many continued to show antisocial behaviour or drug-related problems, but a sizeable minority followed an apparently different pathway, with their prime vulnerability in the late teens most evident in the affective domain. Links between childhood conduct problems and later depressive phenomena have been documented in other prospective studies (e.g. Rutter, 1991) and accord well with retrospective findings that childhood conduct problems are associated with elevated risks for a wide variety of disorders, both internalising and externalising, in adult life (Robins & Price, 1991; Zoccolillo, 1992). Understanding the processes that underlie unexpected, heterotypic continuities of this kind has been among the key challenges posed by longitudinal research.

4 ■

In addition to broadly based epidemiological/longitudinal findings of this kind, recent years have seen important progress in our understanding of developmental trends in many individual disorders (see Rutter, 1996*a,* for an overview). The most extensive advances have probably been made in relation to conduct disorder and antisocial behaviours (Maughan & Rutter, 1998; Rutter *et al*, 1998), hyperactivity (Taylor *et al*, 1996; Mannuzza *et al*, 1998) and depression (Rao *et al*, 1995; Harrington *et al*, 1996; Hankin *et al*, 1998). In addition, important gains have been made in a range of other areas. Follow-back analyses have identified early childhood neurological, cognitive and behavioural precursors of schizophrenia (Jones, 1997), and prospective studies have traced the developmental picture in autism to the middle adult years (Nordin & Gillberg, 1998). Follow-ups of samples with reading disabilities have shown that, although reading difficulties persist, comorbidity with antisocial behaviour may decline in adult life (Maughan *et al*, 1996). By contrast, severe receptive language problems are often followed by serious and persistent social deficits in adulthood (Rutter & Mawhood, 1991), and mild learning disability continues to be associated with poor social conditions and with high rates of psychological distress well beyond the end of schooling (Maughan *et al*, 1999). Childhood behavioural precursors are beginning to be identified for adult personality disorders (Bernstein *et al*, 1996), and temperamental characteristics assessed as early as age 3 years have been found to show modest but interpretable links with disorder almost two decades later (Caspi *et al*, 1996). At this stage, the largest gaps in our understanding of basic developmental trends lie in the field of anxiety disorders. Despite their high prevalence at all developmental periods, reliable pointers to links between anxiety disorders in childhood and their adult counterparts are only now beginning to emerge (Last *et al*, 1997; Pine *et al*, 1998).

Other sequelae of childhood disorder

Much of this first generation of prospective research has been concerned to document risks of persisting vulnerability to psychiatric disorder. However, it is has also revealed that the legacy of childhood disorder extends well beyond vulnerability to psychiatric symptomatology alone. Numerous studies have now confirmed that children with emotional or behavioural problems are likely to face problems in many different aspects of their adult functioning. The widest spectrum of risks seems to follow from early disruptive behaviours: oppositional and conduct disorders and attention-deficit hyperactivity disorder (Offord & Bennett, 1994; Mannuzza *et al*, 1998; Maughan & Rutter, 1998). In comparison with groups without disorders, children with disruptive behavioural problems are more likely to: show poor educational attainments and to drop out of school (Cairns *et al*, 1989; Kessler *et al*, 1995); have poorer early work histories and higher risk of unemployment (Sanford *et al*, 1994; Caspi *et al*, 1998); leave their homes and families at a younger age (Bardone *et al*, 1996); enter romantic and sexual relationships earlier and experience more difficulties and breakdown in those relationships (Stattin & Magnusson, 1996); become pregnant or father children earlier than their peers (Kessler *et al*, 1997*a*); be involved in crime (Farrington *et al*, 1990); and have poorer general health in their early adult lives (Bardone *et al*, 1998). Evidence on the psychosocial sequelae of emotional difficulties is less extensive. At this stage, evidence suggests that problems in social functioning may be less pervasive and somewhat different in form (Turnbull *et al*, 1990). Retrospective studies suggest that early-onset anxiety disorders and depression can also compromise educational achievement (Kessler *et al*, 1995), and there are indications that they may be associated with difficulties in relationship formation and quality (Kandel & Davies, 1986). The limited evidence to date suggests that one characteristic feature may be delayed involvement in adult roles: in the US National Comorbidity Study, for example, early-onset dysthymia and social phobias were both associated with significant delays in age at first marriage, and other emotional diagnoses showed similar trends (Forthofer *et al*, 1996). At this stage, however, we still await a full characterisation of the implications of early emotional difficulties for social functioning in adult life.

The most serious and pervasive problems in adult social functioning – commensurate with many definitions of personality disorder – seem restricted to relatively small groups of children with the most severe childhood difficulties. But taking a less severe definition, much larger groups seem likely to be affected. Zoccolillo *et al* (1992), for example, explored early adult outcomes in a high-risk sample (children raised in institutional care) and an inner-city comparison group, focusing on functioning in four domains: work, intimate relationships, friendships and crime. Not unexpectedly, conduct disorder in childhood predicted antisocial personality disorder in a small subgroup. In addition, however, the great majority of children with conduct disorders showed problems in at least two of these adult domains. Young people without conduct disorders often faced problems in individual aspects of their functioning; what seemed characteristic of groups with previous disorders was the pervasiveness of their difficulties across domains. A similar pattern has now been documented in other studies of socially disadvantaged samples (Quinton *et al*, 1993; Maughan *et al*, 1995). At this stage, it is less clear whether this constitutes an inherent part of the conduct disorder syndrome, a secondary consequence of early impairments, or – as outcomes appear to be better in middle-class samples (Jessor *et al*, 1991) – a result of social disadvantage.

■5

These findings underscore the heavy personal costs that can follow from childhood disorder. Not surprisingly, those costs have other dimensions. Health economic evaluations are now beginning to chart the economic burden of childhood disorder in terms of need for services, dependence on benefits and the cost of lost opportunities (Knapp *et al*, 1999) This group has also estimated the cumulative costs deriving from special educational and mental health service use, substitute parental care, dependence on unemployment benefit and involvement in crime in a longitudinal follow-up of an inner-city epidemiological sample from age 10 to their late 20s (further details available from the author upon request). Teacher ratings of problem behaviour in childhood were strong predictors of later cost differentials, and diagnostic measures even more strikingly so. By comparison with average costs for 10-year-olds without behavioural or emotional problems, cost levels for children with teacher-rated emotional difficulties were 50% higher and those for children with teacher-rated conduct problems were over three times higher. A diagnosis of conduct disorder attracted the highest cost levels, 10 times those expected for children without emotional or behavioural difficulties. Childhood disorder imposes perhaps its heaviest burdens on individuals and their families, but the burden on society is far from negligible.

To conclude this brief overview, we must also note the expanding volume of research examining links between adverse experiences in childhood and outcomes later in life. Historically, much of this work has relied on retrospective studies (e.g. Brown & Harris, 1978), and retrospective methods continue to play a key role (e.g. Fergusson *et al*, 1996;

**Childhood
adversity and
adult functioning**

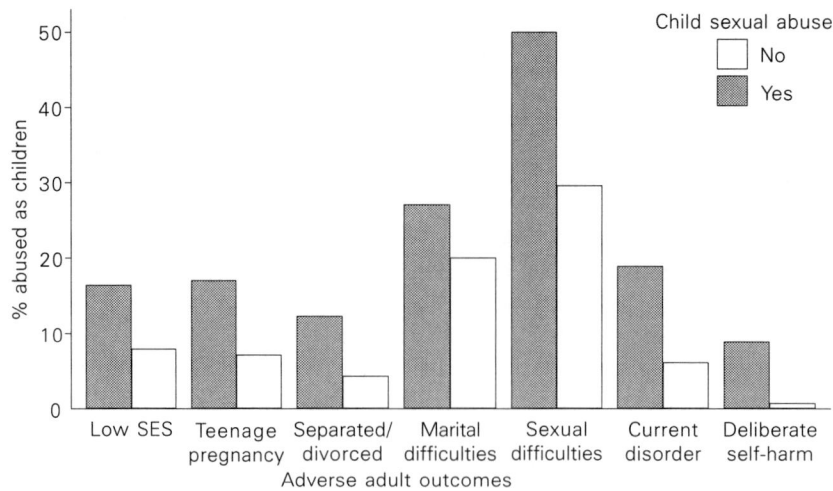

Fig.1.4 Childhood sexual abuse: adverse adult outcomes. SES, socio-economic status. (From Romans et al, 1997.)

Kessler *et al*, 1997*b*; Romans *et al*, 1997). Despite concerns that distressed adults might overreport difficulties in their childhood, methodological investigations suggest that in general, retrospective reporting is unlikely to introduce serious bias (Maughan & Rutter, 1997). None the less, confirmation from prospective studies inevitably provides a more secure basis for conclusions. In some areas – such as the long-term implications of parental divorce – extensive prospective evidence is now available (Amato & Keith, 1991; Rodgers & Pryor, 1998). In others – such as the consequences of physical abuse and neglect – prospective findings remain much more limited (Widom & White, 1997).

Although the specifics of their findings vary in important ways, a number of features have emerged in common across many of these studies. First, although childhood adversities are often associated with increased risks of poor adult outcome, severe adult difficulties affect only a minority of the children exposed. Variations in the severity or pervasiveness of childhood risks, individual differences in susceptibility and interactions with later stressors all seem likely to be important in mediating effects (Maughan & McCarthy, 1997). In general, chronically adverse experiences seem likely to hold stronger implications for later psychopathology than do acute events, and a lack of important positive experiences may have consequences as deleterious as actively negative ones.

Second, if adult functioning is affected, risks of psychiatric disorder once again form only part of a wider spectrum of difficulties that can encompass adult social status, educational and occupational achievements, patterns of relationship formation and child-bearing, and the quality and stability of relationships. Figure 1.4 provides one illustration of this kind, taken from a retrospective study of child sexual abuse (Romans *et al*, 1997).

Third, although it has often been hypothesised that particular types of early adversity are predictors of particular types of adult outcome, current evidence suggests relatively little specificity in the linkages involved. Romans *et al* (1997), for example, found no evidence for a distinctive post-abuse syndrome in their community sample, and concluded that child sexual abuse is best regarded as a non-specific risk for a wide spectrum of psychological and social outcomes. In part, this lack of specificity seems likely to reflect the frequent overlaps between adversities in childhood, and the high rates of comorbidity between disorders and poor functioning in adult life. Few children experience single, severe adversities, and many adults show overlapping patterns of disorder; tracking specific outcomes from particular types of early experience is inevitably a complex task. But it also seems possible that many aspects of early family adversity do indeed have broadly pathogenic implications, and that outcomes vary primarily as a function of individual susceptibilities, intervening circumstances or the severity of early risks.

Individual differences in outcome

Taken together, these findings highlight a series of more general themes. First, the long-term sequelae of early disorder and disadvantage extend well beyond risks of recurrence of psychiatric disorder. Whether as researchers or clinicians, if we confine our attention to diagnostic categories alone we risk overlooking aspects of children's functioning that are important in terms of individual distress and that may also contribute to the perpetuation of disorder. Second, there may be multiple developmental pathways to similar adult outcomes, and divergent sequelae from the same early risks (Cicchetti & Rogosch, 1996). Many developmental pathways are complex and depend on particular configurations of individual and environmental risks. And third, although continuities are strong, they are rarely, if ever, complete. Most studies suggest marked individual differences in risks of adverse adult outcomes, with some young people succumbing to later difficulties, while others follow a more benign outcome course.

How might we begin to understand these varying patterns? A number of different factors seems likely to be important here. First, variability in outcomes may point to heterogeneity in our current concepts of childhood disorder, with different developmental trajectories signalling potentially important aetiological and nosological distinctions. Second, the processes that maintain a disorder may differ in important ways from those involved in its initiation. Tracking exposure to those later risks may be crucial if we are to understand how pathways diverge over time. Third, multiple developmental systems seem likely to be implicated, each of which may prove important targets for research and intervention. And finally, although early models viewed developmental continuities largely in terms of trait persistence, a variety of findings now suggest patterns involving both direct and more indirect links. Some persisting effects may depend on negative chain reactions set off by early risks that subsequently play a key role in perpetuating vulnerability to disorder.

Some of the variability in later outcomes seems likely to signal meaningful heterogeneity in our existing categorisations of disorder. Variations in course are among the key criteria used to validate classificatory schemes (Cantwell & Rutter, 1994), and data on the long-term outcomes of childhood disorders have played a central role in highlighting potentially important distinctions here. Four rather different examples, focusing either on individual disorders or on the comorbidity between them, serve to underscore the importance of long-term follow-up data in this regard.

Heterogeneity in categories of disorder ■ 7

Childhood depression

Concepts of depression in childhood have changed radically over recent years. Initial scepticism that depressive disorders could occur in childhood gave way first to the recognition that syndromes resembling adult depression do indeed occur, and then to the understanding that these syndromes are likely to encompass important heterogeneity (Harrington, 1994; Harrington *et al*, 1996). Findings on long-term outcome have been central to both of these advances. First, adult outcome data have provided strong support for the validity of early-onset depressive disorders: depressed children show a much elevated, and apparently specific, vulnerability to depression in adult life (Harrington *et al*, 1990; Rao *et al*, 1995). Second, both follow-up and other findings have pointed to variability within childhood depression. Risk of adult major depression seems most likely, for example, when the clinical picture in childhood closely resembles adult depression. Childhood-onset dysthymia may also be a marker for recurrent affective illness (Kovacs, 1996). In addition, recent findings suggest that outcomes may also depend in important ways on age at onset. Here, early evidence suggests potentially significant variations between pre- and post-pubertal onset, with continuities to later depression stronger in post-pubertal groups. Family history also seems to vary between age-at-onset groups in potentially informative ways (Harrington *et al*, 1997). At this stage, current models in each of these areas rest on results from just a few follow-up investigations. As more well-characterised childhood samples are tracked to adulthood, we can anticipate further important refinements in our understanding of childhood depressive phenomena.

Depression and conduct disorder

One pattern of particular interest here concerns the co-occurrence of depression and conduct problems. Of the many different forms of apparently heterotypic comorbidity between childhood diagnoses, overlaps between conduct disorder and depression are among the most common: a recent meta-analysis estimated a median joint odds ratio of 6.6 for conduct-disorder–depression comorbidity, little lower than the rate at which depression and anxiety co-occur (Angold *et al*, 1999). The aetiology and meaning of the comorbid pattern, however, has continued to generate debate, with different commentators viewing it as evidence of a separate and distinct syndrome, a subtype of conduct disorder, a consequence of conduct problems, or evidence that conduct disorder itself constitutes a disorder of multiple dysfunction (e.g. Zoccolillo, 1992; Steinhausen & Reitzle, 1996). Although these questions are far from being settled, both prospective and retrospective findings on long-term continuities have contributed to refining the nature of the debate.

A number of different veins of evidence are important here. First, the few data currently available tracing comorbid samples prospectively from childhood to adulthood suggest that the presence of early depressive phenomena does little to moderate the course of antisocial disorders: comorbid groups go on to show levels of adult criminality and social dysfunction quite as marked as those expected in conduct-disorder-only samples (Harrington *et al*, 1991). Second, in well-characterised clinical samples, risks of recurrence of major depression are also high. Fombonne *et al* (2001*a*), tracking samples over a 20-year follow-up period, found closely comparable patterns of relapse in depression-only and comorbid cases, together with an increased risk of minor depression in the comorbid group. We must await data from follow-ups of community samples to assess how far this pattern of pervasively poor outcomes for comorbid cases is paralleled in non-referred groups. The ominous outlook for some young people with comorbid conduct and depressive disorders is, however, already clear: all currently available evidence suggests that risks of suicidality are markedly increased in comorbid groups by contrast with young people with either depression or conduct disorder alone (see, e.g., Lewinsohn *et al*, 1994; Fombonne *et al*, 2001*b*). Whether the developmental mechanisms are similar remains to be determined. I return to these issues later.

Depression and anxiety

Longitudinal findings are also beginning to contribute to our understanding of another key pattern of comorbidity, that between depression and anxiety. High rates of overlap between these disorders have long been observed in both childhood and adult samples, and biological and pharmacological investigations and family history have been used to examine their meaning. More recently, follow-up studies have begun to highlight both some specificity and also potentially important non-specificity in their course. Some of the most illuminating prospective findings to date come from the New York State longitudinal study (Pine *et al*, 1998), tracing a community sample of adolescents over an 11-year period. With well-characterised groups at initial assessment, the investigators identified a series of different developmental trajectories among subgroups in their sample. First, both simple and social phobias showed considerable specificity in their course: each predicted to the same disorder in early adulthood, with no significantly raised risk for other diagnoses. By contrast, other anxiety and mood disorders followed a much less clearly differentiated course. Instead, the findings revealed a broad pattern of conjoint associations between overanxious disorder, generalised anxiety, panic and major depression: adolescent depression was a predictor of generalised anxiety disorder in adulthood, but overanxious disorder was also a predictor of later depression. As the authors note, these findings are consistent with the possibility, also suggested by twin (Kendler *et al*, 1995) and retrospective (Brown *et al*, 1993) studies, that depressive and anxiety disorders may share a common aetiological base.

Age at onset of antisocial behaviours

Finally, knowledge of long-term outcomes has been central to recent proposals for a developmental taxonomy of disruptive and antisocial behaviours (Moffitt, 1993). The heterogeneity of disruptive disorders has long been recognised, yet satisfactory solutions have proved hard to identify. Factor analytic studies have suggested subdivisions based on behavioural dimensions (Loeber & Schmaling, 1985; Frick *et al*, 1993), while successive revisions of the diagnostic criteria have proposed other distinctions: aggressive

8 ■

and non-aggressive, socialised and unsocialised, and differentiations between oppositional-defiant and conduct disorders. Most recently, developmental models focusing on distinctions depending on age at onset have been included in the DSM–IV criteria (American Psychiatric Association, 1994). Among the range of evidence supporting this approach, data on long-term outcomes played a crucial role.

Early onset has long been identified as one of the strongest predictors of the persistence of disruptive behaviours in childhood (Loeber, 1982), and early-onset offending shows similar links with persistence of adult crime (Farrington *et al*, 1990). Genetic studies (DiLalla & Gottesman, 1989; Lyons *et al*, 1995) suggest that antisocial behaviour and criminality in adulthood show higher heritability than adolescent offending, and retrospective studies of antisocial personality disorder (Robins *et al*, 1991) point to early onset of conduct problems as one of the most important childhood predictors. Subsequent studies have highlighted other key distinctions between childhood- and adolescence-onset groups. While early onset of antisocial behaviours is associated with a wide spectrum of risks (cognitive and language deficits, adverse temperamental features, hyperactivity, attentional problems, impulsivity, aggression, family adversity, parenting deficits and poor peer relations), adolescence-onset groups have been found to show fewer individual risks and more adequate peer relations (Moffitt *et al*, 1996). Variations in long-term outcome provided a key impetus for the identification of what promises to be a significant advance in our understanding of the heterogeneity of childhood conduct problems.

In addition to highlighting potentially important nosological distinctions, long-term studies have also begun to identify some of the mechanisms involved in mediating continuity and change. In his 1989 Jack Tizard Lecture, Michael Rutter set out the range of processes that are likely be involved here: genetic mechanisms (both direct and indirect); non-genetic effects on the biological substrate; the impact of cognitive skills, social cognitions and coping strategies; continuities in adverse environments; and the ways in which individuals' behaviour at one stage of development can function to select and shape environments later in the life course (Rutter, 1989). We focus here on the last of these mechanisms – the selection and shaping of environments – to highlight themes that may be especially relevant for practice.

Stability and change: mediating mechanisms ∎ 9

Implicitly or explicitly, much early discussion of continuities in psychopathology assumed that persistence reflected the relatively direct unfolding of pathogenic processes over time. More recent accounts (e.g. Magnusson & Cairns, 1996) suggest a more complex model, arguing that development occurs as a joint function of organismic and environmental forces, with the evolving interplay between the individual and his or her environment playing a key role (Rutter *et al*, 1997*b*). Within this broad framework, particular attention has focused on ways in which individual characteristics influence later life experiences, 'selecting' individuals for settings that are congruent with their dispositions and that may in turn reinforce existing behavioural tendencies (Scarr & McCartney, 1983) or increase exposure to later risks (Rutter *et al*, 1995). Robins's classic follow-up of child guidance patients provided telling illustrations of this kind, with its evidence that childhood conduct problems were followed by much increased risks of unemployment, job instability, divorce and lack of friends in adult life (Robins, 1966). Two equally plausible interpretations could be placed on these findings. On the one hand, they provide clear evidence of the persistence of maladaptive behaviour over time: disruptive behaviour in childhood portends poor functioning in adult life. On the other, they suggest that young people with conduct disorders may be exposed to high levels of stress in adulthood: job losses and relationship breakdowns still constitute adverse life events, and a lack of friends still implies an absence of social support, however they come about. Developmentally, the key question turns on the extent to which processes of this kind contribute in independent ways to the persistence of disorder. The most extensive evidence to date comes from studies of continuities in conduct problems and antisocial behaviour. Here, person–environment interactions likely to reinforce behavioural tendencies have been proposed as central mechanisms for stability from infancy and

Selecting and shaping environments

early childhood onwards (Caspi & Moffitt, 1995). I focus here on mechanisms that may be especially relevant to continuities in poor functioning between adolescence and early adult life.

Associations with deviant peers

In adolescence, one central mechanism of this kind appears to centre on affiliations with deviant peers. Deviant peer relations are among the strongest correlates of conduct problems and delinquency in adolescence (Thornberry & Krohn, 1997), and might reflect both social selection and social causation effects. Social selection processes are well-documented in late childhood and adolescent peer relations (Kandel, 1985; Cairns *et al*, 1988). Aggressive and antisocial young people, boys and girls alike, tend to associate with peers with similar behavioural problems, and age trends in delinquency and in reported involvement with delinquent peers track each other closely over time (Warr, 1993). Birds of a feather do, it seems, flock together; more debated has been the extent, over and above these niche-picking tendencies, to which delinquent affiliations contribute to the persistence of antisocial behaviours over time.

Several longitudinal studies have now provided evidence that relations with behaviourally deviant peers do indeed play an independent role in both the initiation (Keenan *et al*, 1995) and the continuity of delinquency in adolescence (Fergusson & Horwood, 1996). In many instances reciprocal processes seem likely to be involved, with patterns of peer relationships both reinforcing and being reinforced by involvement in delinquency. Equally importantly, there are suggestions that similar processes may continue to operate in adulthood. Men who persist in offending in their 20s and 30s continue to show links with peers showing behaviour deviance (Farrington, 1991), and such friendships have themselves been argued to be especially persistent (Warr, 1993). For some young people, early antisocial tendencies appear to elevate their risks of entering peer networks that then play a key role in reinforcing deviant behaviours.

Early-adult role transitions

More wide-ranging opportunities for selecting and shaping environments come with the social role changes facing all young people in late adolescence and early adulthood: leaving school, leaving home, establishing committed adult relationships and becoming parents. Choices made at this period carry important implications for later life chances (Hogan & Astone, 1986) and, like other developmental transitions, can hold within them sources of both stability and change (Graber & Brooks-Gunn, 1996; Rutter, 1996*b*; Elder, 1998). Under propitious circumstances, the new roles and relationships of early adulthood can hold the potential for escape from adverse early trajectories. Equally clearly, the demands of transitional periods can also evoke less beneficial effects. At the behavioural level, novel and ambiguous situations may reinforce existing behavioural tendencies, accentuating prior dispositions rather than prompting change (Elder & Caspi, 1990; Caspi & Moffitt, 1993). In terms of effects on subsequent environments, a range of findings now suggest that young people with emotional or behavioural difficulties tend to approach the transitions of early adulthood in ways that cut off future opportunities and select them for unsupportive, stress-prone or behaviourally deviant adult worlds.

The timing of transitions provides one simple index of these patterns. As outlined earlier, extensive evidence now suggests that young people with disruptive behaviour problems approach the role changes of early adulthood in a precocious, 'accelerated' fashion, exiting from education, leaving home, beginning sexual and cohabiting relationships and becoming parents significantly earlier than their peers. Figure 1.5 provides one illustration of these trends, using data from the National Child Development Study (Maughan & Taylor, 2001). It shows the ages at which young women in the cohort began their first cohabiting/marital relationships, plotted separately for girls with high and low antisocial behaviour ratings in their mid-teens. Antisocial behaviour in adolescence was strongly associated with higher rates of partnership formation in the teens. By age 20, 44% of girls showing antisocial behaviour had begun cohabiting relationships, by contrast with only 28% of their peers.

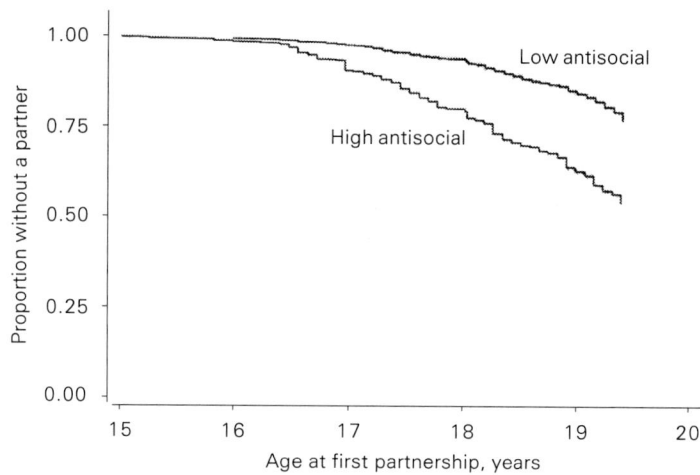

Fig. 1.5 Adolescent conduct problems in women and age at first partnership. (Redrawn with permission from Maughan & Taylor, 2001.)

There is now extensive evidence that early transition patterns of this kind are associated with later difficulty and disadvantage. A variety of different pathways seem likely to be involved here. Dropping out of school, for example, seems likely to constrain employment prospects in relatively direct ways. But the high risks of partnership breakdown associated with early relationship formation (Maughan & Taylor, 2001), and the plethora of adverse consequences of teenage pregnancy and childbearing (Furstenberg *et al*, 1989) may reflect a wider range of processes (Brooks-Gunn *et al*, 1985). Several rather different models have been advanced to account for these effects. First, early or precocious transitions may interrupt the completion of earlier developmental tasks (a 'stage termination' model). Second, from a 'goodness of fit' perspective, the individual may be too immature or unready to take on the demands of the new situation (Lerner, 1985). Third, early transitions in one life domain may pre-empt opportunities in others (so that, for example, early childbearing may cut off opportunities for continued education or for occupational advance). Fourth, individuals entering new roles markedly earlier than their peers may view themselves – or be viewed by others – as deviating in important ways from socially sanctioned patterns of developmental timing, with implications for both self-esteem and sources of support (Neugarten, 1979). And finally, such early transitions may mark the first step in a cumulating pattern of exposure to adverse environmental circumstances, carrying high risks of later stress.

Figure 1.6 illustrates one model of this kind, drawing again on data from the National Child Development Study. It takes as its starting point the heterotypic continuity noted earlier between antisocial behaviour in adolescence and vulnerability to depressed mood in adult life, and explores a range of possible intervening pathways for women in the cohort. The simple bivariate relationship between adolescent antisocial behaviour and adult depressed mood in this sample was clear (odds ratio = 2.06, 95% CI 1.47–2.88). As Fig. 1.6 illustrates, a number of early-adult pathways appeared to mediate these links. The first steps ran through three early-adult role transitions: early motherhood, relationship breakdowns and lack of qualifications. These in turn primarily contributed to low mood through associations with the most proximal risk, socially disadvantaged circumstances at age 33; as Fig. 1.6 shows, teenage motherhood had more direct implications for adult mood. For antisocial girls, life choices made in the teens and early 20s marked the first steps in a pattern of increased exposure to adult stressors that in their turn elevated risks of later depression. Importantly, models focusing on just one of

• 11

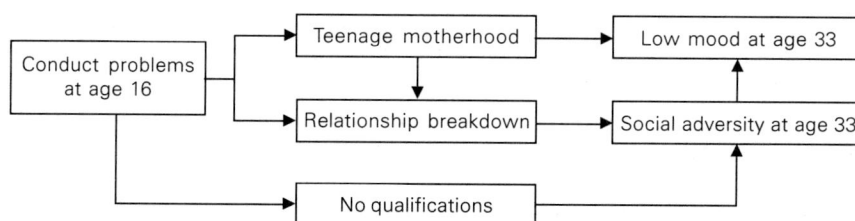

Fig. 1.6 Pathways from adolescent conduct problems to adult low mood in women.

these pathways failed to account for these links; early-adult developments in a number of domains – here including childbearing, interpersonal relationships and social and economic disadvantage – were needed to account for associations between teenage behaviour problems and adult depressed mood.

Close adult relationships

The mediating role of close adult relationships, highlighted in schematic form in these models, has emerged in a wide range of both prospective and retrospective studies. Marital status is among the best-established correlates of psychiatric morbidity in adult life (Bebbington, 1988), with marital disruption associated with increased risks of psychological distress (Bruce & Kim, 1992; Aseltine & Kessler, 1993), and stable relationships, especially perhaps for men, associated with more positive psychological well-being. Lack of a supportive adult relationship has been identified as a key vulnerability factor for depression in women (Harris *et al*, 1990; Bifulco *et al*, 1998) and is associated with poor adult functioning in a range of other domains (e.g. Quinton & Rutter, 1988).

Problems in making or sustaining close adult relationships have consistently been identified as sequelae of childhood disorder and adversity. Adolescent conduct problems (Bardone *et al*, 1996), dysphoric mood (Kandel & Davies, 1986), exposure to sexual abuse (Romans *et al*, 1997) and the experience of parental separation and divorce (Rodgers & Pryor, 1998) are just some of the forms of early distress that show links with later relationship problems. Many different processes might be involved here. Attachment theory (Bowlby, 1973) offers one perspective, arguing that later relationship formation is influenced by internal working models of relationships laid down early in life. Experiences that compromise childhood attachments may thus hold long-term consequences for relationship stability and satisfaction in adulthood. Although yet to be tested in prospective studies, some support is emerging for a model of this kind. Insecure models of attachments in adulthood show strong links with retrospective reports of childhood adversity (Mickelson *et al*, 1997), and one small-scale study has identified a mediating role for attachment representations in links between adverse parenting and problems in marital relationships (McCarthy & Taylor, 2001).

A second route to relationship difficulties may run through assortative mating. Studies of both high-risk (Quinton *et al*, 1993) and general population (Krueger *et al*, 1998) samples have identified clear tendencies for assorting on the basis of behavioural deviance, with antisocial young people showing an increased tendency to form relationships with similarly antisocial partners. It is unclear at this stage how far this reflects active choice processes, a restriction on the 'field of possibles' available to disadvantaged young people and those with disorders, or a lack of support and guidance in making partnership choices. Figure 1.7 illustrates some of the pathways likely to be involved, using data from a study of high-risk and socially disadvantaged girls (Quinton *et al*, 1993). Adolescent conduct problems were associated with markedly increased risks that young women would cohabit with men showing behaviour deviance. Three intervening pathways could be identified here: protective effects of supportive family relationships and an individual disposition to 'planning' key life choices, and risks emanating from affiliations with deviant peers. At each possible branching-point, protective influences reduced risks of deviant first partnerships, adverse factors elevated them. The importance of 'planful competence' for adolescent development has been highlighted in a variety of contexts (Clausen, 1991), and supportive family relationships, along with strong attachments to schooling, have also been identified as protective factors in other high-risk samples (Ensminger & Juon, 1998). Pawlby *et al* (1997), examining very early romantic relationships of high-risk girls, highlighted further issues. Here too, high-risk teenagers began romantic and sexual relationships early, with young men showing behaviour deviance, met casually and known for only limited periods of time. Their investment in these apparently unpropitious relationships, however, was high: they spent more time with boyfriends than with same-gender peers, gave idealised accounts of their dependability and, in a substantial minority of cases, already viewed their boyfriend as their best friend – a development not shown at all in a comparison group of the same age. A range of influences encompassing family, peer group and individual models and expectations of relationships all seem likely to converge to influence early partner choices.

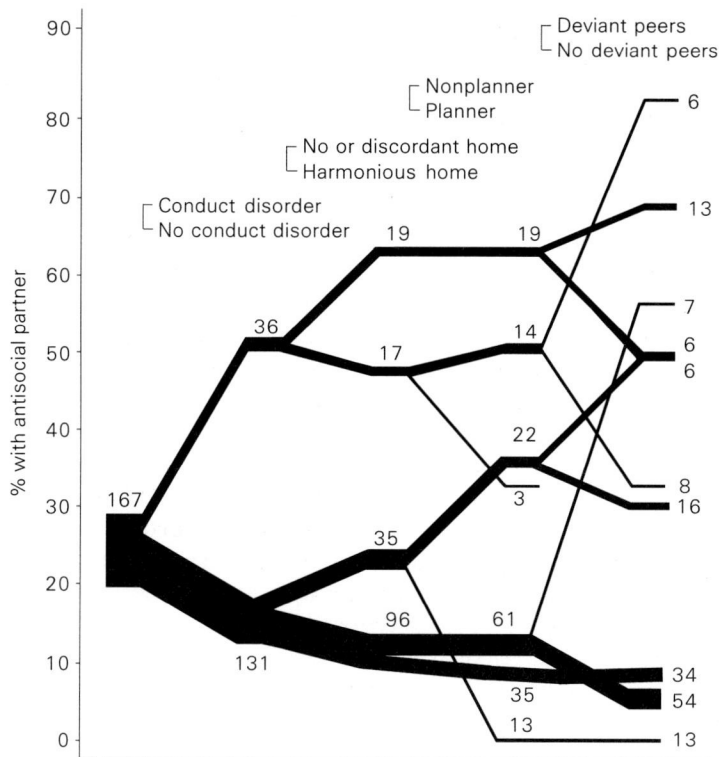

Fig. 1.7 Pathways leading women to relationships with antisocial partners. Frequencies along dividing pathways are shown by the numbers and the line width (redrawn with permission from Quinton et al, 1993). ▪ 13

Cumulating consequences: indirect chains

These and other examples suggest that one important route for the persistence of early disorder may run through its cumulating consequences, elevating risks of exposure to adverse environments in adult life. Models of this kind, variously described as stepping-stone effects (Farrington, 1986), processes of cumulative continuity (Caspi & Moffitt, 1995), indirect chain mechanisms (Rutter, 1997) and processes of social exclusion and marginalisation (Kerner et al, 1995), hold important implications for developmental theory and for practice. From a theoretical perspective, they suggest that continuities in poor functioning not only result from trait persistence, but may also involve more indirect mechanisms, set in train by the effects of early risk. From a practice perspective, the implications are clear: interventions designed to enhance young people's capacities to plan adolescent and early-adult transitions, or to avert them from adverse life pathways at this crucial transitional phase, may hold benefits that extend well beyond the adolescent years.

Perhaps the most compelling support for arguments of this kind comes from studies of early adulthood highlighting the role of positive adult experiences as turning-points away from adverse developmental trajectories (Pickles & Rutter, 1991). Supportive, enduring marital attachments seem especially influential here (Zoccolillo et al, 1992; Quinton et al, 1993; Sampson & Laub, 1993; Farrington & West, 1995), but similar effects have been documented in relation to positive employment experiences, geographical moves and more radical environmental changes such as recruitment into military service (Sampson & Laub, 1996). In each case, previously disadvantaged or delinquent young people exposed to positive experiences later in the life course have shown markedly more adaptive subsequent outcomes.

Turning-points in the life course

Once again, an essential methodological step here has been to test for selection effects: were the young people who encountered these more positive experiences in some way different from those who persisted in less satisfactory functioning? Several studies have now documented effects associated with turning-point experiences that did appear exogenous and could not have been predicted on the basis of individuals' prior characteristics. Farrington & West (1995), for example, chose two carefully matched subgroups of offenders, closely similar in the severity of their prior offending, to examine the effects of marriage. In the 5 years following their marriage, married men committed significantly fewer offences than their single counterparts. Equally important, if marriages broke down, offence rates rose, suggesting reversal effects. Laub *et al* (1998), also exploring the influence of marriage on reduction in offending, used more complex techniques to examine effects of relationships year by year. This more dynamic conceptualisation – also controlling for prior characteristics – suggested that apparent turning-points may be quite gradual in their effects. Reductions in offending were not simply associated with marriage *per se*, nor were they immediate. Instead, they became increasingly evident over time, and occurred in the context of relationships that began early and were characterised by social cohesiveness.

Laub *et al* (1998) also provided explicit tests of one further issue central to developmental models positing both indirect chain and turning-point effects. Each of these conceptualisations assumes that experiences later in the life course play a key role in maintaining or redirecting trajectories. One crucial test here concerns the relative power of early and later factors to predict adult outcomes. Importantly, in this study at least, childhood and adolescent characteristics, powerful predictors of the onset of offending, showed few associations with later criminal trajectories. Instead, more proximal influences – here conceptualised in terms of marital attachments – proved much the more influential factors. Positive adult experiences, when these men encountered them, appeared to provide a much more powerful means of discriminating the later course of offending than many classic and well-established predictors of the onset of delinquent behaviour in childhood and adolescence.

Which aspects of later experiences are most central to these effects? At this stage, findings suggest that experiences that hold the potential to open up new opportunities, that involve environmental change – geographical or interpersonal – and that affect the self-system or social cognitions may be most salient (Rutter, 1996*b*). Sampson & Laub (1993) highlight roles and relationships that foster attachments to social bonds, provide informal social controls and involve a gradual investment in prosocial attachments that, over time, prove inimical to continuance in crime. Just as persistence in behavioural deviance or disorder appears to stem at least in part from the cumulating consequences of early risks, so positive later experiences, when they occur, may contribute to gradually developing preventive effects.

Pointers for practice

Inevitably, this brief overview has been selective, highlighting just some of the key themes to emerge from recent research on childhood–adult links. The focus was chosen to cast light in particular on issues that, in addition to their theoretical significance, may hold messages for practice. Many speak for themselves; I conclude by underscoring two central themes.

First, for many young people suffering from disorders and in distress, problems in social functioning and vulnerability to psychiatric illness seem likely to persist beyond adolescence, and hold important and often wide-ranging implications for their adult lives. Second, although these patterns are common, in many instances they may be neither direct nor inevitable. Although few treatment studies have yet reported on the long-term consequences of their interventions, the 'natural experiments' offered by positive adult experiences suggest that negative chain reactions can be interrupted, and evolving models for the persistence of young people's difficulties emphasise the multiple stages at which intervention may be advantageous. Following these dual threads, several rather different implications appear to follow. First, for the most vulnerable young people, continuing risks may require continuing interventions. Kazdin (2001), for example, argues that currently promising treatments for conduct disorder, most of them time-limited, may need to be supplemented by continuing care or maintenance models, or a 'dental care approach', whereby regular check-ups allow monitoring of progress and provide an early warning that problems may be likely to recur. Second, much early disorder and disadvantage may be reinforced by cumulating later consequences. Offsetting these later risks – especially perhaps those surrounding the key life choices of the adolescent and early adult years – may contribute in significant ways to reducing vulnerability to recurrent disorder. Enhancing family supports, encouraging prosocial attachments and developing young people's own planning and coping skills seem, on the basis of

14 ∎

naturalistic studies, to offer promising routes to protection. The long-term implications of childhood disorder are undoubtedly complex. The studies explored here – in many ways the first generation of long-term longitudinal research – provide some pointers to their amelioration. Future studies, building on these insights, should enable us to target our efforts more precisely.

References

Amato, P. R. & Keith, B. (1991) Parental divorce and adult well-being: a meta-analysis. *Journal of Marriage and the Family*, **53**, 43–58.

American Psychiatric Association (1987) *Diagnostic and Statistical Manual of Mental Disorders* (3rd edn, revised) (DSM–III–R). Washington, DC: APA.

—— (1994) *Diagnostic and Statistical Manual of Mental Disorders* (4th edn) (DSM–IV). Washington, DC: APA.

Angold, A., Costello, E. J. & Erkanli, A. (1999) Comorbidity. *Journal of Child Psychology and Psychiatry*, **40**, 57–87.

Aseltine, R. H. & Kessler, R. C. (1993) Marital disruption and depression in a community sample. *Journal of Health and Social Behavior*, **34**, 237–251.

Bardone, A. M., Moffitt, T. E., Caspi, A., *et al* (1996) Adult mental health and social outcomes of adolescent girls with depression and conduct disorder. *Development and Psychopathology*, **8**, 811–829.

——, ——, ——, *et al* (1998) Adult physical health outcomes of adolescent girls with conduct disorder, depression, and anxiety. *Journal of the American Academy of Child and Adolescent Psychiatry*, **37**, 594–601.

Bebbington, P. E. (1988) The social epidemiology of clinical depression. In *Handbook of Studies on Social Psychiatry* (eds A. S. Henderson & G. Burrows). Amsterdam: Elsevier.

Bernstein, D. P., Cohen, P., Skodol, A., *et al* (1996) Childhood antecedents of adolescent personality disorders. *American Journal of Psychiatry*, **153**, 907–913.

Bifulco, A., Brown, G. W., Moran, P., *et al* (1998) Predicting depression in women: the role of past and present vulnerability. *Psychological Medicine*, **28**, 39–50.

Bowlby, J. (1973) *Attachment and Loss*, vol. 1: *Attachment*. New York: Basic Books.

Brooks-Gunn, J., Petersen, A. C. & Acorn, D. (1985) The study of maturational timing effects at adolescence. *Journal of Youth and Adolescence*, **14**, 149–161.

Brown, G. W. & Harris, T. (1978) *The Social Origins of Depression: A Study of Psychiatric Disorder in Women*. London: Tavistock Publications.

——, —— & Eales, M. J. (1993) Aetiology of anxiety and depressive disorders in an inner city population. 2. Comorbidity and adversity. *Psychological Medicine*, **23**, 155–165.

Bruce, M. L. & Kim, K. M. (1992) Differences in the effects of divorce on major depression in men and women. *American Journal of Psychiatry*, **149**, 914–917.

Cairns, R. B., Cairns, B. D., Neckerman, H. J., *et al* (1988) Social networks and aggressive behavior: peer support or peer rejection? *Developmental Psychology*, **24**, 815–823.

——, ——, ——, *et al* (1989) Early school dropout: configurations and determinants. *Child Development*, **606**, 1437–1452.

Cantwell, D. P. & Rutter, M. (1994) Classification: conceptual issues and substantive findings. In *Child and Adolescent Psychiatry: Modern Approaches* (eds M. Rutter, E. Taylor & L. Hersov) (3rd edn), pp. 3–21. Oxford: Blackwell Scientific Publications.

Caspi, A. & Moffitt, T. E. (1993) When do individual differences matter? A paradoxical theory of personality coherence. *Psychological Inquiry*, **4**, 247–271.

—— & —— (1995) The continuity of maladaptive behaviour: from description to understanding in the study of antisocial behaviour. In *Developmental Psychopathology*, vol. 2 (eds D. Cicchetti & D. Cohen), pp. 472–511. New York: John Wiley & Sons.

——, Newman, D. L., *et al* (1996) Behavioral observations at age 3 years predict adult psychiatric disorders. *Archives of General Psychiatry*, **53**, 1033–1039.

Caspi, A., Wright, B. R., Moffitt, T. E., *et al* (1998) Early failure in the labor market: childhood and adolescent predictors of unemployment in the transition to adulthood. *American Sociological Review*, **63**, 334–451.

Christie, K. A., Burke, J. D., Reiger, D. A., *et al* (1988) Epidemiologic evidence for early onset of mental disorders and higher risk of drug use in young adults. *American Journal of Psychiatry*, **145**, 971–975.

Cicchetti, D. & Rogosch, F. A. (1996) Equifinality and multifinality in developmental psychopathology. *Development and Psychopathology*, **8**, 597–600.

Clausen, J. S. (1991) Adolescent competence and the shaping of the life course. *American Journal of Sociology*, **96**, 805–842.

DiLalla, L. F. & Gottesman, I. I. (1989) Heterogeneity of causes for delinquency and criminality: lifespan perspectives. *Development and Psychopathology*, **1**, 339–349.

Elder, G. H. (1998) The life course and human development. In *Handbook of Child Psychology*, vol. 1: *Theoretical Models of Human Development* (ed. R. M. Lerner), pp. 939–991. New York: John Wiley & Sons.

—— & Caspi, A. (1990) Studying lives in a changing society: sociological and personalogical explorations. In *Studying Persons and Lives* (eds A. I. Rabin, R. A. Zucker, S. Frank, *et al*), pp. 201–247. New York: Springer.

Ensminger, M. E. & Juon, H. S. (1998) Transition to adulthood among high risk youth. In *New Perspectives on Adolescent Risk Behavior* (ed. R. Jessor), pp. 365–391. Cambridge: Cambridge University Press.

Farrington, D. P. (1986) Stepping stones to adult criminal careers. In *Development of Antisocial and Prosocial Behavior* (eds D. Olweus, J. Block & M. R. Yarrow), pp. 359–384. New York: Academic Press.

—— (1991) Antisocial personality from childhood to adulthood. *The Psychologist*, **4**, 389–394.

—— & West, D. J. (1995) Effects of marriage, separation, and children on offending by adult males. In *Current Perspectives on Aging and the Life Cycle: Delinquency and Disrepute in the Life Course* (ed. J. Hagan), pp. 249–281. Greenwich, NJ: JAI Press.

——, Loeber, R., Elliott, D. S., *et al* (1990) Advancing knowledge about the onset of delinquency and crime. In *Advances in Clinical Child Psychology* (eds B. B. Lahey & A. E. Kazdin), pp. 283–342. New York: Plenum Press.

Feehan, M., McGee, R. & Williams, S. M. (1993) Mental health disorders from age 15 to age 18 years. *Journal of the American Academy of Child and Adolescent Psychiatry*, **32**, 1118–1126.

Fergusson, D. M. (1997) Structural equation models in developmental research. *Journal of Child Psychology and Psychiatry*, **38**, 877–887.

—— & Horwood, L. J. (1996) The role of adolescent peer affiliations in the continuity between childhood behavioral adjustment and juvenile offending. *Journal of Abnormal Child Psychology*, **24**, 205–221.

——, Horwood, L. J. & Lynskey, M. T. (1996) Childhood sexual abuse and psychiatric disorder in young adulthood. II. Psychiatric outcomes of childhood sexual abuse. *Journal of the American Academy of Child and Adolescent Psychiatry*, **35**, 1365–1374.

Fombonne, E., Wostear, G., Cooper, V. *et al* (2001*a*) The Maudsley long-term follow-up of child and adolescent depression. I: Psychiatric outcomes in adulthood. *British Journal of Psychiatry* (in press).

——, ——, ——, *et al* (2001*b*)) The Maudsley long-term follow-up of child and adolescent depression. II: Suicidality, criminality and social dysfunction in adulthood. *British Journal of Psychiatry* (in press).

Forthofer, M. S., Kessler, R. C., Story, A. L., *et al* (1996) The effects of psychiatric disorders on the probability and timing of first marriage. *Journal of Health and Social Behaviour*, **37**, 121–132.

Frick, P. J., Lahey, B. B., Loeber, R., *et al* (1993) Oppositional defiant disorder and conduct disorder: a meta-analytic review of factor analyses and cross-validation in a clinic sample. *Clinical Psychology Review*, **13**, 319–340.

Furstenberg, F. F., Brooks-Gunn, J. & Chase-Lansdale, L. (1989) Teenaged pregnancy and child-bearing. *American Psychologist*, **44**, 313–320.

Graber, J. A. & Brooks-Gunn, J. (1996) Transitions and turning points: navigating the passage from childhood through adolescence. *Developmental Psychology*, **32**, 768–776.

Hankin, B. L., Abramson, L. Y., Moffitt, T. E., *et al* (1998) Development of depression from preadolescence to young adulthood: emerging gender differences in a 10-year longitudinal study. *Journal of Abnormal Psychology*, **107**, 128–140.

Harrington, R. (1994) Affective disorders. In *Child and Adolescent Psychiatry: Modern Approaches* (eds M. Rutter, E. Taylor & L. Hersov), pp. 330–350. Oxford: Blackwell Scientific Publications.

——, Fudge, H., Rutter, M., *et al* (1990) Adult outcomes of childhood and adolescent depression. I. Psychiatric status. *Archives of General Psychiatry*, **47**, 465–473.

——, ——, ——, *et al* (1991) Adult outcomes of childhood and adolescent depression: II. Links with antisocial disorders. *Journal of the American Academy of Child and Adolescent Psychiatry*, **30**, 434-439.

——, Bredenkamp, D., Groothues, C., *et al* (1994) Adult outcomes of childhood and adolescent depression. III. Links with suicidal behaviours. *Journal of Child Psychology and Psychiatry*, **35**, 1380–1391.

——, Rutter, M. & Fombonne, E. (1996) Developmental pathways in depression: multiple meanings, antecedents, and endpoints. *Development and Psychopathology*, **8**, 601–616.

——, ——, Weissman, M., *et al* (1997) Psychiatric disorders in the relatives of depressed probands. I. Comparison of prepubertal adolescent and early onset cases. *Journal of Affective Disorders*, **42**, 9–22.

Harris, T., Brown, G. W. & Bifulco, A. (1990) Loss of parent in childhood and adult depression: a tentative overall model. *Development and Psychopathology*, **2**, 311–328.

Hogan, D. P. & Astone, N. M. (1986) The transition to adulthood. *Annual Review of Sociology*, **12**, 109–130.

Jessor, R., Donovan, J. E. & Costa, F. M. (1991) *Beyond Adolescence: Problem Behavior and Young Adult Development*. Cambridge, MA: Harvard University Press.

Jones, P. (1997) The early origins of schizophrenia. *British Medical Bulletin*, **53**, 135–155.

Kandel, D. (1985) On processes of peer influences in adolescent drug use: a developmental perspective. *Alcohol and Substance Abuse in Adolescence*, **4**, 139–163.

—— & Davies, M. (1986) Adult sequelae of adolescent depressive symptoms. *Archives of General Psychiatry*, **43**, 255–262.

Kazdin, A. E. (2001) Treatment of conduct disorders. In *Conduct Disorders* (eds J. Hill & B. Maughan), pp. 408–448. Cambridge: Cambridge University Press.

Keenan, K., Loeber, R., Zhang, Q., *et al* (1995) The influence of deviant peers on the development of boys' disruptive and delinquent behavior: a temporal analysis. *Development and Psychopathology*, **7**, 715–726.

Kendler, K. S., Walters, E. E., Neale, M. C., *et al* (1995) The structure of the genetic and environmental risk factors for six major psychiatric disorders in women: phobia, generalized anxiety disorder, panic disorder, bulimia, major depression, and alcoholism. *Archives of General Psychiatry*, **52**, 374–383.

Kerner, H-J., Weitekamp, E. G. M. & Stelly, W. (1995) From childhood delinquency to adult criminality: first results of the follow-up of the Tuebingen Criminal Behaviour Development Study. *Eurocriminology*, **89**, 127–162.

Kessler, R. C., Foster, C. L., Saunders, W. B., *et al* (1995) Social consequences of psychiatric disorder. I. Educational attainment. *American Journal of Psychiatry*, **52**, 1026–1032.

——, Berglund, P. A., Foster, C. L., *et al* (1997a) Social consequences of psychiatric disorders. II. Teenage parenthood. *American Journal of Psychiatry*, **154**, 1405–1411.

——, David, C. G. & Kendler, K. S. (1997b) Childhood adversity and adult psychiatric disorder in the US National Comorbidity Survey. *Psychological Medicine*, **27**, 1101–1119.

Knapp, M., Scott, S. & Davies, J. (1999) The cost of antisocial behaviour in younger children: a pilot study of economic and family impact. *Clinical Child Psychology and Psychiatry*, **4**, 457–473.

Kovacs, M. (1996) Presentation and course of major depressive disorder during childhood and later years of the life span. *Journal of the American Academy of Child and Adolescent Psychiatry*, **35**, 705–715.

Krueger, R. F., Moffitt, T. E., Caspi, A., *et al* (1998) Assortative mating for antisocial behavior: developmental and methodological implication. *Behavior Genetics*, **28**, 173–186.

Last, C. G., Hansen, C. & Franco, N. (1997) Anxious children in adulthood: a prospective study of adjustment. *Journal of the American Academy of Child and Adolescent Psychiatry*, **36**, 645–652.

Laub, J. H., Nagin, D. S. & Sampson, R. J. (1998) Trajectories of change in criminal offending: good marriages and the desistance process. *American Sociological Review*, **63**, 225–238.

Lerner, R. M. (1985) Adolescent maturational changes and psychosocial development: a dynamic interactional perspective. *Journal of Youth and Adolescence*, **14**, 355–372.

Lewinsohn, P. M., Rohde, P. & Seeley, J. R. (1994) Psychosocial risk factors for future adolescent suicide attempts. *Journal of Consulting and Clinical Psychology*, **62**, 297–305.

Loeber, R. (1982) The stability of antisocial and delinquent child behaviour: a review. *Child Development*, **53**, 1431–1446.

—— & Schmaling, K. (1985) Empirical evidence for overt and covert patterns of antisocial conduct problems. *Journal of Abnormal Child Psychology*, **13**, 337–352.

Lyons, M. J., True, W. R., Eisen, S. A., *et al* (1995) Differential heritability of adult and juvenile antisocial traits. *Archives of General Psychiatry*, **52**, 906–915.

Magnusson, D. & Cairns, R. B. (1996) Developmental science: Towards a unified framework. In *Developmental Science* (eds R. B. Cairns, G. H. Elder & E. J. Costello), pp. 7–30. Cambridge: Cambridge University Press.

Mannuzza, S., Klein, R. G., Bessler, A., *et al* (1998) Adult psychiatric status of hyperactive boys grown up. *American Journal of Psychiatry*, **155**, 493–498.

Maughan, B. & McCarthy, G. (1997) Childhood adversities and psychosocial disorders. *British Medical Bulletin*, **53**, 156–169.

—— & Rutter, M. (1997) Retrospective reporting of childhood adversity: some methodological considerations. *Journal of Personality Disorders*, **11**, 19–33.

—— & —— (1998) Continuities and discontinuities in antisocial behaviour from childhood to adult life. In *Advances in Clinical Child Psychology*, vol. 20 (eds T. H. Ollendick & R. J. Prinz), pp. 1–47. New York: Plenum Press.

—— & Taylor, A. (2001) Adolescent psychological problems, partnership transitions and adult mental health: an investigation of selection effects. *Psychological Medicine* (in press).

——, Pickles, A. & Quinton, D. (1995) Parental hostility, childhood behavior and adult social functioning. In J. McCord (ed.), *Coercion and punishment in long-term perspectives* (pp. 34–58). New York: Cambridge University Press.

■ 17

——, ——, Hagell, M., *et al* (1996) Reading retardation and antisocial behaviour: developmental trends in comorbidity. *Journal of Child Psychology and Psychiatry*, **37**, 405–418.

——, Collishaw, S. & Pickles, A. (1999): Mild mental retardation: psychosocial functioning in adulthood. *Psychological Medicine*, **29**, 351–366.

McCarthy, G. & Taylor, A. (1999) Avoidant/ambivalent attachment style as a mediator between abusive childhood experiences and adult relationship difficulties. *Journal of Child Psychology and Psychiatry*, **40**, 465–478.

Mickelson, K. D., Kessler, R. C. & Shaver, P. R. (1997) Adult attachment in a nationally representative sample. *Journal of Personality and Social Psychology*, **73**, 1092–1106.

Moffitt, T. E. (1993) Adolescence-limited and life-course-persistent antisocial behaviour: a developmental taxonomy. *Psychological Review*, **100**, 674–701.

——, Caspi, A., Dickson, N., *et al* (1996) Childhood-onset versus adolescent-onset antisocial conduct problems in males: natural history from ages 3 to 18 years. *Development and Psychopathology*, **8**, 399–424.

Neugarten, B. L. (1979) Time, age and life cycle. *American Journal of Psychiatry*, **136**, 887–894.

Newman, D. L., Moffitt, T. E., Caspi, A., *et al* (1996) Psychiatric disorder in a birth cohort of young adults: prevalence, comorbidity, clinical significance, and new case incidence from ages 11 to 21. *Journal of Consulting and Clinical Psychology*, **64**, 552–562.

Nordin, V. & Gillberg, C. (1998) The long-term course of autistic disorders: update on follow-up studies. *Acta Psychiatrica Scandinavica*, **97**, 99–108.

Offord, D. R. & Bennett, K. J. (1994) Conduct disorder: long-term outcomes and intervention effectiveness. *Journal of the American Academy of Child and Adolescent Psychiatry*, **33**, 1069–1078.

Pawlby, S. J., Mills, A. & Quinton, D. (1997) Vulnerable adolescent girls: opposite-sex relationships. *Journal of Child Psychology and Psychiatry*, **38**, 909–920.

Pickles, A. & Rutter, M. (1991) Statistical and conceptual models of turning points in developmental processes. In *Problems and Methods in Longitudinal Research: Stability and Change* (eds D. Magnusson, L. R. Bergman, G. Rudinger, *et al*), pp. 131–165. Cambridge: Cambridge University Press.

Pine, D. S., Cohen, P., Gurley, D., *et al* (1998) The risk for early-adulthood anxiety and depressive disorders in adolescents with anxiety and depressive disorders. *Archives of General Psychiatry*, **55**, 56–64.

Quinton, D. & Rutter, M. (1988) *Parenting breakdown: The making and breaking of intergenerational links*. Avebury: Gower.

——, —— & Gulliver, L. (1990) Continuities in psychiatric disorders from childhood to adulthood in the children of psychiatric patients. In *Straight and Devious Pathways from Childhood to Adulthood* (eds L. N. Robins & M. Rutter), pp. 259–277. Cambridge: Cambridge University Press.

——, Pickles, A., Maughan B., *et al* (1993) Partners, peers, and pathways: assortative pairing and continuities in conduct disorder. *Developmental Psychopathology*, **5**, 763–783.

Rao, U., Ryan, N. D., Birmaher, B., *et al* (1995) Unipolar depression in adolescence: clinical outcome in adulthood. *Journal of the American Academy of Child and Adolescent Psychiatry*, **34**, 566–578.

Robins, L. N. (1966) *Deviant Children Grown Up: A Sociological and Psychiatric Study of Sociopathic Personality*. Baltimore, MD: Williams & Wilkins.

—— & Price, R. K. (1991) Adult disorders predicted by childhood conduct problems: results from the NIMH Epidemiologic Catchment Area Project. *Psychiatry*, **542**, 116–132.

——, Tipp, J. & Przybeck, T. (1991) Antisocial personality. In *Psychiatric Disorders in America* (eds L. N. Robins & D. A. Regier), pp. 258–290. New York: Free Press.

Rodgers, B. & Pryor, J. (1998) *Divorce and Separation: The Outcomes for Children*. York: Joseph Rowntree Foundation.

Romans, S., Martin, J. & Mullen, P. (1997) Childhood sexual abuse and later psychological problems: neither necessary, sufficient nor acting alone. *Criminal Behaviour and Mental Health*, **7**, 327–338.

Rutter, M. (1977) Prospective studies to investigate behavioral change. In *The Origins and Course of Psychopathology* (eds J. S. Strauss, H. M. Babigian & M. Roff), pp. 223–247. New York: John Wiley & Sons.

—— (1981) Epidemiological/longitudinal strategies and causal research in child psychiatry. *Journal of the American Academy of Child Psychiatry*, **20**, 513–544.

—— (1988) *Studies of Psychosocial Risk: The Power of Longitudinal Data*. Cambridge: Cambridge University Press.

—— (1989) Pathways from childhood to adult life. *Journal of Child Psychology and Psychiatry*, **30**, 23–51.

—— (1991) Childhood experiences and adult psychosocial functioning. In *The Childhood Environment and Adult Disease* (eds G. R. Bock & J. A. Whelan), CIBA Foundation Symposium no. 156, pp. 189–200. Chichester: John Wiley & Sons.

—— (1993) Cause and course of psychopathology: some lessons from longitudinal data. *Paediatric and Perinatal Epidemiology*, **7**, 105–120.

18

—— (1994) Beyond longitudinal data: causes, consequences, changes and continuity. *Journal of Consulting and Clinical Psychology*, **62**, 928–940.

—— (1996a) Connections between child and adult psychopathology. *European Child and Adolescent Psychiatry*, **5**, 4–7.

—— (1996b) Transitions and turning points in developmental psychopathology: as applied to the age span between childhood and mid-adulthood. *International Journal of Behavioural Development*, **19**, 603–626.

—— (1997) Nature–nurture integration. The example of antisocial behavior. *American Psychologist*, **52**, 390–398.

—— & Mawhood, L. (1991) The long-term psychosocial sequelae of specific developmental disorders of speech and language. In *Biological Risk Factors for Psychosocial Disorders* (eds M. Rutter & P. Casaer), pp. 233–259. Cambridge: Cambridge University Press.

——, Tizard, J., Yule, W., *et al* (1976) Research report: Isle of Wight studies 1964–1974. *Psychological Medicine*, **6**, 313–332.

——, Champion, L., Quinton, D., *et al* (1995) Understanding individual differences in environmental risk exposure. In *Examining Lives in Context: Perspectives on the Ecology of Human Development* (eds P. Moen, G. H. J. Elder & K. Luscher), pp. 61–93. Washington, DC: American Psychological Association.

——, Maughan, B., Pickles, A., *et al* (1997a) Retrospective recall recalled. In *Methods and Models for Studying the Individual* (eds R. B. Cairns, L. R. Bergman & J. Kagan), pp. 219–242. Thousand Oaks, CA: Sage.

——, Dunn, J., Plomin, R., *et al* (1997b) Integrating nature and nurture: implications of person–environment correlations and interactions for developmental psychopathology. *Development and Psychopathology*, **9**, 335–364.

——, Giller, H. & Hagell, A. (1998) *Antisocial Behaviour by Young People*. Cambridge: Cambridge University Press.

Sampson, R. & Laub, J. (1993) *Crime in the Making: Pathways and Turning Points through Life*. Cambridge, MA: Harvard University Press.

—— & —— (1996) Socioeconomic achievements in the life course of disadvantaged men: military service as a turning point, circa 1940–1965. *American Sociological Review*, **61**, 347–367.

Sanford, M., Offord, D., McLeod, K., *et al* (1994) Pathways into the work force: antecedents of school and work force status. *Journal of the American Academy of Child and Adolescent Psychiatry*, **33**, 1036–1046.

Scarr, S. & McCartney, K. (1983) How people make their own environments: a theory of genotype greater than environment effects. *Child Development*, **54**, 424–435.

Silva, P. A. (1990) The Dunedin Multidisciplinary Health and Development Study: a 15-year longitudinal study. *Paediatric and Perinatal Epidemiology*, **4**, 96–127.

Stattin, H. & Magnusson, D. (1996) Antisocial development: a holistic approach. *Development and Psychopathology*, **8**, 617–645.

Steinhausen, H-C. & Reitzle, M. (1996) The validity of mixed disorders of conduct and emotions in children and adolescents: a research note. *Journal of Child Psychology and Psychiatry*, **37**, 339–343.

Taylor, E., Chadwick, O., Heptinstall, E., *et al* (1996) Hyperactivity and conduct disorder as risk factors for adolescent development. *Journal of the American Academy of Child and Adolescent Psychiatry*, **35**, 1213–1226.

Thornberry, T. P. & Krohn, M. D. (1997) Peers, drugs use and delinquency. In *Handbook of Antisocial Behavior* (eds D. Stoff, J. Brieling & J. D. Maser), pp. 218–233. New York: John Wiley & Sons.

Turnbull, J. E., George, L. K., Landerman, R., *et al* (1990) Social outcomes related to age of onset among psychiatric disorders. *Journal of Consulting and Clinical Psychology*, **58**, 832–839.

Warr, M. (1993) Age, peers and delinquency. *Criminology*, **31**, 17–40.

Widom, C. S. & White, H. R. (1997) Problem behaviours in abused and neglected children grown up: prevalence and co-occurrence of substance abuse, crime and violence. *Criminal Behaviour and Mental Health*, **7**, 287–310.

Willett, J. B., Singer, J. D. & Martin, N. C. (1998) The design and analysis of longitudinal studies of development and psychopathology in context: statistical models and methodological recommendations. *Development and Psychopathology*, **10**, 395–426.

Zoccolillo, M. (1992) Co-occurrence of conduct disorder and its adult outcomes with depressive and anxiety disorders: a review. *Journal of American Academy of Child and Adolescent Psychiatry*, **31**, 547–556.

——, Pickles, A., Quinton, D., *et al* (1992) The outcome of childhood conduct disorder: implications for defining adult personality disorder and conduct disorder. *Psychological Medicine*, **22**, 971–986.

■19

2 The significance of genetic variation for abnormal behavioural development

Jim Stevenson

My aim in this chapter is to identify the ways in which genetic studies have cast light on our understanding of the nature of abnormal development in children. I will concentrate on studies that have emerged in the past 10–15 years, a particularly fertile and active period both in quantitative genetic analysis and in the application of molecular genetic methods. However, before concentrating on these developments it is worthwhile briefly considering the history of genetic investigations and theories in child psychiatry research.

Among the first people to introduce genetic ideas into the systematic study of behavioural development in children as it relates to child psychiatry were Alex Thomas and Stella Chess. Their ideas about the origins of temperament in the biology of the child and how this interacts with parental expectations and child-rearing practices to create potential for psychological disturbances were pioneering (Thomas *et al*, 1963, 1968; Thomas & Chess, 1977). It should be noted that Chess and Thomas were also early influences on Michael Rutter, one of whose first papers was on genetic and environmental influences on temperament (Rutter *et al*, 1963). The first large-scale study that Rutter published concerned the children of parents with mental illness (Rutter, 1966). Here he was confronted with the immediate issue of the relative importance of genetic transmission and child-rearing patterns. If adverse consequences arose in the child's development, were they due to biological or to social influences?

The Isle of Wight study is seen as a landmark in the development of an empirical basis for child psychiatry (Rutter *et al*, 1970). This study established the broad features of the epidemiology and natural history of childhood disorders in the general population. It is interesting to reflect on how this study might now be conducted. As I will explain below, genetically informative research has identified a major question concerning differential outcome for children living within the same family. Emphasis is now placed on what is termed the 'non-shared environment'. Differential outcome is a product both of the non-shared environment and of genetic differences between children. I am sure therefore that if Rutter were designing the Isle of Wight study today he would undoubtedly include more than one child from each family, and a major feature of the analysis would be to account for why striking differences emerge in children living within the same family (Plomin & Daniels, 1987).

Rutter's first major study directly testing the role of genetic factors was a twin study undertaken with Susan Folstein (Folstein & Rutter, 1977). This for the first time identified

Based on a paper presented at the Association of Child Psychology and Psychiatry conference 'From research to clinical practice', London, 22 June 1998.

the very significant contribution that genetic factors make to the origins of autism. These findings have now been replicated in a number of subsequent twin and family studies.

It is the conjunction of genetically informative designs with Rutter's abiding concern about differential vulnerability to adverse events in children's lives that set the research agenda for his studies during the 1980s and 1990s. He has now established an extensive set of investigations using genetically informative designs, such as the twin studies with Lindon Eaves in Virginia (e.g., Eaves *et al*, 1997). This is geared to address questions of the mechanisms underlying the joint influence of genetic and experiential factors in determining abnormal development in children.

In many ways I see this to be the research agenda for child psychiatry at the start of this new century. We need no longer approach genetic influences in a vague hand-waving manner: a powerful new set of methodologies now allows the presence of genetic or biological markers to be identified, and this information can be used to quantify the genetic risk carried by an individual child. Increasingly, the focus of research will be the mechanisms whereby genetic loading affects adverse outcome either directly, through impact on the central nervous system, or more indirectly, through the experiential consequences of differences in children's behaviour. This approach centres on the impact of behaviour on the environments experienced and has become central to thinking about biological and social influences on children's development (Plomin *et al*, 1994).

These comments are made by way of introduction, and I hope indicate the crucial role that Rutter has played in bringing about the recognition that the joint action of genetic and environmental influences is central to the research agenda for child psychiatry.

To highlight the issue of the need for us to incorporate genetically informative aspects into our research designs, I want briefly to mention the results of a follow-up of children that Philip Graham, Naomi Richman and I studied some 25 years ago. We published a summary of the findings from our Waltham Forest study in 1982 (Richman *et al*, 1982), identifying the way in which pre-school behavioural difficulties were not transient phenomena. Children showing elevated rates of behavioural difficulties at age 3 years were at an increased risk of educational and behavioural problems some 5 years later. In conjunction with Robert Goodman, I have been attempting to see whether we can, using this sample, identify factors in the early lives of children that might place them at increased risk of later criminality (Stevenson & Goodman, 2001). We have accordingly obtained criminal record information on these 828 children now that they are in their early adult years.

In the Waltham Forest study detailed information was obtained about family relationships, parental mental state and expressed emotion. Incorporating these measures into the data for the risk of adult violent offences for boys, the path analysis throws up an interesting dual route possibility. A model was tested whereby aspects of the family circumstances and parental mental state when the child was 3 years old could influence both marital and parent–child relationships. In turn these could affect the child's behaviour at 3 years (based on parents' report) and behaviour measured by an independent rater at age 8. Finally, all these measures could influence whether the boy had a conviction for adult violent offences.

Figure 2.1 shows a route whereby early behaviour influences later behaviour at age 8 and the risk of later adult violent offences. The father's mental state relates to a number of the measures concerned with the early family relationships experienced by the child at age 3 years. The father's mental state is related to poor marital relationships and increased

■ 21

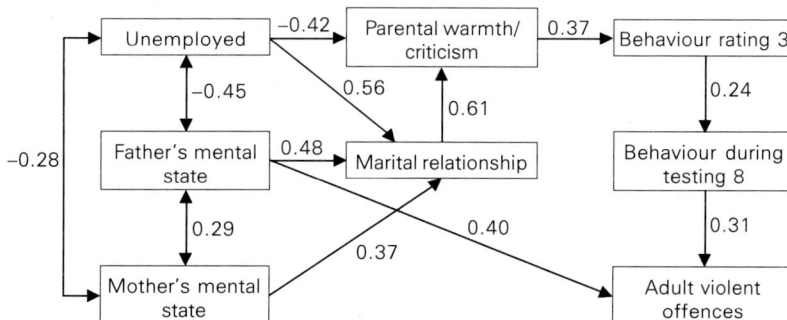

Fig. 2.1 Path diagram of associations between early family characteristics, behaviour and later adult violent offences for boys in the Waltham Forest study.

risk of unemployment, and also to parental lack of warmth and criticism of the child. It has a direct influence on the child's risk of violent offences in adulthood. In the context of the genetic focus of this chapter the key question is whether these two routes represent a social and genetic influence of the father on the child's later behaviour.

The crucial point is that the Waltham Forest study was not designed with this genetic possibility in mind. Therefore it is not possible for us to disentangle the possible role of biological and experiential factors in determining this increased risk. It is precisely this unpicking of the joint effects of genetic and environmental experiential influences on children's abnormal development that I suggest is the new agenda being set by advances in genetic research for child psychiatry.

Evidence for genetic effects on children's behaviour

What is the evidence for genetic influences on children's abnormal behaviour? Genetic research can be broadly divided into that which uses quantitative statistical procedures to identify the relative contributions of genetic and environmental influences on individual differences in development, and molecular genetic investigations that attempt to identify the specific genes that affect behavioural development.

The quantitative approach has been important not only in identifying the basic heritability of different kinds of condition, but also in highlighting the importance of different kinds of environmental influence on psychopathology in children. As Plomin and his colleagues have emphasised, the striking thing about contemporary genetic research has been that the insights gained into the environment have been just as important as those gained into the biology (Plomin & Bergeman, 1991). In particular, for personality and psychopathology the environmental influence that is most salient is that described as non-shared. These are circumstances and experiences that generate differences between children living in the same family. Under this formulation, shared environmental influences, which are those that engender similarities between children living in the same family, are seen to be far less significant. These shared environmental influences have been the mainstay of previous investigations into child socialisation.

Going back to the Isle of Wight study, its design allowed the rates of psychiatric disturbance to be compared between social classes. This allowed some estimate to be made of the impact of what would be called a shared environmental influence in elevating the rates of disturbances within these groups. What the current genetically informative designs have indicated is that between-family influences such as social class are minor compared to within-family influences that impinge on children's development.

The main tool for quantitative genetic research has been the study of twins (Bouchard & Propping, 1993). Here the assumption is made that there are just two classes of twin. The first is monozygotic (identical) pairs and the second is dizygotic (fraternal). Monozygotic twins are identical in their genetic make-up. It must be remembered that many genes show little variation between people, and indeed many of us are genetically identical to each other for most of our genes. There are nevertheless some genes that show variability, and this variability is the essential influence of interest in the genetic approach to behaviour. It addresses individual differences rather than species-typical aspects of behaviour.

Dizygotic twins share on average 50% of those genes that show variability between people. We can therefore look at the relative similarities within monozygotic and dizygotic twin pairs to identify the relative contribution of genetic and environmental influences on individual differences. The estimate that emerges from these quantitative analyses is referred to as 'heritability'. It is important to recognise some of the limitations on this statistic. The first is that heritability refers to the proportion of a phenotypical characteristic that is attributable to genetic differences within a population. If at any given historical time different populations were studied, for example populations with different cultures or different gene pools, then there would be differences in the value of heritability obtained. Similarly, within a population heritability estimates obtained at different times may well differ. For example, the relative contribution of genetic and environmental influences on height is likely to change as a population shifts from having a generally poor level of nutrition to one that is more adequate (Tizard, 1975).

The second feature of a heritability estimate is that it is a population statistic. It tells us to what extent genetic variation between people within a population is important in

Table 2.1 Selected twin heritabilities for psychiatric disorders with childhood onset (based on LaBuda et al, 1993)

Condition	Heritability
Autism	1.00
Anorexia nervosa	0.78
Obsessive–compulsive disorder	0.68
Hyperactivity	0.64
Tourette's syndrome	0.64

influencing a characteristic. It does not by itself tell us anything about the circumstances for a particular individual. A heritability estimate might indicate that on average half the variation in a characteristic is determined by genetic differences between people. Nevertheless, the features of one individual within that population might be determined solely by their genetic make-up, whereas those of another might result purely from environmental influences. Thus, rather than being the end-point of genetic analysis, the heritability estimate is the starting point for a more clinically interesting and relevant exploration of how this heritability arises.

LaBuda *et al* (1993) reviewed twin studies of disorders originating in childhood. Some conditions, such as autism, show a remarkably high degree of genetic influence, while in others, such as conduct disorder, the role of genetic factors is very much lower (Table 2.1). It is important to note that in none of these cases are we dealing with disorders that are affected by a single major gene. When we first learn about genetic influences and mechanisms we are introduced to Mendel's laws regarding the ways in which dominant and recessive effects are transmitted across generations. These influences are single major gene effects. They show distinctive patterns of transmission and by studying a family history one can see the nature of the genetic mechanism involved.

None of the psychiatric disorders displayed in Table 2.1 is of this kind. The most heritable condition identified on this list is autism. Pickles *et al* (1995) have estimated by that between four and ten genes are involved in its transmission: what is referred to as an oligogenic mechanism. This explains why, although the heritability might be 1, a study of first-degree relatives of a child with autism shows that the vast majority of siblings do not show autism itself. Taking the base rate of autism in the general population to be about 5 per 10 000, the rate of autism in the brothers and sisters of children who have autism is about 5%. This represents a rate some 100 times that in the general population, but it still means that the vast majority of the siblings of children with autism do not have the disorder. What this clearly implies is that the individual must have the full complement of the 4–10 genes involved in order to show autism. Brothers and sisters will be at risk of having one or two of these genes, but only 5% of them will actually have exactly the same complement as that of their affected brother or sister.

Anorexia nervosa is rather surprising in the level of genetic influence that seems to be implicated by these twin results. Many people would look on anorexia as a response to experiences in early adolescence that put undue stress on the child to achieve, to conform to or to meet expectations about body size and shape. It would appear from the work of Holland *et al* (1988) and Rutherford *et al* (1993) that genetic influences on attitudes towards eating and body shape are quite marked.

Next I want to consider the genetic research of a number of specific conditions in a little more detail.

Affective disorder

There are now good family data on the extent to which children of parents with major depressive disorders are at risk of an increased rate of depression. Equally, studies that have looked at the parents of children with depression have also found an higher rate of affective disorders. For example, Beardslee *et al* (1996) found that the rate of depression in these at-risk children was three times higher than that in children of well parents. Harrington *et al* (1993) also found a three-fold increased risk of depression in parents of children with depression compared to parents of children with non-affective disorders. As always, this evidence of familiality could be consistent with either genetic or environmental transmission. We therefore have to turn to genetically informative designs to try to tease apart these two effects.

A number of twin studies have now been published concerned with the heritability of affective disorders, both depression and anxiety (Rende *et al*, 1993; Thapar & McGuffin, 1995; Eaves *et al*, 1997; Eley, 1997). The estimates of heritability for depression range from 60% (Eaves *et al*, 1997) to 34% (Rende *et al*, 1993). However, these indices of a moderate level of heritability disguise a more complex picture.

First, the evidence for genetic factors in parents' reports on their child's depressive symptomatology seems somewhat stronger than in child's own reports (e.g. Eaves *et al*, 1997). Second, it has been established for some time that heritability measures changes with age. The most striking finding in this regard is the increase in the heritability measure of IQ with age. Affective disorders also show an increase in the importance of genetic factors with age, especially in girls (Silberg *et al*, 1999). Third, one of the important features of genetic research is the ability to test for changes in the mix of genetic and environmental influences using different definitions and different degrees of severity of child disorders. In childhood affective disorders, there is some evidence that the shared environment may be more important in extreme depressive symptomatology than in less severe forms. I will return to this issue of testing for changes in genetic influences with severity when I discuss attention-deficit hyperactivity disorder (ADHD). Fourth, evidence is now emerging that genetic liability for both anxiety and depression is shared in children, as it appears to be in adults (Eley & Stevenson, 1999). This parallels Kendler *et al*'s (1995) suggestion that in adults there may be a common genetic influence for both anxiety and depression, with experience determining which form of affective disorder would be shown.

Thalia Eley has recently completed a study looking at anxiety and depressive symptomatology in child and adolescent twins (Eley & Stevenson, 1999). One of the difficulties in this area is the problem of symptom overlap between anxiety and depression, and in an attempt to overcome this difficulty she factor-analysed the State Trait Anxiety Inventory (Spielberger, 1972) and the Child Depression Inventory (Kovacs, 1985) to identify more clearly separate indicators. Figure 2.2 shows the results obtained. In the diagram the numbers against A, C and E (representing the significance of genetic, shared-environmental and non-shared environmental influences respectively) have to be squared to obtain the heritability estimates.

It can be seen that genetic factors appear more important in depression than they do in anxiety. Similarly, shared environmental influences are slightly more important for anxiety than they are for depression. For the present purposes it is the correlations at the top of the diagram that are of particular interest. These show a value of 1 connecting the genetic influences on anxiety and depression. This indicates a perfect genetic correlation between the genes influencing anxiety and those influencing depression. However, the correlation for the non-shared environmental influences is zero. This indicates that the non-shared influences on anxiety are completely different from those influencing depression. Similarly, the shared environmental influences on the two conditions are separate. From this data alone we cannot tell which environmental influences lead to anxiety and which lead to depression. However, another facet of Eley's work was to measure life events in these children. This showed that the life events involving some form of loss were associated with depression, whereas those involving some form of threat were related to anxiety (Eley & Stevenson, 2000).

This twin research therefore suggests quite a complex pattern of age- and gender-related differences in the role of genes and environments in affective disorders. Moreover,

Fig. 2.2 Bivariate genetic analysis of anxiety and depressive symptoms in child and adolescent twins. A, C and E respectively represent the significance of genetic, shared and non-shared environmental influences (based on Eley & Stevenson, 1999).

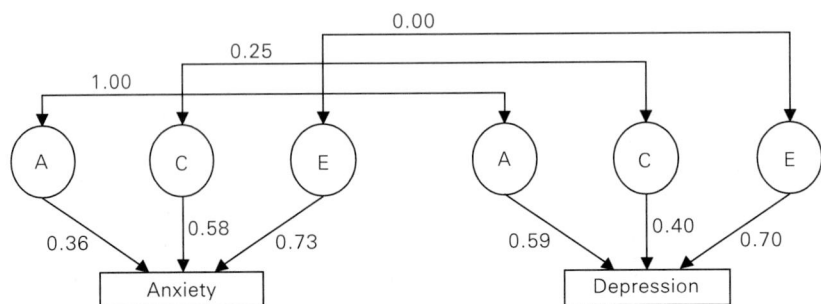

it seems that genetic factors (perhaps a substantial proportion) are shared between anxiety and depression. Shared factors experienced within families and non-shared environmental influences (such as life events) both play a role in the realisation of the genetic risk and the particular form of affective disorder that might be shown.

As yet there have been no molecular genetic studies looking specifically at child and adolescent affective disorders.

Autism

Following the landmark study by Susan Folstein & Michael Rutter (1977), autism has been a major focus for genetic research in child psychiatry. As discussed above, there is a striking degree of familiality and an increased risk in the siblings of probands some 100 times that in the general population. This 5% incidence of autism in the siblings of probands is very similar to the degree of concordance found in dizygotic twins at least one of whom has autism.

There have now been three major studies using twin methods applied to autism and they find concordance rates for monozygotic twins of 60–90% (Folstein & Rutter, 1977; Steffenberg *et al*, 1989; Bailey *et al*, 1995). The marked discrepancy between concordance rates for monozygotic and dizygotic twins is consistent with a very strong genetic influence on autism. It is important to recognise that the pattern of inheritance within families with autism is not consistent with any simple major gene effect. That is, there is no simple pattern of recessive or dominant transmission nor is there a gender-linked mechanism. As mentioned above, Pickles *et al* (1995) have estimated that between four and ten genes are involved in the autistic condition, and others have suggested that as many as 15 might be implicated (Risch *et al*, 1999). The direct risk of autism arising from obstetric or perinatal complications is less than was originally proposed. Twin research has brought to the fore the notion that what is influenced in autism is a broader phenotype that includes both communication and social deficits, accompanied by obsessive patterns of behaviour and circumscribed interests.

The search for the genes involved in autism is now reaching a stage where the localisation of susceptibility genes is starting to be reported. An important step in this was the publication of a paper demonstrating linkage to a region on chromosome 7 (International Molecular Genetic Study of Autism Consortium, 1998). Chromosome 7 was also the site of a gene identified by Fisher *et al* (1998) as contributing to a specific form of language impairment within the large three-generational pedigree of the KE family. The regions being identified in these two studies are distinct and therefore there is no indication that this represents a replication. However, the linkage to chromosome 7 has been replicated by Philippe *et al* (1999). This group also confirmed that genes at 15q11–q12 are involved in autism. This finding has also been replicated (Bass *et al*, 2000). The current understanding of the role of genetic factors has been reviewed by Rutter (2000).

■ 25

Attention-deficit hyperactivity disorder

Autism is a relatively rare disorder with a large genetic contribution to its aetiology. A much more common condition is attention-deficit hyperactivity disorder (ADHD), which has also consistently been shown to have a strong genetic component. Biederman and colleagues have conducted a number of studies looking at the families of children with ADHD. They have found, for example, odds ratios of the order of 4–5 in terms of the risk to first-degree relatives of children with ADHD (Biederman *et al*, 1990). This familial loading appears to be higher in children with ADHD comorbid with antisocial behaviour (Faraone *et al*, 1995). ADHD therefore runs in families, but we need to turn to twin research to identify whether this is a genetic or an environmental mechanism.

The first twin studies, which Goodman and I conducted, suggested a moderate level of heritability for ADHD, the magnitude of which depended on the definition applied (Goodman & Stevenson, 1989; Stevenson, 1992). Since this initial work on the London Twin Study, the finding has been replicated in a substantial number of twin studies around the world (Gillis *et al*, 1992; Thapar *et al*, 1995; Silberg *et al*, 1996; Levy *et al*, 1997; Sherman *et al*, 1997; Coolidge *et al*, 2000). On occasion the heritability measures for ADHD or hyperactivity have been as high as 90%. However, an average figure is 60–70%. An adoption study has confirmed the genetic influences on ADHD (Sprich *et al*, 2000).

One striking feature of the twin research on ADHD has been the very low values obtained for the correlations between dizygotic twin pairs. This could arise through two major influences. The first is the possibility that the twins develop behaviours that emphasise the contrast between them: one twin becomes more hyperactive while the other becomes less so. This effect reduces the dizygotic twin correlations relative to that between siblings. The other possibility is that parents are introducing a rating bias: they rate one twin as more hyperactive in contrast to the other, even though this contrast does not reflect actual differences in behaviour. An extensive effort has been made to try to disentangle these two possibilities in relation to ADHD, and the evidence is now most consistent for there being a rating bias effect rather than a true sibling contrast effect.

A pattern found in population studies of twins is that the genetic influence on individual differences in the symptoms of hyperactivity within the normal range is just as great as its influence on more extreme forms. Using a national cohort of twins Helena Gjone showed that when attention problems were identified at 0.5, 1, and 1.5 standard deviations above the mean, the heritability measure of the condition remained relatively constant, at about 0.8 (Gjone et al, 1996). This suggests that even for more extreme forms of hyperactivity, the relative mix of genetic and environmental influences remains relatively constant. This does not preclude the possibility that more extreme proband definitions, at perhaps just 1% of the population, would identify a condition where either genetic or environmental factors have a strikingly different role to play. Unfortunately, the population studies that have been conducted to date are simply too small to allow such extreme definitions to be examined.

An obvious alternative is to use twin pairs in which one member has been referred to services with ADHD or hyperactivity. There are a number of methodological problems with such clinic-based twin samples. In particular, the level of comorbidity is especially high among them. Therefore, although this represents an attractive alternative for identifying twin samples with a more substantial number of extremely hyperactive children, it does not represent an optimal solution to the problem.

Attention-deficit hyperactivity disorder has been a particular focus for molecular genetic studies, some of the findings of which are summarised in Table 2.2. It can be seen that a consistent feature of the genes thought to be involved in ADHD is that they are implicated in the functioning of the dopamine system, although one study (Quist et al, 2000) points to the serotonin system. It should also be recognised that a number of studies have not been able to replicate some of the associations presented here (Sullivan et al, 1998). One finding that has provoked particular interest is the potential association between variation at the dopamine D4 receptor gene and ADHD. Swanson and his colleagues have demonstrated in two samples that a particular form of the DRD4 gene is found more commonly in children with ADHD than in controls (LaHoste et al, 1996; Swanson et al, 1998; Holmes et al, 2000). It has also been suggested that this allele (a version of the gene) is associated with an elevation in the personality dimension of novelty-seeking – which is conceptually related to facets of ADHD (Benjamin et al, 1996; Ebstein et al, 1996). Another version of the DRD4 gene (120-base-pair repeat) has been reported by McCracken et al (2000) to be associated with ADHD.

LaHoste et al's (1996) data on allelic frequency in ADHD are presented in Fig. 2.3. It can be seen that the 7-repeat allele is more common in children with ADHD than in controls. However, it is important to note that the large majority of children with ADHD

Table 2.2 Summary of molecular genetic studies on attention-deficit hyperactivity disorder (ADHD)

Genes implicated in ADHD	Study
Dopamine transporter locus (DAT1)	Cook et al (1995); Gill et al (1997)
Dopamine D2 receptor gene (DRD2)	Comings et al (1991); Blum et al (1995)
Dopamine D4 receptor gene (DRD4):	
7-fold repeat allele	LaHoste et al (1996); Swanson et al (1998)
120-base-pair repeat allele	McCracken et al (2000)
Dopamine D5 receptor gene	Barr et al (2000)
Serotonin HTR2A receptor gene	Quist et al (2000)

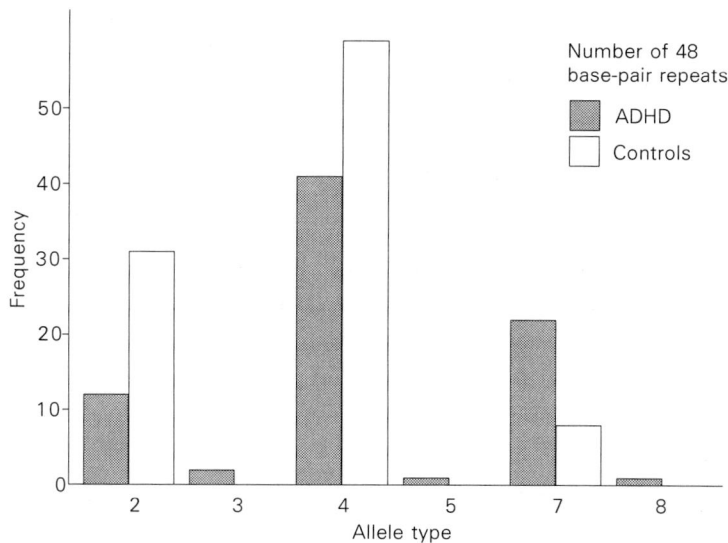

Fig. 2.3 Allelic frequency in attention-deficit hyperactivity disorder (ADHD) and control subjects (from LaHoste et al, 1996).

do not show this particular allelic form. Whatever the involvement of this allele in influencing the functioning of the dopamine system it cannot alone be carrying the genetic influences on ADHD: a number of genes are likely to be involved. This polygenic mix, along with environmental factors, produces a distribution of liability within the population, which the twin evidence suggests is best considered as a continuum of risk.

■ 27

Conduct disorders

Turning now to a broad group of conduct disorders, well-replicated evidence from a number of epidemiological studies suggests that conduct disorders show familiality. The classic work of Farrington and colleagues in the Cambridge longitudinal study, for example, showed that delinquency or criminality in parents increased the risk of similar problems in their sons by 3–4 times (Farrington, 1995). Danish adoption studies in particular have thrown light on the complexity of genetic and environmental influences on conduct disorder (e.g. Bohman,1996). Using criminality as the measure, Bohman showed that the base rate in the population was 3%, whereas it rose to 6% for boys adopted into a home in which there was an environmental risk of criminality. Where risk derived from a biological parent, the rate increased to 12%. The most striking feature of these findings was the interaction between environmental and genetic risk, where if both risk factors were present, the rates of criminality in the sons rose to 40%.

Twin research has consistently shown heritability measures in childhood to be lower than in adolescence, and those in adolescence to be lower than in adulthood (e.g., Gjone & Stevenson,1997). The high heritability measure for antisocial behaviour in adulthood is consistent with the pattern that lifelong antisocial behaviour is more strongly influenced by genetic factors than is adolescent antisocial behaviour (although the prevalence of antisocial behaviour peaks in the general population during adolescence, it does so for reasons that are primarily environmental, not genetic).

Different forms of antisocial behaviour also seem to be influenced differentially by genetic and environmental factors (Simonoff et al, 1998). For example, it has been quite consistently reported that the heritability measure is more marked for aggressive antisocial behaviour than for delinquent activities. This was confirmed by analysis of twin data from Sweden and Britain (Eley et al, 1999).

Dividing antisocial behaviour into aggressive and non-aggressive forms, Eley et al found that in both Britain and Sweden, genetic factors were more important (with the heritability measure of about 70%) in aggressive than in non-aggressive behaviours. The pattern of results was very similar for Britan and Sweden in relation to aggression. For aggressive antisocial behaviour, the pattern of results was identical for males and females. Some differences emerged in the significance of genetic and environmental factors in non-aggressive antisocial behaviour. As well as the genetic contribution being lower overall it was markedly lower for males, and in particular for delinquent activity in British males. In contrast, the shared environmental influences were more important for these non-aggressive antisocial behaviours.

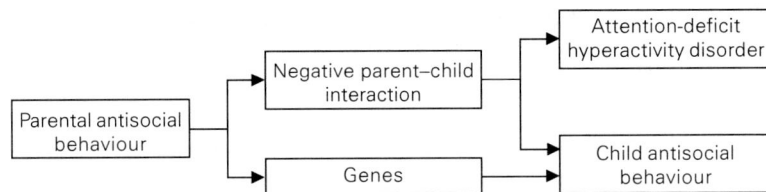

Fig. 2.4 Homotypic and heterotypic transmission.

To date there have been no molecular genetic studies directly concerned with conduct disorder, although the previously mentioned work linking the DRD4 allele to novelty-seeking may have some relevance. There have also been studies on the molecular genetics of drug and alcohol problems, which are clearly related to conduct disorder (Slutske et al, 1998).

Thus far I have reviewed the evidence in relation to transmission of the same problem from parent to child. However, the conduct disorders considered illustrate that this is too simple a picture. Here, we have both transmission of the same problem across generations (what I will call homotypic transmission) and also a possible increased risk that other disorders might develop (heterotypic transmission). For example, a parent showing antisocial behaviour is likely to pass genes on to the child, which will in turn be promoting homotypic transmission of child antisocial behaviour (see Fig. 2.4). However, at the same time such a parent will be at increased risk of presenting the child with negative parent–child interactions. These conflict-laden relationships between parent and child will feed back as an environmental influence to increase the risk of child antisocial behaviour (Reid & Patterson,1989); they are also thought to be important in the development of other externalising problems such as ADHD (Moffitt, 1990). We therefore have the possibility that a problem present in the parental generation represents a risk through both homotypic and heterotypic transmission. The joint action of environmental and genetic factors in mediating the transmission of conduct disorders has been investigated within twin (Meyer et al, 2000) and adoption (O'Connor et al, 1998) studies. For an integrative overview of this research see Lahey et al (1999).

Reading disability

I wish to finish this review by making some comments about the genetics of a specific learning disability. I have chosen the issue of reading disability to illustrate this, partly because I have been concerned with research in this area myself, but also because it represents a condition for which there has been a very fruitful convergence of evidence from molecular and quantitative genetics.

It has been recognised since the early part of the 20th century that reading disability tends to run in families. Probably the most extensive data-set on which to judge the extent of the risk is that available from the Colorado Family Reading study (Vogler et al, 1985). This revealed an elevated risk for a child with an affected parent, and the risk was slightly higher for girls than it was for boys.

Two major twin studies looking at the genetics of reading disability are the Colorado and the London studies. These were planned independently of each other and were started during the 1980s. The Colorado study is directed by John DeFries and the London study by Philip Graham and myself. We have undertaken a number of combined analyses of our data-sets both to enhance the statistical power of the analysis and to establish whether the findings replicate across samples. The results show that for spelling disability there is a substantial heritability, at around 60% (DeFries et al,1991). The Colorado study found more substantial heritabilities for reading disability, which it was suggested was due to the age difference between the two samples. Indeed, the decline in heritability of reading disability with age has subsequently been demonstrated by DeFries et al (1997).

Both these twin studies were able to test which aspects of the reading process were most strongly influenced by genetic factors. Using a two-route approach, in which reading can be achieved either by whole-word recognition or by the use of the regular link between letters and sounds, it was found that non-word reading (a measure of the use of the letter-to-sound route) was most strongly influenced by genetic factors (Stevenson,1991).

28

Table 2.3 Summary of molecular genetic studies on reading disability

Locus	Ability	Study
1(s199)	Phonological decoding	Pauls (1998)
2p15-16	Dyslexia	Fagerheim *et al* (1999)
6p21.3	Word recognition	Cardon *et al* (1994)
6p21.3	Phonological segmentation	Grigorenko *et al* (1997)
6p21.3	Orthographic and phonological ability	Gayan *et al* (1999)
6p21.3	Irregular word and non-word reading	Fisher *et al* (1999)
15q21	Word recognition	Smith *et al* (1983)
15q21	Single-word reading	Grigorenko *et al* (1997)
15q21	Spelling disability	Schulte Korne *et al* (1997)
15q15	Reading disability	Morris *et al* (2000)
15q21	Dyslexia	Nopola-Hemmi *et al* (2000)

Finally, the twin studies were used to address the issue of the origins of comorbidity between specific learning disabilities, such as with reading and spelling, and other behaviour problems such as ADHD. In a joint analysis of data from both the Colorado and London studies I was able to show that the risk of showing the combined condition stemmed primarily from shared genetic aetiology (Stevenson *et al*, 1993).

The agreement between the Colorado and London studies was quite striking given the fact that they had very different designs. The Colorado study relied on the identification of twins with reading disabilities within the education system, whereas the London study was based on a total population sample.

Reading disability is one of the first complex psychological phenotypes to which molecular genetic techniques have been successfully applied. After some early work suggesting that word recognition disability might be linked to a locus on chromosome 15 (Smith *et al*,1983), chromosome 15 was implicated in reading disability in four other studies (Grigorenko *et al*, 1997, in the USA; Schulte Korne *et al*, 1997, in Germany; Morris *et al*, 2000, in the UK; Nopola-Hemmi *et al*, 2000, in Finland). The chromosome that has generated greatest interest in terms of its involvement in reading disability is chromosome 6. After an initial publication of linkage by Cardon *et al* (1994), three other teams found linkage to a site on chromosome 6 at 6p21.3: Grigorenko *et al* (1997), in a separate large-family study; Gayan *et al* (1999), in a new sample of sibs; and Fisher *et al* (1999), again using an affected sib-pair technique. There has been at least one non-replication of the linkage to chromosome 6 by Field & Kaplan (1998). The Yale group have found linkage to a locus on chromosome 1 (Pauls, 1998), and there has been one report of a gene influencing dyslexia on chromosome 2 (Fagerheim *et al*, 1999). These molecular genetic findings have been summarised in Table 2.3.

One important feature of all these molecular genetic studies is the way in which different aspects of the reading phenotype seem to be associated differentially with the various loci. This is shown at its most striking in the findings from the Grigorenko group at Yale. They found that phonological segmentation (a measure of phonological awareness) was most strongly associated with a locus on chromosome 6; phonological decoding (based on the measure of non-word reading discussed above) showed the strongest linkage to chromosome 1; and finally single-word reading as a global skill was most strongly linked to chromosome 15. It is a real puzzle to work out why the reading phenotype should fractionate in this way.

I have tried to represent the complex relationships involved in Fig. 2.5. There are clearly pleiotropic effects whereby the same gene may be affecting more than one aspect of the reading phenotype. Indeed, the gene on chromosome 6 has been found to be linked to phonological awareness, phonological decoding and whole-word recognition. These abilities themselves show a degree of developmental interdependence. For example, phonological decoding is thought to arise as a result of developing phonological awareness. It is possible that the reverse is also taking place: developing literacy skills may be feeding back into sensitivities about the sound properties of language (Wagner *et al*,1994).

It is probably as well at this stage to reflect on what the identification of a susceptibility gene actually means. In terms of the biological processes involved, genes are very remote from the psychological skill of being able to pronounce a written word. Genes influence biological systems by producing and regulating the production of proteins. It is the way

■29

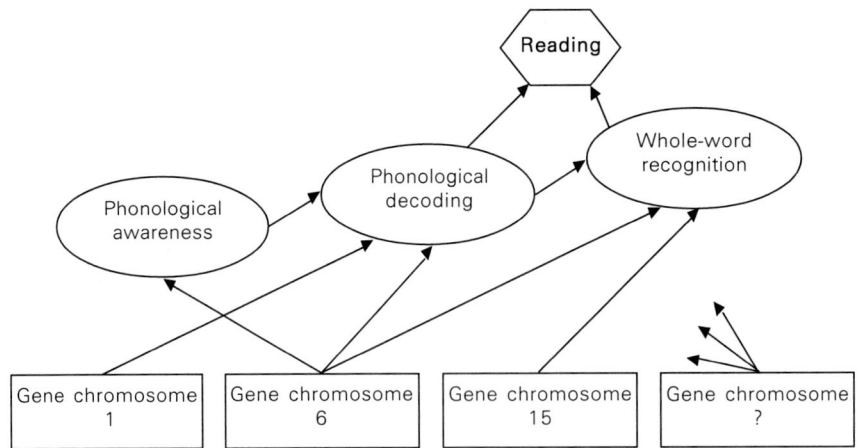

Fig. 2.5 Complex
pleiotropic effects in
reading development.

in which these proteins combine that influences both developing brain structure and brain function. It is important to recognise that even though a number of loci have been suggested as influential in reading, we have not yet identified the actual genes involved, let alone identified the gene product that might lead to variations in brain function.

The complexity at the molecular genetic level in the influences on reading is reflected in the quantitative analyses that have been made. Bettina Hohnen and I have been attempting to identify the role of genetic factors in influencing differences in aspects of language function and early-developing literacy skills (Hohnen & Stevenson, 1999). Figure 2.6 represents the best-fit model that arose from our research, which identifies four separate genetic influences on these abilities. The first (labelled A_1) is a general genetic influence that affects both performance IQ and all the language and literacy measures; the second (A_2) impinges on all the language and literacy scores; the third and fourth (A_3 and A_4) are two specific genetic effects restricted to phonological awareness and to literacy respectively. These findings represent something of the complexity of the genetic architecture at the phenotypic level (there is a parallel architecture for the role of environmental influences), which for many conditions we are only just beginning to understand.

Models of genetic and environmental influence

Finally, I want to make some general comments about the ways in which we can conceptualise the significance of genetic and environmental risk factors in influencing childhood disorders. In many ways the questions currently being addressed are the old ones concerning the role of nature and nurture in child development. However, we are now in a position to specify the genetic and environmental risk factors in much greater detail. We have both molecular and quantitative methodologies that allow us to test alternative models in this framework with a precision that was not possible until very recently. The terminology therefore is a familiar one concerning genetic and environmental influences, their interactions and correlations, but the possibilities of testing these effects directly within genetically informative designs make the precision with which answers can be provided that much greater.

Fig. 2.6 Genetic influences
on reading and language
abilities at age 6 years
(based on Hohnen &
Stevenson, 1999).

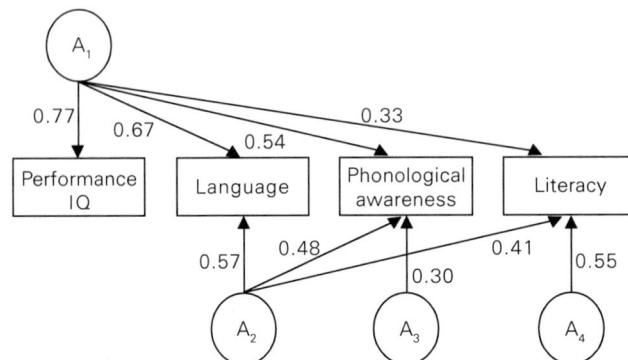

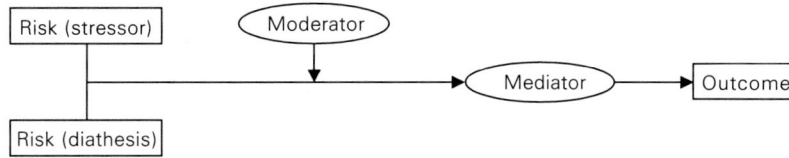

Fig. 2.7 Model of the realisation of risk.

A very general model of the way in which risk factors operate is shown in Fig. 2.7. A traditional formulation of such a model is in terms of a diathesis risk factor, which is often conceptualised as a biologically or genetically based factor interacting with a stressor, usually an environmental factor that co-acts to influence outcome. I would like to extend this terminology to include factors that increase the likelihood of an adverse outcome. These are either biological or environmental moderating factors that change the likelihood of an adverse outcome in the presence of a risk factor. Mediators are the processes by which the risk factors have their impact on the outcome. Risk and moderating factors can be either genetic or environmental.

Let us consider as an example ADHD. Table 2.4 shows various risks and moderating and mediating factors for this disorder. We have seen previously that the 7-repeat DRD4 allele is a candidate as a genetic risk factor for ADHD. There is evidence that disrupted early care is also related to an elevated incidence of hyperactivity in children (Schachar & Wachsmuth, 1991). Examples of moderating variables can be divided into those that seem to increase the probability of an adverse outcome (vulnerability factors) and those that have the opposite effect (protective factors). A long history of research indicates that aspects of temperament act as vulnerability factors for environmental or genetic risk factors (Caspi *et al*, 1995), and poor peer relationships also seem to increase vulnerabilities to adverse outcome (Dodge *et al*, 1990). A protective factor that tends to be overlooked is high IQ (Goodman *et al*, 1995). There is a striking relationship between the risk of psychopathology and IQ in children, and I have conceptualised it here as being a protective factor. I have perhaps controversially labelled this as a genetically based moderator, but the breakdown I am making between genetic and environmental variables is simplistic. We know that roughly half the variance in IQ is due to genetic factors and half to environmental influences. I have chosen consistent parenting as an example of a protective moderating factor. The division of influences into genetic and environmental ones is fairly arbitrary. It makes no sense to try to make this distinction for mediators, which are the net effect of a whole range of genetic and environmental effects and cannot be classified as one or the other. Here, I have simply given an example of delay aversion and behavioural inhibition deficit as psychologically based mediators of the effects of risk factors on outcomes.

Figure 2.8 is an attempt to put this together and it shows two possible routes through to ADHD symptomatology. I should emphasise that this is a hypothetical diagram, and in particular the designation of delay aversion as a mediator of the effects of disruptive care and behavioural inhibition deficits as a mediator of the genetic effects is speculative. However, we have recently obtained evidence from a twin study of hyperactivity that is consistent with this formulation (Kuntsi & Stevenson, 2001).

Figure 2.8 illustrates the nature of the issues that we will be able to address concerning the co-action of genetic and environmental influences. Of the two routes, one mediates

Table 2.4 Examples of risks and moderating and mediating factors for attention-deficit hyperactivity disorder

Factor	Basis	
	Genetic	*Environmental*
Risk	7-repeat DRD4 allele	Disrupted care
Moderators		
Vulnerability	Temperament	Poor peer relationships
Protective	High IQ	Consistent parenting
Mediators	Delay aversion	
	Behavioural inhibition	

■31

Risk   Moderator   Mediator   Outcome

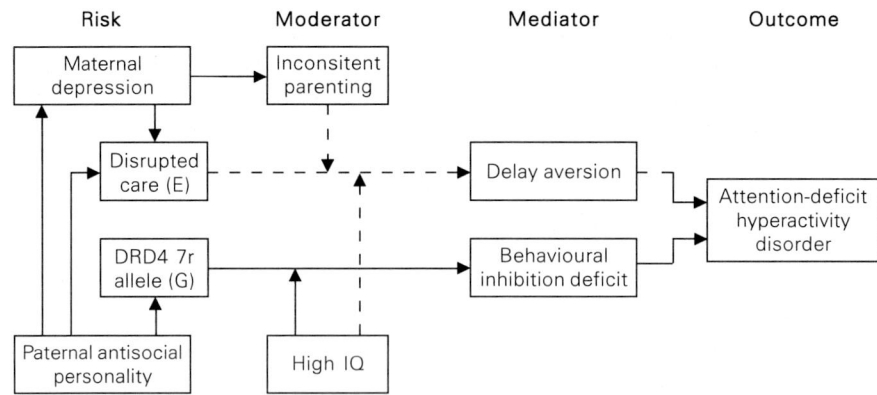

Fig. 2.8 Two routes leading to attention-deficit hyperactivity disorder (broken line indicates environmental transmission). E, environmental; G, genetic.

a primarily environmental effect and the other a primarily genetic one. In both cases there are moderating factors, with inconsistent parenting acting to increase the risk of delay aversion resulting from early disruptive care. High IQ is given as a protective factor for both routes. The real situation is, as always, more complicated. If we look at the more distal causes of disruptive care and the putative genetic factor we can see ways in which the risk factors and the moderating factors may be correlated. Paternal antisocial personality will be an influence that both increases the risk of disruptive care and may also be associated with the transmission of a genetic influence to the child. It in turn may be correlated with maternal depression, which both increases the risk of disruptive care and also the likelihood of a vulnerability factor (inconsistent parenting) being present. All of these influences introduce the possibility of gene–environment correlations, which may be present both for risk factors and also between risk factors and moderating factors.

This already complicated diagram does not include the possibilities of gene–environment interactions, which are difficult to represent diagrammatically. They would arise, for example, if the impact of disruptive care were more marked for those children carrying the 7-repeat DRD4 allele. It is the possibilities raised by developments in molecular and quantitative genetics that allow models such as this one to be tested, which represents the real excitement in the research agenda for child psychiatry (Plomin & Rutter, 1998). Most crucially we can now use the DNA obtained from a mouthwash to identify whether an individual is carrying the genetic risk factor (Freeman *et al*, 1997) and use this, together with information on experiences, to examine the joint action of genetic and social risk factors on the child's behavioural development.

Conclusions

Let me draw some conclusions from this overview of recent genetic research in child psychiatry. Most aspects of abnormal development in children are influenced to some extent by genetic variation, but the ways in which genes and environments interact are extremely complex. However, we should be able to use molecular and quantitative approaches to identify specific gene–environment interactions and correlations and indeed the co-actions of the main effects of genes and environments.

At present the clinical implications of genetic studies must be seen to be somewhat limited. There are a number of reasons why we need to be cautious. First, with the exception of some rare conditions, no childhood disorders are likely to be caused by a single major gene effect. Second, I would argue that many childhood disorders are simply the extremes of a normally distributed liability. The contributions of genes and environments to this liability are known only at the population level, and we cannot say to what extent an individual's condition is determined by genetic or environmental factors. Third, even when genetic and environmental risk factors are known, the complexity with which they interact with each other and with other moderating factors makes the application of this knowledge to the individual case very complex.

However, it seems very likely that future research will attempt to explain these mechanisms. We already have the genetic technology to enable us to start to tease apart the kind of model that I described in relation to ADHD. This technology will increasingly influence the way in which we conceptualise and diagnose childhood disorders. It may lead to a further fractionation of different disorders according to the nature of the genetic

32

and environmental risk factors involved. There may well be implications for the way in which we approach prevention, for example, by environmental interventions during the development of children who are genetically at risk. We might also develop a new range of pharmacological interventions based on our developing understanding of the molecular biology of childhood disorders.

I think it is no exaggeration to say that Michael Rutter has been the leading figure in setting this new agenda for child psychiatry in the 21st century. His contributions to our understanding of both the genetic mechanisms and environmental influences pertinent to child psychiatric disorders have been unsurpassed. Even more important is his vision of the way in which we can come to understand the joint action of these influences on developing children and through that knowledge plan more rational and effective ways of intervening to support and help vulnerable children.

References

Bailey, A., Le Couteur, A., Gottesman, I., *et al* (1995) Autism as a strongly genetic disorder – evidence from a British twin study. *Psychological Medicine*, **25**, 63–77.

Barr, C. L., Wigg, K. G., Feng, Y., *et al* (2000) Attention-deficit hyperactivity disorder and the gene for the dopamine D5 receptor. *Molecular Psychiatry*, **5**, 548–551.

Bass, M. P., Menold, M. R., Wolpert, C. M., *et al* (2000) Genetic studies in autistic disorder and chromosome 15. *Neurogenetics*, **2**, 219–226.

Beardslee, W. R., Keller, M. B., Seifer, R., *et al* (1996) Prediction of adolescent affective disorder: effects of prior parental affective disorders and child psychopathology. *Journal of the American Academy of Child and Adolescent Psychiatry*, **35**, 279–288.

Benjamin, J., Li, L., Patterson, C., *et al* (1996) Population and familial association between the d4 dopamine-receptor gene and measures of novelty seeking. *Nature Genetics*, **12**, 81–84.

Biederman, J., Faraone, S. V., Keenan, K., *et al* (1990) Family-genetic and psychosocial risk-factors in DSM–III attention deficit disorder. *Journal of the American Academy of Child and Adolescent Psychiatry*, **29**, 526–533.

Blum, K., Sheridan, P. J., Wood, R. C., *et al* (1995) Dopamine d2 receptor gene variants – association and linkage studies in impulsive–addictive–compulsive behaviour. *Pharmacogenetics*, **5**, 121–141.

Bohman, M. (1996) Predisposition to criminality: Swedish adoption studies in retrospect. In *Genetics of Criminal and Antisocial Behaviour* (eds G. R. Bock & J. A. Goode), pp. 99–114). Chichester: John Wiley & Sons.

Bouchard, T. J. & Propping, P. (1993) *Twins: A Tool of Behavioral Genetics*. Chichester: John Wiley & Sons.

Cardon, L. R., Smith, S. D., Fulker, D. W., *et al* (1994) Quantitative trait locus for reading-disability on chromosome-6. *Science*, **266**, 276–279.

Caspi, A., Henry, B., McGee, *et al* (1995) Temperamental origins of child and adolescent behavior problems – from age 3 to age 15. *Child Development*, **66**, 55–68.

Comings, D. E., Comings, B. G., Muhleman, D., *et al* (1991) The dopamine-d2 receptor locus as a modifying gene in neuropsychiatric disorders. *Journal of the American Medical Association*, **266**, 1793–1800.

Cook, E. H., Stein, M. A., Krasowski, M. D., *et al* (1995) Association of attention-deficit disorder and the dopamine transporter gene. *American Journal of Human Genetics*, **56**, 993–998.

Coolidge, F. L., Thede, L. L. & Young, S. E. (2000) Heritability and the comorbidity of attention deficit hyperactivity disorder with behavioral disorders and executive function deficits: a preliminary investigation. *Developmental Neuropsychology*, **17**, 273–287.

DeFries, J. C., Stevenson, J., Gillis, J. J., *et al* (1991) Genetic etiology of spelling deficits in the Colorado and London twin studies of reading-disability. *Reading and Writing*, **3**, 271–283.

——, Alarcon, M. & Olson, R. C. (1997) Genetic aetiologies of reading and spelling deficits: developmental differences. In *Dyslexia: Biology, Cognition and Intervention* (eds C. Hulme & M. Snowling), pp. 20–37. London: Whurr.

Dodge, K., Coie, J., Pettit, G., *et al* (1990) Peer status and aggression in boys' groups: developmental and contextual analyses. *Child Development*, **61**, 1289–1309.

Eaves, L. J., Silberg, J. L., Meyer, J. M., *et al* (1997) Genetics and developmental psychopathology. 2. The main effects of genes and environment on behavioral problems in the Virginia twin study of adolescent behavioral development. *Journal of Child Psychology and Psychiatry*, **38**, 965–980.

Ebstein, R. P., Novick, O., Umansky, R., *et al* (1996) Dopamine D4 receptor (D4DR) exon III polymorphism associated with the human personality trait of novelty seeking. *Nature Genetics*, **12**, 78–80.

Eley, T. C. (1997) Depressive symptoms in children and adolescents: aetiological links between normality and abnormality. *Journal of Child Psychology and Psychiatry*, **38**, 861–865.

■33

—— & Stevenson, J. (1999) Using genetic analysis to clarify the distinction between depressive and anxious symptoms in children. *Journal of Abnormal Child Psychology*, **27**, 105–114.

—— & —— (2000) Specific life events and chronic experiences differentially associated with depression and anxiety in young twins. *Journal of Abnormal Child Psychology*, **28**, 383–394.

——, Lichtenstein, P. & Stevenson, J. (1999) Sex differences in the etiology of aggressive and non-aggressive antisocial behaviour: results from two twin studies. *Child Development*, **70**, 155–168.

Fagerheim, T., Raeymaekers, P., Tonnessen, F. E., *et al* (1999) A new gene (DYX3) for dyslexia is located on chromosome 2. *Journal of Medical Genetics*, **36**, 664–669.

Faraone, S. V., Biederman, J., Chen, W., *et al* (1995) Genetic heterogeneity in attention-deficit hyperactivity disorer (ADHD): gender, psychiatric comorbidity, and maternal ADHD. *Journal of Abnormal Psychology*, **104**, 334–345.

Farrington, D. P. (1995) The Twelfth Jack Tizard Memorial Lecture. The development of offending and antisocial behaviour from childhood: key findings from the Cambridge Study in Delinquent Development. *Journal of Child Psychology and Psychiatry*, **36**, 929–964.

Field, L. L. & Kaplan, B. J. (1998) Absence of linkage of phonological coding dyslexia to chromosome 6p23-p21.3 in a large family data set. *American Journal of Human Genetics*, **63**, 1448–1456.

Fisher, S. E., Vargha-Khadem, F., Watkins, K. E., *et al* (1998) Localisation of a gene implicated in a severe speech and language disorder. *Nature Genetics*, **18**, 168–170.

——, Marlow, A. J., Lamb, J., *et al* (1999) A quantitative-trait locus on chromosome 6p influences different aspects of developmental dyslexia. *American Journal of Human Genetics*, **64**, 146–156.

Folstein, S. & Rutter, M. (1977) Infantile autism: a genetic study of 21 twin pairs. *Journal of Child Psychology and Psychiatry*, **18**, 297–321.

Freeman, B., Powell, J., Ball, D., *et al* (1997) DNA by mail: an inexpensive and noninvasive method for collecting DNA samples from widely dispersed populations. *Behavior Genetics*, **27**, 251–257.

Gayan, J., Smith, S. D., Cherny, S. S., *et al* (1999) Quantitative-trait locus for specific language and reading deficits on chromosome 6p. *American Journal of Human Genetics*, **64**, 157–164.

Gill, M., Daly, G., Heron, S., *et al* (1997) Confirmation of association between attention deficit hyperactivity disorder and a dopamine transporter polymorphism. *Molecular Psychiatry*, **2**, 311–313.

Gillis, J. J., Gilger, J. W., Pennington, B. F., *et al* (1992) Attention deficit disorder in reading-disabled twins: Evidence for a genetic etiology. *Journal of Abnormal Child Psychology*, **20**, 303–315.

Gjone, H. & Stevenson, J. (1997) The association between internalising and externalising behaviour in childhood and early adolescence: genetic and environmental common influences. *Journal of Abnormal Child Psychology*, **25**, 277–286.

——, —— & Sundet, J. M. (1996) Genetic influence on parent-reported attention-related problems in a Norwegian general-population twin sample. *Journal of the American Academy of Child And Adolescent Psychiatry*, **35**, 588–596.

Goodman, R. & Stevenson, J. (1989) A twin study of hyperactivity. 2. The etiological role of genes, family relationships and perinatal adversity. *Journal of Child Psychology and Psychiatry*, **30**, 691–709.

——, Simonoff, E. & Stevenson, J. (1995) The impact of child IQ, parent IQ and sibling IQ on child behavioral-deviance scores. *Journal of Child Psychology and Psychiatry*, **36**, 409–425.

Grigorenko, E. L., Wood, F. B., Meyer, M. S., *et al* (1997) Susceptibility loci for distinct components of developmental dyslexia on chromosomes 6 and 15. *American Journal of Human Genetics*, **60**, 27–39.

Harrington, R. C., Fudge, H., Rutter, M., *et al* (1993) Child and adult depression: a test of continuities with data from a family study. *British Journal of Psychiatry*, **162**, 627–633.

Hohnen, B. & Stevenson, J. (1999) The structure of genetic influences on general cognitive, language, phonological and reading abilities. *Developmental Psychology*, **35**, 590–603.

Holland, A. J., Sicotte, J. & Treasure, J. (1988) Anorexia nervosa: evidence for a genetic basis. *Journal of Psychosomatic Research*, **32**, 561–571.

Holmes, J., Payton, A, Barrett, J. H., *et al* (2000) A family-based and case-control association study of the dopamine D4 receptor gene and dopamine transporter gene in attention deficit hyperactivity disorder. *Molecular Psychiatry*, **5**, 523–530.

International Molecular Genetic Study of Autism Consortium (1998) A full genome screen for autism with evidence for linkage to a region on chromosome 7q. *Human Molecular Genetics*, **7**, 571–578.

Kendler, K. S., Walters, E. E., Neale, M. C., *et al* (1995) The structure of the genetic and environmental risk-factors for six major psychiatric disorders in women: phobia, generalised anxiety disorder, panic disorder, bulimia, major depression and alcoholism. *Archives of General Psychiatry*, **52**, 374–383.

Kovacs, M. (1985) The Children's Depression Inventory (CDI). *Psychopharmacology Bulletin*, **21**, 995–1124.

Kuntsi, J. & Stevenson, J. (2001) Psychological mechanisms in hyperactivity. II. The role of genetic factors. *Journal of Child Psychology and Psychiatry* (in press).

LaBuda, M. C., Gottesman, I. I. & Pauls, D. L. (1993) Usefulness of twin studies for exploring the etiology of childhood and adolescent psychiatric disorders. *American Journal of Medical Genetics*, **48**, 47–59.

Lahey, B. B., Waldman, I. D. & McBurnett, K. (1999) Annotation: the development of antisocial behavior: an integrative causal model. *Journal of Child Psychology and Psychiatry*, **40**, 669–682.

LaHoste, G. J., Swanson, J. M., Wigal, S. B., *et al* (1996) Dopamine D4 receptor gene polymorphism is associated with attention deficit hyperactivity disorder. *Molecular Psychiatry*, **1**, 121–124.

Levy, F., Hay, D. A., McStephen, M., *et al* (1997) Attention-deficit hyperactivity disorder: a category or a continuum? Genetic analysis of a large-scale twin study. *Journal of the American Academy of Child and Adolescent Psychiatry*, **36**, 737–744.

McCracken, J. T., Smalley, S. L., McGough, J. J., *et al* (2000) Evidence for linkage of a tandem duplication polymorphism upstream of the dopamine D4 receptor gene (DRD4) with attention deficit hyperactivity disorder (ADHD). *Molecular Psychiatry*, **5**, 531–536.

Meyer, J. M., Rutter, M., Silberg, J. L., *et al* (2000) Familial aggregation for conduct disorder symptomatology: the role of genes, marital discord and family adaptability. *Psychological Medicine*, **30**, 759–774.

Moffitt, T. E. (1990) Juvenile-delinquency and attention deficit disorder – boys' developmental trajectories from age 3 to age 15. *Child Development*, **61**, 893–910.

Morris, D. W., Robinson, L., Turic, D., *et al* (2000) Family-based association mapping provides evidence for a gene for reading disability on chromosome 15q. *Human Molecular Genetics*, **9**, 843–848.

Nopola-Hemmi, J., Taipale, M., Haltia, T., *et al* (2000) Two translocations of chromosome 15q associated with dyslexia. *Journal of Medical Genetics*, **37**, 771–775.

O'Connor, T. G, Deater-Deckard, K., Fulker, D., *et al* (1998) Genotype–environment correlations in late childhood and early adolescence: antisocial behavioral problems and coercive parenting. *Developmental Psychology*, **34**, 970–981.

Pauls, D. (1998) Yale study of genetics of reading disability. Paper presented at a meeting on "Molecular genetic studies of reading and spelling disability". University of Marburg, Germany.

Philippe, A., Martinez, M., Guilloud-Bataille, M., *et al* (1999) Genome-wide scan for autism susceptibility genes. *Human Molecular Genetics*, **8**, 805–812.

Pickles, A., Bolton, P., Macdonald, H., *et al* (1995) Latent class analysis of recurrence risk for complex phenotypes with selection and measurement error: a twin and family history study of autism. *American Journal of Human Genetics*, **57**, 717–726.

Plomin, R. & Bergeman, C. S. (1991) The nature of nurture: genetic influence on 'environmental' measures. *Behavior and Brain Sciences*, **14**, 373–427.

—— & Daniels, D. (1987) Why are children in the same family so different from one another? *Behavioral and Brain Sciences*, **10**, 1–60.

—— & Rutter, M. (1998) Child development, molecular genetics, and what to do with genes once they are found. *Child Development*, **69**, 1223–1242.

——, Reiss, D., Hetherington, E. M., *et al* (1994) Nature and nurture: genetic contributions to measures of the family environment. *Developmental Psychology*, **30**, 32–43.

Quist, J. F., Barr, C. L., Schachar, R., *et al* (2000) Evidence for the serotonin HTR2A receptor gene as a susceptibility factor in attention deficit hyperactivity disorder (ADHD). *Molecular Psychiatry*, **5**, 537–541.

Reid, J. B. & Patterson, G. R. (1989) The development of antisocial-behavior patterns in childhood and adolescence. *European Journal of Personality*, **3**, 107–119.

Rende, R. D., Plomin, R., Reiss, D., *et al* (1993) Genetic and environmental-influences on depressive symptomatology in adolescence – individual-differences and extreme scores. *Journal of Child Psychology and Psychiatry*, **34**, 1387–1398.

Richman, N., Stevenson, J. & Graham, P. J. (1982) *Preschool to School: A Behavioural Study*. London: Academic Press.

Risch, N., *et al* (1999) A genomic screen of autism: evidence for a multilocus etiology. *American Journal of Human Genetics*, **65**, 493–507.

Rutherford, J., McGuffin, P., Katz, R. J., *et al* (1993) Genetic influences on eating attitudes in a normal female twin population. *Psychological Medicine*, **23**, 425–436.

Rutter, M. (1966) *Children of Sick Parents: An Environmental and Psychiatric Study*. Oxford: Oxford University Press.

—— (2000) Genetic studies of autism: from the 1970s into the millennium. *Journal of Abnormal Child Psychology*, **28**, 3–14.

■35

—, Korn, S. & Birch, H. G. (1963) Genetic and environmental factors in the development of 'primary reaction patterns'. *British Journal of Social and Clinical Psychology*, **2**, 161–173.

—, Tizard, J. & Whitmore, K. (1970) *Education, Health and Behaviour*. London: Longman.

Schachar, R. J. & Wachsmuth, R. (1991) Family dysfunction and psychosocial adversity – comparison of attention-deficit disorder, conduct disorder, normal and clinical controls. *Canadian Journal of Behavioural Science. Revue Canadienne des Sciences du Comportement*, **23**, 332–348.

Schulte Korne, G., Grimm, T., Nothen, M. M., *et al* (1997) Evidence for linkage of spelling disability to chromosome 15. *American Journal of Medical Genetics*, **74**, 661.

Sherman, D. K., Iacono, W. G. & McGue, M. K. (1997) Attention-deficit hyperactivity disorder dimensions: a twin study of inattention and impulsivity–hyperactivity. *Journal of the American Academy of Child and Adolescent Psychiatry*, **36**, 745–753.

Silberg, J., Meyer, J., Pickles, A., *et al* (1996) Heterogeneity among juvenile antisocial behaviors – findings from the Virginia twin study of adolescent behavioral-development. *Ciba Foundation Symposia*, **194**, 76–86.

—, Pickles, A., Rutter, M., *et al* (1999) The influence of genetic factors and life stress on depression among adolescent girls. *Archives of General Psychiatry*, **56**, 225–232.

Simonoff, E., Pickles, A., Meyer, J., *et al* (1998) Genetic and environmental influences on subtypes of conduct disorder behavior in boys. *Journal of Abnormal Child Psychology*, **26**, 495–509.

Slutske, W. S., Heath, A. C., Dinwiddie, S. H., *et al* (1998) Common genetic risk factors for conduct disorder and alcohol dependence. *Journal of Abnormal Psychology*, **107**, 363–374.

Smith, S. D., Kimberling, W. J., Pennington, B. F., *et al* (1983) Specific reading disability: identification of an inherited form through linkage analysis. *Science*, **219**, 1345–1347.

Spielberger, C. (1972) *Preliminary Test Manual for the State–Trait Anxiety Inventory for Children*. Palo Alto, CA: Consulting Psychologists Press.

Sprich, S., Biederman, J., Crawford, M. H., *et al* (2000) Adoptive and biological families of children and adolescents with ADHD. *Journal of the American Academy of Child and Adolescent Psychiatry*, **39**, 1432–1437.

Steffenberg, S., Gillber, C., Hellgren, L., *et al* (1989) A twin study of autism in Denmark, Finland, Iceland, Norway and Sweden. *Journal of Child Psychology and Psychiatry*, **30**, 405–416.

Stevenson, J. (1991) Which aspects of processing text mediate genetic effects? *Reading and Writing: An Interdisciplinary Journal*, **3**, 249–269.

—— (1992) Evidence for a genetic etiology in hyperactivity in children. *Behavior Genetics*, **22**, 337–344.

—— & Goodman, R. (2001) The association between behaviour at three years and adult criminality. *British Journal of Psychiatry*, in press.

—, Pennington, B. F., Gilger, J. W., *et al* (1993) Hyperactivity and spelling disability – testing for shared genetic etiology. *Journal of Child Psychology and Psychiatry*, **34**, 1137–1152.

Sullivan, P. F., Fifield, W. J., Kennedy, M. A., *et al* (1998) No association between novelty seeking and the type 4 dopamine receptor gene (drd4) in two New Zealand samples. *American Journal of Psychiatry*, **155**, 98–101.

Swanson, J. M., Sunohara, G. A., Kennedy, J. L., *et al* (1998) Association of the dopamine receptor d4 (drd4) gene with a refined phenotype of attention deficit hyperactivity disorder (ADHD): a family-based approach. *Molecular Psychiatry*, **3**, 38–41.

Thapar, A. & McGuffin, P. (1995) Are anxiety symptoms in childhood heritable? *Journal of Child Psychology and Psychiatry*, **36**, 439–447.

—, Hervas, A. & McGuffin, P. (1995) Childhood hyperactivity scores are highly heritable and show sibling competition effects – twin study evidence. *Behavior Genetics*, **25**, 537–544.

Thomas, A. & Chess, S. (1977) *Temperament and Development*. New York: Brunner/Mazel.

—, ——, Birch, H., *et al* (1963) *Behavioral Individuality in Early Childhood*. New York: New York University Press.

—, —— & ——. (1968) *Temperament and Behavioural Disorders in Childhood*. New York: New York University Press.

Tizard, J. (1975) Race and IQ: the limits of probability. *New Behaviour*, **1**, 6–9.

Vogler, G. P., Defries, J. C. & Decker, S. N. (1985) Family history as an indicator of risk for reading disability. *Journal of Learning Disabilities*, **18**, 419–421.

Wagner, R. K., Torgesen, J. K. & Rashotte, C. A. (1994) Development of reading-related phonological processing abilities: new evidence of bidirectional causality from a latent variable longitudinal study. *Developmental Psychology*, **30**, 73–87.

36 ▪

3 Reflections on the past and future of developmental psychopathology

Dante Cicchetti

Developmental psychopathology is an evolving inter-disciplinary scientific perspective whose main focus involves elucidating the interplay between the biological, psychological, and social-context aspects of normal and abnormal development across the life course (Zigler & Glick, 1986; Mednick *et al*, 1991; Cicchetti, 1993; Rutter, 1996*a;* Keshavan & Murray, 1997; Cicchetti & Toth, 1998*a*). In an early statement concerning its goals, I wrote,

> "Developmental psychopathology should bridge fields of study, span the life cycle, and aid in the discovery of important new truths about the processes underlying adaptation and maladaptation, as well as the best means of preventing or ameliorating psychopathology. Moreover, this discipline should contribute greatly to reducing the dualisms that exist between the clinical study of and research into childhood and adult disorders, between the behavioural and biological sciences, between developmental psychology and psychopathology, and between basic and applied science." (Cicchetti, 1990: p. 20)

Indeed, during the quarter-century that has elapsed since its emergence, theory and research in the field of developmental psychopathology have contributed to dramatic knowledge gains in the multiple domains of child and adult development (see Cicchetti & Cohen, 1995*a,b*). In particular, there has been an emphasis on increasingly specific process-level models of normal and abnormal development, an acknowledgement that multiple pathways exist to the same outcome and that the effects of a component's value may vary in different systems, and an intensification of interest in biological and genetic factors, as well as in social and contextual factors related to the development of maladaptation and psychopathology (e.g., Cicchetti & Tucker, 1994*b*; Cicchetti & Rogosch, 1996*b*; Cicchetti & Richters, 1997; Cicchetti & Aber, 1998; Cicchetti & Cannon, 1999).

In recognition of scientific achievements in this young field, the Steering Committee of the Institute of Medicine (1989) adopted the principles of developmental psychopathology as the organising framework for its report *Research on Children and Adolescents with Mental, Behavioral, and Developmental Disorders*. Likewise, the National Institute of Mental Health's *National Plan for Research on Child and Adolescent Mental Disorders* (National Advisory Mental Health Council, 1990), an outgrowth of the work of the Institute of Medicine's report, embraced developmental psychopathology as its overarching paradigm for organising future research priorities. Furthermore, the Institute

■ 37

of Medicine (1994) highlighted developmental psychopathology as one of four core sciences considered essential for expanding the frontiers of prevention and intervention efforts into reducing the risk factors for mental disorders and their sequelae throughout the life course.

Although some advances have been made in breaking down the barriers that exist between basic and applied research and between practitioners and researchers, a great deal of work remains to be completed before true progress is achieved. As Neal Miller (1995) wrote,

> "Clinical observations can direct the attention of laboratory workers to significant new problems and laboratory experiments can refine and correct clinical observations [p. 901] ... All of the different specialties – ranging from the basic to the applied and from the biological to the social and cultural – are needed to advance our common goal of better understanding human behavior." (p. 910)

Despite the fact that Miller was discussing the importance of basic and applied research, and a multi-domain and interdisciplinary perspective for the field of neuroscience, his recommendations echo the basic principles and philosophical beliefs of developmental psychopathologists.

Prior to its relatively recent crystallisation as an integrative framework for examining the links between the study of psychopathology and the study of normal development, the field of developmental psychopathology must acknowledge a long ancestry, dating back to the beginning of Western thought (Kaplan, 1967; Cicchetti, 1990; Overton & Horowitz, 1991). It is interesting to note that every one of the ideas that are central to the major developmental theories of the 20th century, including Freudian psychoanalytic theory, Wernerian organismic developmental theory and Piagetian structural developmental theory, can be identified in the writings of Plato and Aristotle (Kaplan, 1967).

For example, the notion of the role of integration of multiple domains of behaviour for the harmonious functioning of the individual was anticipated by the Platonic concept of the triune character of the soul. In Plato, one also can find the idea of hierarchically integrated domains of functioning within his conceptualisation of the dominance of reason (a higher function) over passion (a lower function). Moreover, in Plato's view of the dynamic role of the individual one discovers another historical root of the organismic perspective.

Likewise, Aristotle was one of the first to argue that individuation, differentiation and self-actualisation were the characteristic aspects of developmental transformations. He also stressed the interdependence between the environment and the individual. A believer in the concept of the multiple determination of behaviour, Aristotle contended that different levels of behavioural organisation exist in humans. Further, one also can find in Aristotle an emphasis on a holistic understanding of behaviour – the part must be viewed in relation to the whole in order to understand its true meaning. Although neither Plato nor Aristotle focused on the interrelation between these ideas and the psychopathological condition, none the less they built a potent theoretical and philosophical orientation for the field of developmental psychopathology (see e.g., Kaplan, 1967; Overton & Horowitz, 1991).

More broadly, developmental psychopathology owes its emergence and coalescence to many historically based endeavours within a variety of disciplines, including cultural anthropology, embryology, epidemiology, genetics, the neurosciences, philosophy, psychiatry, psychoanalysis, psychobiology, clinical, developmental and experimental psychology, and sociology (see Cicchetti, 1990, for a review of these historical forces). The influence of these disciplines on the field of developmental psychopathology illustrates the manner in which advances in our knowledge of developmental processes and progress within particular scientific disciplines can mutually inform each other. To provide one example, the work of embryologists since the 19th century has provided a rich empirical foundation for the emergence of organismic theories of development of great significance for understanding normal and abnormal human behaviour (Fishbein, 1976; Sameroff, 1983). From their efforts to learn about normal embryological functioning, early embryologists derived the principles of a dynamically active organism and of a hierarchically integrated system that were later used in investigations of the processes of abnormal development not only within embryology, but also within the neurosciences, clinical neurology, clinical and experimental psychology, and psychiatry (see, e.g., Jackson, 1884; Goldstein, 1939; Weiss, 1961, 1969; Kuo, 1967; Shakow, 1968; Teitelbaum, 1971, 1977).

Before the emergence of developmental psychopathology, the efforts of those working in these areas had been largely separate and distinct. Notably, a number of the major theoretical systematisers in these diverse scientific fields conceptualised psychopathology as a distortion or exaggeration of the normal condition and reasoned that the study of normal biological, psychological and social processes could be more clearly understood through the investigation of pathological phenomena (Cicchetti & Cohen, 1995c). The Medical Research Council Unit in Child Psychiatry, opened in 1984, and the Social, Genetic and Developmental Psychiatry Research Centre at the Institute of Psychiatry in London, both directed by Michael Rutter, aim to advance the understanding of the developmental processes involved in psychopathology and exemplify the multi-disciplinary perspective that should characterise developmental psychopathology research. At these sites, collaboration occurs between an unusually wide variety of scientists, ranging from behavioural geneticists, to developmental and clinical psychologists, to social anthropologists and psychiatrists.

Although the field of developmental psychopathology grew in importance during the 1970s, predominantly through its identification as an important perspective by researchers conducting prospective longitudinal studies of children at risk for schizophrenia (Garmezy & Streitman, 1974; for a review of findings from these high-risk studies, see Watt *et al*, 1984), it was not until the 1980s that the field began to exert a major influence on the manner in which researchers investigated the mental disorders and high-risk conditions of children and adults (Rutter & Garmezy, 1983; Cicchetti, 1984a,b; Rutter, 1986; Zigler & Glick, 1986). During the past two decades, conceptualisations of the nature of mental disorder, aetiological models of risk and pathology, the scientific questions posed, and the sampling, design, measurement and data-analysis strategies utilised in traditional research on psychopathology have been re-examined, challenged and cast into a new light by developmental psychopathologists (Sameroff & Chandler, 1975; Sroufe & Rutter, 1984; Sroufe, 1990; Richters & Cicchetti, 1993; Cicchetti & Cohen, 1995a,b; Cicchetti & Richters, 1997; Richters, 1997; Wakefield, 1997).

■ 39

Sroufe & Rutter (1984) originally defined developmental psychopathology as

> "*the study of the origins and course of individual patterns of behavioral maladaptation*, whatever the causes, whatever the transformations in behavioral manifestation, and however the course of the developmental pattern may be". (p. 18; italics theirs)

The authors of the Institute of Medicine's (1989) report on child and adolescent behaviour and mental disorders elaborated on this definition, stating that the developmental psychopathology perspective should incorporate

> "the emerging behavioral repertoire, cognitive, and language functions, social and emotional processes, and changes occurring in anatomical structures and physiological processes of the brain". (p. 14)

Theorists and researchers in the field of developmental psychopathology seek to unify, within a life-span framework, the many contributions to the study of individuals at high risk for, or suffering from, mental disorders. Developmental psychopathologists strive to engage in a comprehensive evaluation of biological, psychological and social factors and to ascertain how these multiple levels of functioning may influence individual differences, the continuity or discontinuity of adaptive and maladaptive behavioural patterns and the pathways by which the same developmental outcomes may be reached. In practice, this entails a comprehension of and an appreciation for the developmental

What is developmental psychopathology?

transformations and reorganisations that occur in neurobiological, cognitive, socio-emotional, linguistic and representational development over time, an analysis of the risk and protective factors operating in the individual and his or her environment, investigation of how emergent functions, competencies and developmental tasks modify the expression of a disorder or lead to new symptoms and difficulties, and the recognition that a particular stressor, set of stressful circumstances or underlying mechanism may result in different biological and psychological problems, depending on when in the developmental course they occur (Cicchetti & Aber, 1986; Rutter, 1987; Institute of Medicine, 1989). Moreover, as noted by Rutter (1990), various difficulties will have different meanings for an individual depending on cultural considerations, as well as on the individual's current level of psychological and biological functioning. The interpretation of the experience, in turn, will affect the adaptation or maladaptation that ensues.

Developmental psychopathologists stress that individuals with disorders may move between pathological and non-pathological forms of functioning (Zigler & Glick, 1986). Moreover, even in the midst of pathology, individuals may display adaptive coping mechanisms. It is only through the consideration of both adaptive and maladaptive processes that it becomes possible to delimit the presence, nature and boundaries of the underlying psychopathology. Furthermore, developmental psychopathology is a perspective that is especially applicable to the investigation of critical transitional points in development across the life span (Rutter, 1996c). With respect to the emergence of psychopathology, all periods of life are consequential, in that the developmental process may take a pernicious turn towards mental disorder at any phase. Developmental psychopathologists acknowledge that disorders may appear at any point in the life span (Cicchetti, 1993; Rutter, 1996b; Keshavan & Murray, 1997) and advocate the importance of examining the course of disorders once manifest, including their phases and sequelae (cf. Zigler & Glick, 1986; Post et al, 1996). Rutter (1996c) has theorised that key transitional or turning points may be times when the presence of protective mechanisms could help individuals redirect themselves from a risk trajectory onto a more adaptive developmental pathway. In contrast to the often dichotomous world of mental disorder/non-disorder in traditional psychiatric and psychological approaches, developmental psychopathology recognises that normality often fades into abnormality, that adaptive and maladaptive may take on differing definitions depending on whether one's time referent is immediate circumstance or long-term development, and that processes within the individual can be characterised as having shades or degrees of psychopathology.

Principles of developmental psychopathology

To elaborate more completely the principles that underpin the field of developmental psychopathology, I turn next to an explication of its tenets. This delimitation of the principles is not presented in any presumed order of importance, nor is it meant to be an all-inclusive list. Furthermore, I wish to stress that, if taken in isolation, many components of a developmental psychopathology perspective are equally applicable to other disciplines or fields of inquiry. However, the incorporation and integration of previously discrete concepts serve to set developmental psychopathology apart as a unique approach for understanding processes contributing to adaptation and maladaptation across the life course.

Normal and abnormal

A focus on the boundary between normal and abnormal development is central to a developmental psychopathology perspective. Such a viewpoint emphasises not only how knowledge from the study of normal development can inform the study of high-risk conditions and psychopathological disorders, but also how the investigation of risk and pathology can enhance our comprehension of normal development. Even before a psychopathological disorder emerges, certain pathways signify adaptational failures in normal development that probabilistically forebode subsequent maladaptation and psychopathology (Sroufe, 1989; Cicchetti & Rogosch, 1996a). Similarly, information obtained from investigating psychopathology can augment the comprehension of normal development.

The central focus of developmental psychopathology involves the elucidation of developmental processes and how they function, as indicated and elaborated by the examination of extremes in the distribution (i.e., individuals with mental disorders). Developmental psychopathologists also direct attention towards variations in the continuum between the mean and the extremes. These variations may represent individuals who are currently not divergent enough to be considered to have a disorder, but who may progress to further extremes as development continues. Such individuals may be vulnerable to developing future disordered outcomes, or developmental deviations may, for some individuals, reflect either the earliest signs of an emerging dysfunction or an already existing dysfunction that is partially compensated for by other processes within or outside the individual.

Because of the interrelations between the investigation of normal and abnormal development, developmental psychopathologists must be cognisant of normal pathways of development within a given cultural context (Garcia-Coll *et al*, 1996), uncover deviations from these pathways, articulate the developmental transformations that occur as individuals progress through these deviant developmental courses, and identify the processes and mechanisms that may divert an individual from a particular pathway onto a more or less adaptive course (cf. Cicchetti & Aber, 1986; Sroufe, 1989).

Despite the importance of undertaking work that can elucidate the interface between normality and abnormality, investigations of the determinants of human behaviour are greatly hampered by the ethical impossibility of conducting experiments that will compromise the integrity of biological and psychological ontogenetic processes. Therefore, attention must be directed towards 'experiments of nature' to elucidate our understanding of developmental processes and mechanisms. These so-called natural experiments "are especially important for the purpose of dissociating possible (causal) mechanisms that offer competing explanations" (Rutter, 1994: p. 935). Moreover, the examination of individuals with high-risk conditions and mental disorders can provide a natural opportunity for the study of system organisation, disorganisation and reorganisation that is otherwise not possible owing to constraints associated with human participants. Because there are limits to experimental manipulations that can be invoked with humans, utilisation of individuals who are experiencing difficulties is frequently the only way to examine developmental processes in their full complexity.

Often, the investigation of a system in its smoothly operating normal or healthy state does not afford the opportunity to comprehend the interrelations between its component subsystems. Noam Chomsky (1968) reflected on this state of affairs when he asserted:

■41

> "One difficulty in the psychological sciences lies in the familiarity of the phenomena with which they deal. [...] One is inclined to take them for granted as necessary or somehow 'natural'. [...] We also lose sight of the need for explanation when phenomena are too familiar and 'obvious.' We tend too easily to assume that explanations must be transparent and close to the surface." (p. 21)

Because pathological conditions such as brain damage, mental disorder and residing in a malignant environment (such as is the case with child maltreatment or growing up in a Romanian institution) enable scientists to isolate the components of the integrated system, their investigation sheds light on the normal structure of the system and prevents us from falling prey to the problems identified by Chomsky. Consequently, examinations of developmental extremes and imperfections must be conducted. The anthropologist Stephen Gould (1980) has articulated the central role that the discovery of anomalies can play in elucidating the history of evolution. Gould noted that whereas 'good fits' between organisms and their ecological niches generate so great an array of interpretations as to be uninformative, the identification of anomalies greatly decreases the number of explanations possible. As Gould (1986) stated,

> "We must look for imperfections and oddities because any perfection in organic design or ecology obliterates the paths of history and might have been created as we find it." (p. 63)

I agree with Michael Scriven's view (cited in Kaplan, 1964) that one can learn more from studying disarray than from disregarding it. If we choose simply to ignore or bypass the study of these atypical phenomena, then the eventual result is likely to be the construction of theories that are contradicted by the revelation of critical facts in risk and psychopathology (cf. Lenneberg, 1967). Similar to genetic research on pathological embryos and to neurobiological and genetic linkage studies on psychopathology, investigations of the ecological, biological and psychological factors that cause development to go awry can help to inform our understanding of more normative ontogenetic processes. When extrapolating from non-typical populations with the goal of informing developmental theory, it is critical to investigate a range of individuals at high risk for, or suffering from, mental disorders. The study of a single pathological or risk process may result in spurious conclusions if generalisations are made based solely on that condition or disorder. However, if a given biological or behavioural pattern is viewed in the light of an entire spectrum of disordered modifications, then it may be possible to attain significant insight into the processes of development not generally achieved through sole reliance on studies of relatively non-disordered populations (Lenneberg, 1967).

Diversity in process and outcome

Diversity in process and outcome are hallmarks of the developmental psychopathology perspective (Cicchetti & Rogosch, 1996a; Garcia Coll & Vasquez Garcia, 1996). With the acquisition of more knowledge about diversity in development, it has become increasingly recognised that the same rules of normal development do not necessarily exist for, or apply to, all children and families (e.g., Baldwin et al, 1990; Garcia Coll et al, 1996). In this regard, the principles of equifinality and multifinality, derived from general systems theory, are germane (von Bertalanffy, 1968; Cicchetti & Rogosch, 1996a). Equifinality refers to the observation that a diversity of paths may lead to the same outcome (Sroufe, 1989). Accordingly, the breakdown, as well as the maintenance, of a system's function can occur in many ways, especially when taking into account environment–organism interactions and transactions. Thus, instead of a singular primary pathway, a variety of developmental progressions may eventuate in a given disorder. In contrast, multifinality suggests that single pathways can lead to multiple outcomes. Thus, a particular adverse event should not necessarily be seen as contributing to the same adaptive or maladaptive outcome in every individual.

With regard to multifinality, a major reason for the finding that any given pathway will eventuate in an array of outcomes rather than in a single end-point is the concept of differentiation in development (Werner, 1957). Thus, for example, as Robins (1966) reported, children diagnosed with conduct disorder may, as adults, develop antisocial personality, alcoholism, depression or schizophrenia, or manifest normal functioning. Likewise, investigations of the correlates and consequences of maltreatment in childhood have consistently revealed diversity in process and outcome, despite similarities in the occurrence of abuse (Cicchetti & Toth, 1995). In discussing depressive disorder in childhood, Harrington et al (1996) concluded that there are several different kinds of depressive syndrome in children, with some being related to depressive disorders in adulthood and others better conceptualised as components of another psychopathological disorder.

Self-organisation

Although more remote historical factors and immediate influences are both seen as important to the process of development, the individual is not merely a passive recipient of environmental input. Rather, active individual choice and self-organisation increasingly have been viewed as exerting critical influences on development (Cicchetti & Tucker, 1994a). The concept of self-organisation, drawn from non-linear dynamic systems theory, conveys how individuals maintain continuity despite changing environmental circumstances, as well as how new features of the self, which appear discontinuous with prior adaptation, may emerge (Schore, 1997). Early experience and prior levels of adaptation neither doom the individual to continued maladaptive functioning nor inoculate the individual from future problems in functioning. Thus, for example, Cicchetti & Rogosch's

(1997*b*) finding that, over time, most maltreated children evidence at least some self-righting tendencies in the face of the extreme adversity experienced in their lives, attests to the strong biological/genetic and psychological self-strivings toward resilience that all living organisms should possess (Cicchetti & Rogosch, 1997a; Waddington, 1957). In contrast, the absence of such resilient self-strivings in a not insignificant number of maltreated children attests to the deleterious and pernicious impact that traumatic experiences can exert on the biological and psychological processes of self-organisation (Cicchetti & Rogosch, 1997b).

Moreover, it has been demonstrated not only that biological factors can affect psychological processes, but also that social and psychological experiences can modify gene expression and brain structure, organisation and functioning (Cicchetti & Tucker, 1994a; Post *et al*, 1994; Eisenberg, 1995; Nelson & Bloom, 1997; Bremner & Narayan, 1998), and therefore across the life course developmental plasticity can take place through both biological and psychological self-organisation. Alterations in gene expression induced by social and psychological experiences produce changes in patterns of neuronal and synaptic connections (Kandel, 1998). These changes not only contribute to the biological basis of individuality, but also play a prominent role in initiating and maintaining the behavioural abnormalities that are induced by social and psychological experiences (Post *et al*, 1994, 1996; Ciaranello *et al*, 1995; Kandel, 1998).

Early stresses, either physiological or emotional, may condition or sensitise young neural networks to produce cascading effects through later development, possibly constraining the child's flexibility to adapt to new challenges with new strategies rather than with old conceptual and behavioural prototypes. There has been remarkable evidence that early psychological trauma may result not only in emotional sensitisation, but also in pathological sensitisation of neurophysiological reactivity (Pollak *et al*, 1997, 1998; Teicher *et al*, 1997).

In a temperamentally sensitive brain in particular, less severe forms of psychological insult may create emotional sensitisations that ripple through the developmental process with effects that are neuropsychological more than neurophysiological, but that none the less compound themselves into relatively enduring forms of psychopathology. The process by which this occurs may be so complex that, as the dynamics of the brain's maturation unfold, it may be impossible to predict the eventual outcome of each psychological insult. In these instances, the best predictions ultimately may be made on the basis of the more immediate causal mechanisms, the homeostatic, feedback-regulated mechanisms of self-organisation, through which the child spontaneously strives for consistency and order in a chaotic self-and-world matrix. The self in this context is not just an abstract psychological entity. It may represent the configuration of adaptive homeostatic mechanisms that strive to achieve organisational coherence within the massively distributed, dynamically differentiating neural networks of the human cortex. Whether or not they cohere to form an integrated self, the homeostatic, self-regulatory structures of the mind are the major stabilisers in the chaotic dynamics of psychological and biological development.

■43

Resilience

Developmental psychopathologists are as interested in individuals at high risk for developing psychopathology who do not manifest it over time, as they are in individuals who develop an actual disorder (Sroufe & Rutter, 1984). Therefore they are committed to understanding pathways to competent adaptation despite exposure to conditions of adversity (Skuse, 1984; Masten *et al*, 1990; Rutter, 1990; Cicchetti & Garmezy, 1993; Masten & Coatsworth, 1998; Luthar *et al*, 2000). In addition, developmental psychopathologists emphasise the need to understand the functioning of individuals who, after having diverged onto deviant developmental pathways, resume more positive functioning and achieve adequate adaptation (Cicchetti & Rogosch, 1997b).

Resilience has been operationalised as the individual's capacity for adapting successfully and functioning competently despite experiencing chronic adversity, or following exposure to prolonged or severe trauma (Masten *et al*, 1990). The roots of work on resilience can be traced back to earlier research in diverse areas, including investigations of individuals with schizophrenia and their offspring, studies of the effects of persistent poverty, and work on coping with acute and chronic stressors (Cicchetti & Garmezy, 1993; Haggerty *et al*, 1994). By uncovering the mechanisms and processes that lead to competent adaptation despite the presence of adversity, developmental psychopathologists have helped to enhance the understanding of both normal development and psychopathology. I agree with Rutter (1996*b*) that resilience does not exist statically in the "psychological chemistry of the moment" (p. 210). Resilience is a dynamic process, and both biological and psychological processes of self-organisation exert a vital role in how individuals fare when they are exposed to adversity.

Within this perspective, it is important that resilient functioning be conceptualised not as a static or trait-like condition, but as being in dynamic transaction with intra- and extra-organismic forces (Cicchetti *et al*, 1993; Egeland *et al*, 1993). Furthermore, research on the processes leading to resilient outcomes offers great promise as an avenue for facilitating the development of prevention and intervention strategies (Cicchetti & Toth, 1992*a*; Toth & Cicchetti, 1999). Through the examination of the proximal and distal processes and mechanisms that contribute to positive adaptation in situations that more typically eventuate in maladaptation, researchers and clinicians will be better prepared to devise ways of promoting competent outcomes in high-risk populations.

Cultural and contextual influences

Developmental psychopathologists are devoting increasing attention to cultural and contextual issues (Garcia Coll *et al*, 1996; Boyce *et al*, 1998; Cicchetti & Aber, 1998; Garcia Coll *et al*, 2000). Despite the fact that there is growing awareness that contextual factors play an important role in defining phenomena as 'psychopathological' (Richters & Cicchetti, 1993), there are vast differences in how the contexts for human development are conceptualised. To date, researchers interested in context tend to examine contextual influences at one (or perhaps two) level(s) of analysis, usually within the family. In charting children's and adults' trajectories along various developmental pathways, it is necessary to examine their functioning in multiple domains of development and across multiple settings (Luthar, 1991). Consequently, community-, institution-, and society-level influences on individual development are now beginning to be examined systematically (Cicchetti & Aber, 1998).

For example, Luthar & McMahon (1996) discovered that inner-city youths whose peer reputations were aggressive none the less were popular with their peers. Thus, in addition to the more typical pathway to peer popularity (e.g., prosocial behaviours, academic success), Luthar & McMahon identified a less typical pathway characterised by disruptive and aggressive behaviours and poor academic functioning. Congruent with Richters & Cicchetti's (1993) theoretical position, Luthar & McMahon hypothesised that within the crime-, violence-, and poverty-laden disenfranchised communities in which these youths reside, aggressive behaviours that are viewed as deviant by the mainstream may be associated with prestige and high status among particular sociocultural groups.

Empirical work also demonstrates that social-context experiences can affect neurobiological structure and functioning (Cicchetti & Tucker, 1994*a*; Eisenberg, 1995; Bremner & Narayan, 1998). For example, a number of investigators have demonstrated that a mother's emotional condition and, implicitly, her interactions with her infant may affect developing patterns of brain organisation in the early years of life, when sensitive periods for neurobiological growth most likely occur (Edelman, 1987; Dawson *et al*, 1992; Cicchetti & Tucker, 1994*a*; Nelson & Bloom, 1997). Infants of mothers suffering from depression have been shown to exhibit frontal-lobe electroencephalogram asymmetries suggestive of an emerging propensity towards greater negative affectivity (Field *et al*, 1995); quality of attachment among 14-month-old offspring of mothers with depressive symptomatology also has been related to hemispheric activation asymmetries (Dawson *et al*, 1992). Similarly, among adults, exposure to severe trauma has been shown to influence brain structure, as evidenced by altered hippocampal volume in patients with combat-related post-traumatic stress disorder (Bremner *et al*, 1995) and in adult females who have been sexually and/or physically abused during childhood (Gurvits *et al*, 1996; Stein *et al*, 1997).

Research methods

Given the broad and integrative features of the developmental psychopathology perspective, encompassing transactions between multiple domains from diverse levels of functioning over the life course, no single study can capture completely the complexity involved in specifying the developmental process in its entirety. As a result, explicit choices must be made by researchers regarding the specific questions they wish to address in their research, the processes that they seek to investigate, the assessment and measurement of those processes (particularly over time), and the adequacy of strategies utilised to analyse their data. Employing precision and parsimony of design at the outset to address specific questions will most likely yield more straightforward findings than reliance on statistical procedures to control for extraneous or confounding challenges to interpretation.

Ideally, research should be grounded solidly in a strong theoretical conceptualisation. In turn, there must be fidelity between the theory the researcher is attempting to evaluate and the research methods and analyses employed in the study design. Research designs will be particularly strong if alternative theoretical predictions can be pitted against each other in the same study. Care must be taken that both positions are adequately conceptualised and measured for this comparison to be meaningful. Given the multiple systems involved in development and the emergence of psychopathology, it is also beneficial for research to incorporate more than one level of analysis into the study design. Exclusive focus within one domain or developmental system does not allow for an examination of how development may be affected across domains. For example, attention to phenomena at the cognitive level alone, without consideration of affective processes, may result in an incomplete appraisal of the phenomena under study (Cicchetti & Sroufe, 1976; Schneider-Rosen & Cicchetti, 1991; Cicchetti et al, 1997). Research incorporating assessment at both the psychological and biological level is particularly important. Understanding the biological effects of psychological experience or the psychological impact of biological processes will result in a more integrative perspective of development (Cicchetti & Tucker, 1994a; Nelson & Bloom, 1997).

Developmental psychopathology research must be concerned with differentiating variation over time that is due to development from variation that results from emerging individual differences. Ascertainment of disturbances in functioning needs to be considered within the context of what is normative for individuals within different developmental periods of interest; some measures may lose their usefulness as children progress to more advanced levels, and researchers need to plan for how comparable, developmentally appropriate measurements of a construct will be obtained across the time span under study.

■45

Implications for practice

Although it might be assumed that logical connections exist between the provision of psychotherapeutic interventions to children and adolescents and developmental theory and research, far too few bridges have been built between these areas of knowledge (Cicchetti et al, 1988; Shirk, 1988; Cicchetti & Toth, 1992b; Noam, 1992; Shirk & Russell, 1996). Because non-developmental adult-derived classification guidelines have historically been applied to formulating diagnoses of the mental disorders of childhood, it is not surprising that adevelopmental approaches to intervention, frequently drawn from the adult literature, have often been the norm when providing interventions to children and adolescents. The perpetuation of the "developmental uniformity myth" (Kendall et al, 1984) to interventions for children, wherein it is assumed that mental disorders manifest themselves similarly regardless of age and, therefore, do not require therapeutic techniques that are sensitive to developmental change, has impeded efforts to provide theoretically guided and developmentally appropriate services to children and adolescents. Further, decision-making regarding what constitutes an action that is in a child's best interest cannot be made adequately unless the child's level of functioning across an array of developmental domains (e.g., cognition, social-cognition, emotion and language) and the concomitant capacity to comprehend the meaning of certain events are considered. Moreover, different incidents can have different meanings depending on when they occur in the developmental period. The individual's history, temperament, and current supports and resources all play a role in helping a child to construct an 'individual' meaning from a given event, thereby further contributing to the overall impact on the child.

Fortunately, in recent years an increased dialogue has occurred among theorists, basic researchers and professionals interested in providing developmentally guided prevention and intervention for children and adolescents. A major impetus to this process has emanated from the field of developmental psychopathology, which advocates the importance of an active, bidirectional interchange between theoreticians, researchers and practitioners interested in normal and pathological development (Cicchetti, 1984b, 1990; Rutter, 1986; Cicchetti & Toth, 1991). As a growing number of research investigations have illustrated how the study of the interface between normal and abnormal development is mutually enriching for scientists of each persuasion, so the application of findings conceptualised within developmental psychopathology to intervention efforts has similarly increased (Cicchetti & Toth, 1998a).

The hierarchical nature of development possesses important implications for prevention and intervention efforts. Because all stage-salient issues are life-span issues, ongoing differentiation, integration and organisation occur. Of special note for purposes of intervention, each point of reorganisation and the resultant disequilibrium may make the individual more amenable to change. In view of the disequilibrium generated during periods of transition, providing prevention and intervention efforts during such transitions might be especially effective in initiating change (Cicchetti & Toth, 1992a). Moreover, at times it may be useful to generate a state of disequilibrium to afford the opportunity for the provision of an intervention that could result in the attainment of a higher level of organisation (Futterweit & Ruff, 1993). Naturally occurring events that result in disequilibration of the individual may also provide timely opportunities for initiating intervention. For example, although a therapist may be reluctant to confront a patient during times of stress, deciding to provide a more supportive function, such an approach could result in the loss of a prime period for providing a more growth-promoting intervention.

At least partially as an outgrowth of a developmental psychopathology perspective, those interested in understanding atypical development and in applying this knowledge to the prevention and treatment of psychopathology have become increasingly sensitive to the developmental dimensions of therapy. Psychotherapists, for example, have become more cognisant of the fact that no particular treatment is likely to be effective throughout the life course. Moreover, even children of similar ages cannot be viewed as a unitary group. For example, adolescents' world views are defined by the meaning systems that they use to understand themselves, their peers and their parents. Accordingly, different methods of therapy must be provided that account for differences in symptomatology, cognition, self-understanding, biological maturation and patterns of recovery from illness. To provide effective psychotherapeutic interventions, an in-depth understanding of each individual's developmental organisation is necessary.

Assessment of factors such as when during the life course and why a disorder occurred, how long it has continued and what precursors to the disordered functioning can be identified requires a developmental approach to ensure that prevention and intervention strategies are appropriately timed and guided. The effect of an intervention will be enhanced or inhibited in relation to its sensitivity and responsivity to factors associated with the developmental period during which the intervention is provided.

Similarly, interventions may need to take into consideration the developmental period during which a pathology-inducing insult occurred, even if the actual referral for treatment is initiated years later. For example, in cases of sexual abuse that may have occurred when a child was preverbal, verbally mediated intervention strategies may not be as effective as more experiential approaches because the memory of the abuse may never have been encoded verbally (Cicchetti & Toth, 1998b; Toth & Cicchetti, 1998). To provide another example, in instances of childhood depression, the developmental period during which a stressor occurred that may have contributed to the initiation of an affective disorder must be considered. If a child suffered the loss of a parent during toddlerhood, a period when individuation and autonomy are central, then the loss may have ramifications that are more significant than they would have been had it occurred in later childhood.

In contemplating the implications of a hierarchical model of development for intervention, questions arise regarding the way in which intervention should proceed.

Research in clinical neurology and developmental psychobiology has shown that recovery of function after an insult follows a sequential appearance of competencies that is consistent with that observed during ontogeny, that is, from simple to complex and from lower to higher brain centres (Sherrington, 1906; Denny-Brown et al, 1949; Teitelbaum, 1977). Similarly, it might be that the achievement of competent functioning on stage-salient developmental issues that have been unsuccessfully resolved follows the same emergence after intervention as that observed in children who successfully resolve their developmental issues without intervention. If so, then important conclusions could be drawn regarding the identification of precursors to recovered functioning in children and adolescents who have a psychiatric disorder or who have been exposed to significant adversity. Such information could be incorporated into the psychotherapeutic arena.

Specifically, the issue of whether later stage-salient issues can be positively reworked without addressing earlier issues becomes a critical question. For example, is it possible to help an individual gain a positive sense of self without addressing the origins of a negative self-view that may have derived from an insecure attachment to the caregiver in childhood? Conversely, might it be possible that attention to a current salient issue could reverberate to earlier issues, resulting in an overall reorganisation of early issues as well? Because the concept of hierarchical integration posits that early issues become coordinated with later issues, one might argue that a similar reverse process would occur, wherein earlier issues could benefit from positive resolution of currently salient developmental issues.

Aspects of the developmental course of illness also possess implications for intervention. The previously discussed concepts of equifinality and multifinality should alert all clinicians to the importance of using multiple strategies of treatment. For example, children's developmental histories, stage in the life cycle, current functioning and developmental organisation across psychological and biological domains, and the characteristics that define a given disorder all must be factored into the process of treatment planning. Likewise, interventions should be directed at a range of developmental domains (e.g., cognition, language, emotion and representation), rather than assuming that a given psychopathological disorder can be addressed by focusing exclusively on a single domain of development. This perspective holds true even for conditions that might be considered the outgrowth of a predominantly biological insult or characteristic, as maladaptation in one domain is likely to affect function in other domains. Thus, interventions must address the broader matrix of causal influences and sequelae if successful and sustained progress is to occur.

In considering the influence of the course of illness on the type of intervention that is provided, Post (1992) suggests that different interventions are likely to be more or less effective at various points during the illness. Specifically, he argues that in treating mood disorders, psychodynamic therapies may be more effective when provided for an initial depressive episode, whereas recurrent episodes might be more responsive to behavioural and cognitive techniques. This premise is based on findings of behavioural sensitisation and electrophysiological kindling in individuals with histories of repeated mood disorders. Post further maintains that because most psychodynamic therapeutic techniques require the reworking of cortical control using the limbic and cortically based representational memory systems, depressed patients with hypoactive cortical systems may not be amenable to such insight-oriented therapies. Finally, he believes that different pharmacological interventions are differentially effective during various stages of disease evolution. Although his research is based on work with adults with mood disorders, Post's findings also are compelling in relation to children, because he applies a developmental perspective when describing aspects of the progression, course and treatment of mental illness. Because developmental changes during childhood can be quite rapid, therapeutic strategies must be evaluated continually in relation to the developmental process and to the course of illness.

Since development is viewed as a naturally unfolding process that emerges from the individual and his or her biological and psychological characteristics, in combination with the context in which he or she lives, issues related to whether or not to intervene also require careful evaluation. This may be especially relevant for prevention efforts, where intervention is provided before the crystallisation of a mental disorder. Although it is often assumed that prevention can do no harm, this premise is not necessarily true

■47

(cf. Rutter, 1982). The importance of fully understanding development so as not to intervene unnecessarily or in an iatrogenic manner is stressed by Thomas (1979), who argues that intervention for one component of a complex system contains a significant risk of unanticipated negative consequences for other parts of the system. A similar position that is relevant to practice is discussed by Howitt (1992), who examines how a desire to protect children from abuse can actually lead to harm if intervention into families is misguided. Although seemingly a quite negative perspective, these positions underscore the risks of initiating intervention without fully considering its potential impact on the developing system. Such issues assume special relevance in cases of child maltreatment, where decisions regarding the adequacy of parenting and possible placement of children in foster care arise routinely. Particularly disconcerting is the failure to incorporate any data on developmental processes into this decision-making process. Decision-making related to the development and provision of prevention and intervention services that is not theory-informed and data-driven is all too frequently the norm.

Future directions

A number of challenges face developmental psychopathologists as they plan an agenda for the 21st century. Several, although by no means all, are highlighted below.

First, the field of developmental psychopathology must become increasingly interdisciplinary in nature. An inherent advantage of the developmental psychopathology perspective is that it is not constrained by a rigid adherence to existing methods and interdisciplinary boundaries, which can impede the discovery of new and unexpected phenomena. It is clear that progress towards a process-level understanding of normal and abnormal development will require research designs that allow for the simultaneous consideration of multiple domains of social (e.g., culture, community), psychological and biological variables. Thus, collaborations between researchers from different disciplines and the implementation of cross-sectional and prospective longitudinal investigations that examine normal and atypical biological and psychological development at multiple levels of analysis, especially as these variables change across contexts and influence one another over developmental time, are essential. The organisational perspective on development (Sroufe, 1979; Cicchetti & Schneider-Rosen, 1986), with its emphasis on understanding the differentiation, integration and organisation of biological and psychological development and its focus on studying the whole person in context, will play an important role in framing the questions as we seek to elucidate the relations between environmental, psychological and biological factors in the aetiology, course, sequelae, prevention and treatment of various high-risk conditions and mental disorders.

Second, investigations must strive for enhanced fidelity between the elegance and complexity of the theoretical models embraced by developmental psychopathologists and the measurement and data-analysis strategies employed in studies using them (Richters, 1997). The existence of equifinality and multifinality in development requires that researchers increasingly endeavour to discover the multiplicity of processes and outcomes that may be articulated at the individual person-oriented level as opposed to the prevailing variable-oriented strategies that dominate the field (cf. Bergman & Magnusson, 1997; Cairns *et al*, 1998). In the future, scientists must conceptualise and design research with these differential pathway concepts as a foundation (Cicchetti & Rogosch, 1996*a*). Doing so will assist investigators in achieving the unique goals of developmental psychopathology as defined by Sroufe & Rutter (1984) – to explain the development of individual patterns of adaptation and maladaptation. Along these lines, the theoretical models that reflect the complexity of normal and abnormal developmental processes warrant the implementation of new methodologies (Richters, 1997).

Third, technological advances that have occurred in non-invasive neuroimaging techniques and molecular genetics (e.g., functional magnetic resonance imaging and mice 'knockout' genes) should enable exciting collaborations to occur with scientists who possess expertise in neuroanatomy, various domains of normal and abnormal biological and psychological development, and cognitive neuroscience. An existing problem with neuroimaging technology is that it can be extremely difficult to obtain sound data from children because of the developmental limitations that hamper their ability to comply with the procedural demands of these techniques. Additionally, we do not yet possess an adequate neuroimaging knowledge base of normal brain changes at different developmental periods of infancy and childhood against which to compare abnormal brain development (Thatcher *et al*, 1996; Cicchetti & Cannon, 1999). Investigations of normal and abnormal development are mutually informing, and it is therefore imperative that normative information on brain developmental changes over time increasingly be ascertained in future neuroimaging research. Moreover, research in the field of developmental psychopathology should not be guided solely by technological advances. It is crucial that sophisticated theory and sound research knowledge be used to frame the questions that are examined through the use of these neuroimaging procedures.

Finally, research obtained through investigations in the field of developmental psychopathology must be disseminated more widely. A critical area in fostering improvements for the delivery of mental health services to children and adolescents is improved dissemination of research findings on childhood psychopathology and treatment outcome. Currently, the flow of information from the academic research arena into the policy forum is a trickle at best. Although a great deal of research in the area of childhood psychopathology possesses policy implications, far too little reaches the desks of those in positions to implement change. This failure is not a unidirectional occurrence, as researchers and formulators of policy are equally responsible for communication failure. Researchers too often conceive their questions without giving sufficient thought to the real-world issues with which child advocates are grappling. The results from many potentially informative investigations are buried in inaccessible scientific journals. Researchers must become increasingly skilled and interested in framing and disseminating their findings so that they can be incorporated into the policy arena. Similarly, child advocates must increase their efforts to seek out information that may not be readily available to them.

■49

To provide an example, there is an urgent need for scientists to educate the media, the lay public and policy makers concerning what is known about resilience, as well as the limitations of this knowledge. Researchers need to convey the incorrect nature of views such as "resilience implies invincibility" or "if only children tried harder, then they, too, could be resilient". Unless scientists take an active stance in communicating accurate knowledge about resilience, the perpetuation of such inaccurate views could impede the development of social policies that could foster the promotion of competent adaptation in children experiencing significant adversity.

As the field of developmental psychopathology ushers in its next era of scientific and clinical challenges, opportunities for fascinating collaborations on pressing theoretical, empirical and social issues will abound and afford chances for informing the urgent socio-political issues of our time. We have not yet succeeded in educating society about the importance of research in the area of mental health. It is imperative that we become more effective in conveying the benefits that can be derived from developmentally informed research conducted with populations at high risk for, or suffering from, mental disorder.

In conclusion, despite its relatively brief history, the field of developmental psychopathology has contributed significantly to the understanding of risk, disorder and adaptation across the life course. Although numerous challenges lie ahead, we must have the courage to continue a critical examination of the implicit as well as the explicit conceptual and scientific assumptions that exist in the field to sustain our momentum and to foster new advances and further opportunities to influence society more broadly.

References

Baldwin, A., Baldwin, C. & Cole, R. (1990) Stress-resistant families and stress-resistant children. In *Risk and Protective Factors in the Development of Psychopathology* (eds J. Rolf, A. Masten, D. Cicchetti, *et al*), pp. 257–280. New York: Cambridge University Press.

Bergman, L. R. & Magnusson, D. (1997) A person-oriented approach in research on developmental psychopathology. *Development and Psychopathology*, **9**, 291–319.

Boyce, W. T., Frank, E., Jensen, P. S., *et al* (1998) Social context in developmental psychopathology: recommendations for future research from the MacArthur network on psychopathology and development. *Development and Psychopathology*, **10**, 143–164.

Bremner, J. D. & Narayan, M. (1998) The effects of stress on memory and the hippocampus throughout the life cycle: implications for childhood development and aging. *Development and Psychopathology*, **10**, 871–885.

—, Randall, P., Scott, M., *et al* (1995) MRI-based measurement of hippocampal volume in patients with combat-related post traumatic stress disorder. *American Journal Psychiatry*, **152**, 973–981.

Cairns, R. B., Bergman, L. R. & Kagan, J. (eds) (1998) *Methods and Models for Studying the Individual*. Thousand Oaks, CA: Sage.

Chomsky, N. (1968) *Language and Mind*. New York: Harcourt Brace Jovanovich.

Ciaranello, R., Aimi, J., Dean, R., *et al* (1995) Fundamentals of molecular neurobiology. In *Developmental Psychopathology. Vol. 1. Theory and Methods* (eds D. Cicchetti & D. Cohen), pp. 109–160. New York: John Wiley & Sons.

Cicchetti, D. (ed.) (1984*a*) *Developmental Psychopathology*. Chicago: University of Chicago Press.

—— (1984*b*) The emergence of developmental psychopathology. *Child Development*, **55**, 1–7.

—— (1990) An historical perspective on the discipline of developmental psychopathology. In *Risk and Protective Factors in the Development of Psychopathology* (eds J. Rolf, A. Masten, D. Cicchetti, *et al*), pp. 2–28. New York: Cambridge University Press.

—— (1993) Developmental psychopathology: reactions, reflections, projections. *Developmental Review*, **13**, 471–502.

—— & Aber, J. L. (1986) Early precursors to later depression: an organizational perspective. In *Advances in Infancy. Vol. 4* (eds L. Lipsitt & C. Rovee-Collier), pp. 81–137. Norwood, NJ: Ablex.

—— & —— (eds) (1998) Contextualism and developmental psychopathology (special issue). *Development and Psychopathology*, **10**, 137–141.

—— & Cannon, T. D. (1999) Neurodevelopmental processes in the ontogenesis of psychopathology. *Development and Psychopathology*, **11**, 375–393.

—— & Cohen, D. (eds) (1995*a*) *Developmental Psychopathology. Vol. 1. Theory and Methods*. New York: John Wiley & Sons.

—— & —— (eds) (1995*b*) *Developmental Psychopathology. Vol. 2. Risk, Disorder and Adaptation*. New York: John Wiley & Sons.

—— & —— (1995*c*) Perspectives on developmental psychopathology. In *Developmental Psychopathology. Vol. 1. Theory and Method* (eds D. Cicchetti & D. Cohen), pp. 3–20. New York: John Wiley & Sons.

—— & Garmezy, N. (eds) (1993) Milestones in the development of resilience (special issue). *Development and Psychopathology*, **5**, 497–774.

—— & Richters, J. E. (eds) (1997) The conceptual and scientific underpinnings of research in developmental psychopathology (special issue). *Development and Psychopathology*, **9**, 189–471.

—— & Rogosch, F. A. (1996*a*) Equifinality and multifinality in developmental psychopathology. *Development and Psychopathology*, **8**, 597–600.

—— & —— (eds) (1996*b*) Developmental pathways (special issue). *Development and Psychopathology*, **8**, 597–896.

—— & —— (1997*a*) Self-organization (special issue). *Development and Psychopathology*, **9**, 797–815.

—— & —— (1997*b*) The role of self-organization in the promotion of resilience in maltreated children. *Development and Psychopathology*, **9**, 799–817.

—— & Schneider-Rosen, K. (1986) An organizational approach to childhood depression. In *Depression in Young People, Clinical and Developmental Perspectives* (eds M. Rutter, C. Izard & P. Read), pp. 71–134. New York: Guilford.

—— & Sroufe, L. A. (1976) The relationship between affective and cognitive development in Down's Syndrome infants. *Child Development*, **47**, 920–929.

—— & Toth, S. L. (1991) The making of a developmental psychopathologist. In *Child Behavior and Development: Training for Diversity* (eds J. Cantor, C. Spiker & L. Lipsitt), pp. 34–72. Norwood, NJ: Ablex.

—— & —— (eds) (1992*a*) Developmental approaches to prevention and intervention (special issue). *Development and Psychopathology*, **4**, 489–728.

—— & —— (1992*b*) The role of developmental theory in prevention and intervention. *Development and Psychopathology*, **4**, 489–493.

—— & —— (1995) A developmental psychopathology perspective on child abuse and neglect. *Journal of the American Academy of Child and Adolescent Psychiatry*, **34**, 541–565.

—— & —— (1998*a*) Perspectives on research and practice in developmental psychopathology. In *Handbook of Child Psychology. Vol. 4* (ed W. Damon) (5th edn), pp. 479–583. New York: John Wiley & Sons.

—— & —— (eds) (1998*b*) Risk, trauma, and memory (special issue). *Development and Psychopathology*, **10**, 589–898

—— & Tucker, D. (1994*a*) Development and self-regulatory structures of the mind. *Development and Psychopathology*, **6**, 533–549.

—— & —— (eds) (1994*b*) Neural plasticity, sensitive periods, and psychopathology (special issue). *Development and Psychopathology*, **6**, 531–814.

—, Toth, S. L. & Bush, M. (1988) Developmental psychopathology and incompetence in childhood: suggestions for intervention. In *Advances in Clinical Child Psychology. Vol. 11* (eds B. Lahey & A. Kazdin), pp. 1–71. New York: Plenum.

——, Rogosch, F. A., Lynch, M. & Holt, K. (1993) Resilience in maltreated children: processes leading to adaptive outcome. *Development and Psychopathology*, **5**, 629–647.

——, ——, Toth, S. L. & Spagnola, M. (1997) Affect, cognition, and the emergence of self-knowledge in the toddler offspring of depressed mothers. *Journal of Experimental Child Psychology*, **67**, 338–362.

Dawson, G., Grofer Klinger, L., Panagiotides, H., *et al* (1992) Frontal lobe activity and affective behavior of infants of mothers with depressive symptoms. *Child Development*, **63**, 725–737.

Denny-Brown, D., Twitchell, T. E. & Saenz-Arroyo, I. (1949) The nature of spasticity resulting from cerebral lesions. *Transactions of the American Neurological Association*, **74**, 108–113.

Edelman, G. (1987) *Neural Darwinism*. New York: Basic Books.

Egeland, B., Carlson, E. & Sroufe, L. A. (1993) Resilience as process. *Development and Psychopathology*, **5**, 517–528.

Eisenberg, L. (1995) The social construction of the human brain. *American Journal of Psychiatry*, **152**, 1563–1575.

Field, T. M., Fox, N., Pickens, J., *et al* (1995) Relative right frontal EEG activation in 3- to 6-month old infants of 'depressed' mothers. *Developmental Psychology*, **31**, 358–363.

Fishbein, H. (1976) *Evolution, Development, and Children's Learning*. Pacific Palisades, CA: Goodyear Publishing Co.

Futterweit, L. R. & Ruff, H. A. (1993) Principles of development: implications for early intervention. *Journal of Applied Developmental Psychology*, **14**, 153–173.

Garcia Coll, C. & Vazquez Garcia, H. A. (1996) Definitions of competence during adolescence: lessons from Puerto Rican adolescent mothers. In *Rochester Symposium on Developmental Psychopathology. Vol. 7. Adolescence: Opportunities and Challenges* (eds D. Cicchetti & S. Toth), pp. 283–308. Rochester, NY: University of Rochester Press.

——, Lamberty, G., Jenkins, R., *et al* (1996) An integrative model for the study of developmental competencies in minority children. *Child Development*, **67**, 1891–1914.

——, Akerman, A. & Cicchetti, D. (2000) Cultural influences on developmental processes and outcomes: implications for the study of development and psychopathology. *Development and Psychopathology*, 333–356.

Garmezy, N. & Streitman, S. (1974) Children at risk: conceptual models and research methods. *Schizophrenia Bulletin*, **9**, 55–125.

Goldstein, K. (1939) *The Organism*. New York: American Book Co.

Gould, S. (1980) *The Panda's Thumb*. New York: Norton.

—— (1986) Evolution and the triumph of homology, or why history matters. *American Scientist*, **74**, 60–69.

Gurvits, T. V., Shenton, M. E., Hokama, H., *et al* (1996) Magnetic resonance imaging study of hippocampal volume in chronic, combat-related posttraumatic stress disorder. *Biological Psychiatry*, **40**, 1091–1099.

Haggerty, R., Sherrod, L., Garmezy, N., *et al* (eds) (1994) *Stress, Risk, and Resilience in Children and Adolescents*. New York: Cambridge University Press.

Harrington, R., Rutter, M. & Fombonne, E. (1996) Developmental pathways in depression: multiple meanings, antecedents, and endpoints. *Development and Psychopathology*, **8**, 601–616.

Howitt, D. (1992) *Child Abuse Errors: When Good Intentions Go Wrong*. New Brunswick, NJ: Rutgers University Press.

Institute of Medicine (1989) *Research on Children and Adolescents with Mental, Behavioral, and Developmental Disorders*. Washington, DC: National Academy Press.

—— (1994) *Reducing Risks for Mental Disorders: Frontiers for Preventive Intervention Research*. Washington, DC: National Academy Press.

Jackson, J. H. (1884) Evolution and dissolution of the nervous system. Reprinted 1958 in *The Selected Writings of John Hughlings Jackson. Vol. 2* (ed. J. Taylor), pp. 45–75. New York: Basic Books.

Kandel, E. (1998) A new intellectual framework for psychiatry. *American Journal of Psychiatry*, **155**, 457–469.

Kaplan, A. (1964) *The Conduct of Inquiry*. San Francisco, CA: Chandler Publishing Co.

Kaplan, B. (1967) Meditations on genesis. *Human Development*, **10**, 65–87.

Kendall, P., Lerner, R. & Craighead, W. E. (1984) Human development and intervention in childhood psychopathology. *Child Development*, **55**, 71–82.

Keshavan, M. & Murray, R. (eds) (1997) *Neurodevelopment and Adult Psychopathology*. New York: Cambridge University Press.

Kuo, Z.-Y. (1967) *The Dynamics of Behavior Development*. New York: Random House.

Lenneberg, E. (1967) *Biological Foundations of Language*. New York: John Wiley & Sons.

Luthar, S. S. (1991) Vulnerability and resilience: a study of high-risk adolescents. *Child Development*, **62**, 600–616.

—— & McMahon, T. (1996) Peer reputation among inner city adolescents: structure and correlates. *Journal of Research on Adolescence*, **6**, 581–603.

■51

——, Cicchetti, D. & Becker, B. (2000) The construct of resilience: a critical review and guidelines for future work. *Child Development*, **71**, 543–562.

Masten, A. & Coatsworth, D. J. (1998) The development of competence in favorable and unfavorable environments: lessons from research on successful children. *American Psychologist*, **53**, 205–220.

——, Best, K. & Garmezy, N. (1990) Resilience and development: contributions from the study of children who overcome adversity. *Development and Psychopathology*, **2**, 425–444.

Mednick, S., Cannon, T., Barr, C., *et al* (eds) (1991) *Fetal Neural Development and Adult Schizophrenia*. New York: Cambridge University Press.

Miller, N. E. (1995) Clinical–experimental interactions in the development of neuroscience: a primer for nonspecialists and lessons for young scientists. *American Psychologist*, **50**, 901–911.

National Advisory Mental Health Council (1990) *National Plan for Research on Child and Adolescent Mental Disorders* (Publication 90-1683). Rockville, MD: US Department of Health and Human Services.

Nelson, C. A. & Bloom, F. E. (1997) Child development and neuroscience. *Child Development*, **68**, 970–987.

Noam, G. G. (1992) Development as the aim of clinical intervention. *Development and Psychopathology*, **3**, 679–696.

Overton, W. & Horowitz, H. (1991) Developmental psychopathology: Integration and differentiations. In *Rochester Symposium on Developmental Psychopathology. Vol. 3. Models and Integrations* (eds D. Cicchetti & S. L. Toth), pp. 1–42. Rochester, NY: University of Rochester Press.

Pollak, S., Cicchetti, D. & Klorman, R. (1997) Cognitive brain event-related potentials and emotion processing in maltreated children. *Child Development*, **68**, 773–787.

——, ——, ——, *et al* (1998) Stress, memory, and emotion: developmental considerations from the study of child maltreatment. *Development and Psychopathology*, **10**, 811–828.

Post, R. (1992) Transduction of psychosocial stress into the neurobiology of recurrent affective disorder. *American Journal of Psychiatry*, **149**, 999–1010.

——, Weiss, S. & Leverich, G. (1994) Recurrent affective disorder: roots in developmental neurobiology and illness progression based on changes in gene expression. *Development and Psychopathology*, **6**, 781–814.

——, ——, ——, *et al* (1996) Developmental neurobiology of cyclic affective illness: implications for early therapeutic interventions. *Development and Psychopathology*, **8**, 273–305.

Richters, J. E., (1997) The Hubble hypothesis and the developmentalist's dilemma. *Development and Psychopathology*, **9**, 193–229.

—— & Cicchetti, D. (1993) Mark Twain meets DSM–III–R: Conduct disorder, development, and the concept of harmful dysfunction. *Development and Psychopathology*, **5**, 5–29.

Robins, L. (1966) *Deviant Children Grown Up*. Baltimore, MD: Williams & Wilkins.

Rutter, M. (1982) Prevention of children's psychosocial disorders: myth and substance. *Pediatrics*, **70**, 883–894.

—— (1986) Child psychiatry: the interface between clinical and developmental research. *Psychological Medicine*, **16**, 151–160.

—— (1987) Psychosocial resilience and protective mechanisms. *American Journal of Orthopsychiatry*, **57**, 316–331.

—— (1990) Psychosocial resilience and protective mechanisms. In *Risk and Protective Factors in the Development of Psychopathology* (eds J. Rolf, A. S. Masten, D. Cicchetti, *et al*), pp. 181–214). New York: Cambridge University Press.

—— (1994) Beyond longitudinal data: causes, consequences, and continuity. *Journal of Consulting and Clinical Psychology*, **62**, 928–940.

—— (1996a) Developmental psychopathology as an organizing research construct. In *The Lifespan Development of Individuals: Behavioral Neurobiological, and Psychosocial Perspectives* (ed. D. Magnusson), pp. 394–413. New York: Cambridge University Press.

—— (1996b) Developmental psychopathology: concepts and prospects. In *Frontiers of Developmental Psychopathology* (eds M. F. Lenzenweger & J. J. Haugaard), pp. 209–237. New York: Oxford University Press.

—— (1996c) Transitions and turning points in developmental psychopathology: as applied to the age span between childhood and mid-adulthood. *International Journal of Behavioral Development*, **19**, 603–626.

—— & Garmezy, N. (1983) Developmental psychopathology. In *Handbook of Child Psychology. Vol. IV* (ed. E. M. Hetherington) (4th edn), pp. 774–911. New York: John Wiley & Sons.

Sameroff, A. J. (1983) Developmental systems: contexts and evolution. In *Handbook of Child Psychology. Vol. 1* (ed. P. Mussen), pp. 237–294. New York: John Wiley & Sons.

—— & Chandler, M. J. (1975) Reproductive risk and the continuum of caretaking casualty. In *Review of Child Development Research. Vol. 4* (ed. F. D. Horowitz), pp. 187–244. Chicago, IL: University of Chicago Press.

Schneider-Rosen, K. & Cicchetti, D. (1991) Early self-knowledge and emotional development: visual self-recognition and affective reactions to mirror self-image in maltreated and nonmaltreated toddlers. *Developmental Psychology*, **27**, 481–488.

Schore, A. N. (1997) Early organization of the nonlinear right brain and development of a predisposition to psychiatric disorders. *Development and Psychopathology*, **9**, 595–631.

Sherrington, C. (1906) *The Integrative Action of the Nervous System*. New York: Scribner's.

Shakow, D. (1968) Contributions from schizophrenia to the understanding of normal psychological function. In *The Reach of Mind: Essays in Memory of Kurt Goldstein* (ed. M. Simmel), pp. 173–199. New York: Springer.

Shirk, S. (1988) Causal reasoning and children's comprehension of therapeutic interpretations. In *Cognitive Development and Child Psychotherapy* (ed. S. Shirk), pp. 53–90. New York: Plenum.

—— & Russell, R. (1996) *Change Processes in Child Psychotherapy*. New York: Guilford Press.

Skuse, D. (1984) Extreme deprivation in early childhood. II. Theoretical issues and comparative review. *Journal of Child Psychology and Psychiatry*, **25**, 543–572.

Sroufe, L. A. (1979) The coherence of individual development: early care, attachment, and subsequent developmental issues. *American Psychologist*, **34**, 834–841.

—— (1989) Pathways to adaptation and maladaptation: psychopathology as developmental deviation. In *Rochester Symposium on Developmental Psychopathology. Vol. 1. The Emergence of a Discipline* (ed. D. Cicchetti), pp. 13–40. Hillsdale, NJ: Lawrence Erlbaum Associates.

—— (1990) Considering normal and abnormal together: the essence of developmental psychopathology. *Development and Psychopathology*, **2**, 335–347.

—— & Rutter, M. (1984) The domain of developmental psychopathology. *Child Development*, **55**, 17–29.

Stein, M. B., Koverola, C., Hanna, C., *et al* (1997) Hippocampal volume in women victimized by childhood sexual abuse. *Psychological Medicine*, **27**, 951–959.

Teicher, M., Ito, Y., Glod, C., *et al* (1997) Preliminary evidence for abnormal cortical development in physically and sexually abused children using EEG coherence and MRI. *Annals of the New York Academy of Sciences*, **821**, 162–175

Teitelbaum, P. (1971) The encephalization of hunger. In *Progress in Physiological Psychology. Vol. 4* (eds E. Stellar & J. Sprague), New York: Academic Press.

—— (1977) Levels of integration of the operant. In *Handbook of Operant Behavior* (eds W. K. Horig & J. Staddon), pp. 7–27. Englewood Cliffs, NJ: Prentice Hall.

Thatcher, R., Lyon, G., Rumsey, J., *et al* (eds) (1996) *Developmental Neuroimaging: Mapping the Development of Brain and Behavior*. San Diego, CA: Academic Press.

Thomas, L. (1979) *The Medusa and the Snail: More Notes of a Biology Watcher*, pp. 110–111. New York: Viking Press.

Toth, S. L. & Cicchetti, D. (1999) Developmental psychopathology and child psychotherapy. In *Handbook of psychotherapies with children and families* (eds S. Russ & T. Ollendick), pp. 15–44. New York: Plenum Press.

—— & —— (1998) Remembering, forgetting, and the effects of trauma on memory: a developmental psychopathology perspective (editorial). *Development and Psychopathology*, **10**, 589–605.

von Bertalanffy, L. (1968) *General System Theory*. New York: Braziller.

Wadddington, C. H. (1957) *The Strategy of Genes*. London: Allen and Unwin.

Wakefield, J. (1997) When is development disordered? Developmental psychopathology and the harmful dysfunction analysis of mental disorder. *Development and Psychopathology*, **9**, 269–290.

Watt, N., Anthony, E. J., Wynne, L. *et al* (eds) (1984) *Children at Risk for Schizophrenia: A Longitudinal Perspective*. New York: Cambridge University Press.

Weiss, P. (1961) Deformities as cure to understanding development of form. *Perspectives in Biology and Medicine*, **4**, 133–151.

—— (1969) *Principles of Development*. New York: Hafner.

Werner, H. (1957) The concept of development from a comparative and organismic point of view. In *The Concept of Development* (ed. D. B. Harris), pp. 125–148. Minneapolis, MN: University of Minnesota Press.

Zigler, E. & Glick, M. (1986) *A Developmental Approach to Adult Psychopathology*. New York: John Wiley & Sons.

■ 53

4 Autism

Two-way interplay
between research and clinical work

Michael Rutter

Research is the lifeblood of clinical practice in all fields of medicine, including child psychiatry (Rutter, 1998). It has become generally accepted that all of us, as clinicians, need to base what we do on solid empirical research findings. This is reflected, for example, in the growing ascendancy of evidence-based medicine. It is appropriate that we are challenged to demonstrate that we are using methods that work and that we are not neglecting approaches that are even more effective (Goodman, 1997). Nevertheless, there are dangers if we adopt too mechanical, and too simplistic, an interpretation of evidence-based medicine. Of course, we need to know which treatments are most effective for which problems in which circumstances, and research has a crucial role to play in finding that out. Where, then, do the dangers lie?

Several points need to be made. First, the essence of research lies in the process of problem-solving and not in the mere provision of a set of factual answers. Medawar (1982) brought this out well in his essays about the nature of scientific enquiry. A creative imagination is as fundamental as the rigorous testing of hypotheses. Research comprises the telling of stories about how mechanisms in nature might be operating, then using experimental-type strategies to test the ideas expressed in the stories, to compare alternative explanations and gradually, in iterative fashion, to move progressively closer to what might be the truth.

Second, as an extension of that same point, the most important thing is not to know which of our current methods are best but, rather, to have a means of moving forward to develop even better methods in the future. That can only happen if the research is devised to determine *why* methods work in particular circumstances and not just whether they are better than alternative approaches.

Third, major improvements in clinical practice are even more reliant on basic research into the nature of causal processes than on studies of treatment. By basic causal processes, of course, I mean not just the neural processes that underlie the workings of the mind, but also the psychological and social mechanisms that are crucial for the understanding of multi-factorial disorders as they arise in social beings. Many of the greatest clinical advances have relied on research from the past that, at the time, seemed to have little clinical relevance (Dollery, 1978). Often, it takes many years to bring together findings that have arisen in disparate fields and to recognise how they may be employed for clinical benefit.

Fourth, it would be a mistake to portray the picture as a one-way traffic from research to clinical practice. The reality is a more complex interplay, with each feeding into the other and each serving to correct the other's mistakes (Rutter, 1990).

Reprinted, with amendments and with permission, from Rutter (1999).

Finally, it is necessary to appreciate that progress does not consist of a smooth consistent moving forward, in which each step taken constitutes an improvement on what had been the situation before. Instead, it tends to proceed in a series of fits and starts with occasional false claims, mistaken inferences and misleading enthusiasms taking the field in the wrong direction. That is as evident in research as it is in clinical practice. This need for research and clinical practice to move ahead together was clearly evident in Emanuel Miller's (1960, 1968) writings on child psychiatry.

In this chapter I seek to illustrate the ongoing interplay between research and clinical practice by considering the disorder of autism. As we shall see, progress has often been possible only through the results of basic research far removed from child psychiatry. The reliance of genetic research on advances in molecular biology and the reliance of functional brain imaging on technological advances in physics constitute two obvious cases in point. Here, however, I will take these for granted, crucially important though they are, and stick to the research/clinical practice interface as it has operated in relation to studies of patients.

The story starts with Kanner's delineation of the syndrome of autism in a seminal paper in 1943. The paper has rightly become a classic. It is quite remarkable how successful he was in identifying the key clinical features, and even in many of the inferences drawn from them. In an era that has sometimes been thought of representing 'epidemic environmentalism', he was astute in suggesting that autism represented some kind of inbuilt deficit. A year later, in 1944, there was a somewhat comparable independent account by Asperger (see Frith, 1991), but it did not make the same impact and it does not compare with Kanner's account in either incisiveness of observation or conceptual clarity.

The first delineation of the syndrome

■ 55

The beginning, therefore, was provided by a set of clinical observations. In essence, Kanner was putting forward the hypothesis that autism represented a meaningfully distinctive disorder that differed from other psychiatric conditions and that might well prove to have a different aetiology, course and response to treatment. The first question had to be whether Kanner's observations could be repeated in other patient samples. It took a little time for this to happen, but other confirmatory reports began to come in from many other centres. There was no doubt, therefore, that the pattern of behaviour described by Kanner did indeed exist and could be recognised by others.

The first research step with respect to syndrome definition, however, took longer. That is, it was necessary to undertake systematic studies to determine whether Kanner's hypothesis that the syndrome was meaningfully different from other psychiatric conditions could be confirmed. Three further research avenues (beyond syndrome delineation) that would have to be explored concerned the nature of the disorder, its aetiology and response to interventions. In telling the story of the interplay between research and clinical practice in the period between 1943 and the present, I shall organise the issues and findings in relation to those four themes, considering developments as they have taken place over four broad time periods: the 1950s and 1960s, the 1970s into the mid-1980s, the late 1980s and early 1990s, and the late 1990s. In placing areas of research within a particular time period, greater weight has been attached to when the research ideas and approaches first came to the fore than when papers were published, which was sometimes several years later.

Before turning to the research, a word is necessary on the clinical concepts as represented in Kanner's writings, as well as in those of others. Like all of us, Kanner, remarkable clinician though he was, was a creature of his times, and, inevitably, his thinking was influenced by the *Zeitgeist* within which he had to operate. Accordingly, during the late 1940s the clarity of Kanner's vision was eroded in some respects. Autism came to be viewed as an unusually early manifestation of schizophrenia, with its aetiology including the environmentally mediated effects of rearing by 'refrigerator' parents (Kanner, 1949). It should be noted that these clinical assumptions were not based on research. Thus, there had been no attempt at that time to consider how one might test the notion that autism was part of schizophrenia. Similarly, there were no tests of the environmental causation hypothesis and, indeed, no consideration at all of the possibility that, in so far as the parents showed particular personality characteristics, these might reflect genetic factors rather than environmental risks. Nevertheless, undeterred by the lack of research evidence, therapists were galloping down the road of interventions designed to ameliorate the supposed damage of adverse parenting (Bettelheim, 1967), a strategy widely perceived by families as blaming them for causing their children's problems (Rimland, 1965).

Phase 1: the 1950s and 1960s

Against that background, let me now turn to consider the first phase, the 1950s and 1960s, beginning with studies on diagnosis and syndrome definition.

Diagnosis and syndrome delineation

During this first time period, there were various attempts by committees, such as the Creak working party (1961), to produce lists of symptoms by which autism might be recognised (except by then it had come to be called 'schizophrenic syndrome of childhood'). The first attempt to use empirical research findings to determine diagnostic criteria, however, came from the Maudsley Hospital study (Rutter, 1966; Rutter *et al*, 1967; Lockyer & Rutter, 1969, 1970). Children who had been diagnosed as suffering from autism (or 'infantile psychosis', the synonym used at that time) were systematically compared with children attending the same clinic who received some other diagnosis and who were matched for age, gender and IQ level (features all known to be associated with variations in symptomatology – see, e.g., Rutter *et al*, 1970). Note the importance of having a comparison group with some other psychiatric disorder. The question was not how to differentiate autism from normality. The relevant question was how to differentiate autism from other psychiatric disorders.

Using direct observations of the children, as well as systematic accounts from caregivers, the Maudsley Hospital study showed that there were only three domains of behaviour that were present in nearly all children with autism and that were significantly more frequent in the autistic group than in the control group. These were: (i) a general failure to develop social relationships, together with various specific abnormalities in interpersonal functioning; (ii) language retardation, with impaired comprehension, echolalia and pronominal reversal; and (iii) ritualistic and compulsive phenomena associated with repetitive stereotyped play patterns. A systematic follow-up into adolescence and early adult life, in which the children were seen in person, confirmed that these characteristics continued to differentiate the autistic group many years after clinic referral. These features, together with an onset before 30 months (as also emphasised by Kanner), were then taken as the defining characteristics of the syndrome.

So far, so good. However, the validation of diagnoses has to go beyond the features used to define the syndrome. It is necessary that validation test whether the syndrome differs from other conditions with respect to features other than symptomatology, such as aetiology, epidemiological characteristics, course of disorder, or response to treatment (Rutter, 1965). That first study provided preliminary evidence of this kind. The diagnosis of autism was associated with a distinctive pattern of scores on IQ tests, with persisting language delay and with poor employment prospects. In each of these respects, the children with autism differed significantly from their matched controls. Autism also differed from the general run of emotional and conduct disorders in terms of the high frequency with which epileptic fits developed in adolescence (Rutter, 1970). The clinical benefit that derived from this and comparable studies was both the availability of applicable diagnostic criteria and also the knowledge that the diagnosis carried clinical meaning and prognostic value.

Nature of the disorder

During this first phase of research, a greater understanding of the nature of autism derived primarily from three main types of research: follow-up studies, psychological studies and comparative studies. Long-term follow-ups were undertaken of Kanner's cases (Eisenberg, 1956; Kanner, 1971; Kanner *et al*, 1972), Creak's cases (1963a,b), Lotter's cases (1974a,b, 1978) and children seen at the Maudsley Hospital (Rutter *et al*, 1967; Rutter, 1970). All showed considerable consistency in the broad pattern of behaviour from early childhood into adult life but, equally, all showed a remarkable heterogeneity in the degree of social impairment whenever outcome was assessed. Although the majority remained severely handicapped, about one in six went on to obtain regular paid employment. Much the most important predictor of outcome was the children's initial level of non-verbal IQ. When this was in the severely retarded range, a good outcome was highly unlikely. The overall level of language impairment also proved to be quite important, especially at the top end of the range. Good social functioning in adult life, even in those without mental retardation, was unlikely if the child had not developed useful speech by the age of 5 years. The overall level of disturbance was of some slight prognostic importance, but non-viable IQ and language were far more influential.

Before these studies were undertaken, the general clinical view was that children with autism were not testable for IQ and language, and also that even if scores could be obtained, they carried little meaning because of the children's social impairment. The studies were influential in showing that both views were wrong. Given an appropriate choice of tests and administration by skilled and experienced clinical psychologists, the great majority of children with autism were testable. Moreover, the stability of their IQ scores over time was much the same as that of any other group of children, and the scores were good predictors of clinical outcome. The findings made an impact on clinical practice in showing the importance of skilled psychological assessment, and this came, over time, to be accepted as a necessary part of any diagnostic appraisal.

The follow-up studies were also crucially important in producing what was, at that time, an entirely unexpected finding. About a quarter of children with autism who had not shown neurological abnormalities when assessed in early childhood developed epilepsy during the follow-up period, with an onset most often during adolescence (Rutter, 1970). This finding did much to bring about a change of concept from the view that autism was an acquired psychogenic disorder to a view that it might constitute a neurodevelopmental disorder based on organic brain dysfunction. This led clinicians to pay more attention to the possibility of an organic aetiology, and it came to be accepted that an adequate clinical assessment had to include a systematic medical evaluation, together with the use of special tests where there were indications that they might be of value.

Psychological studies undertaken during the 1960s were informative in showing the very considerable extent to which children with autism showed distinctive and unusual patterns of scores on cognitive tests. Even on tests that did not involve any use of speech, children with autism performed badly when verbal or sequencing skills were required (Lockyer & Rutter, 1970). It was concluded that the problem was not lack of speech as such, but rather a serious deficit in cognitive skills involving sequencing, abstraction and other language-related functions. A series of well-planned, systematic experimental studies by Hermelin & O'Connor (1970) took things very much further, in showing that children with autism made relatively little use of *meaning* in their memory and thought processes. Both sets of findings indicated that the social and behavioural abnormalities of autism might arise on the basis of a cognitive deficit that involved some aspect of abstraction, or conceptual inference. The further implication was that it might be desirable for treatment strategies to shift from insight-oriented psychotherapy to educational and behavioural approaches that sought to help children cope better with what might prove to be basic cognitive handicaps.

Comparative studies in the 1960s mainly focused on the differentiation from learning disability ('mental retardation') (because children with autism had been shown to have low IQ scores) and schizophrenia (because of the severe abnormalities in relationships in both conditions and because of the supposition that autism might be an early manifestation of schizophrenia). The experimental studies undertaken by Hermelin & O'Connor (1970) were decisive in showing the host of ways in which children with autism differed from well-matched groups of children with learning disability but without the syndrome of autism. Kolvin (1971) and his colleagues in England and Makita (1966) in Japan each showed that the age of onset of psychoses in childhood followed a markedly bipolar pattern – with peaks under the age of 3 years and over the age of 11 years, and a very decided trough in between. The findings suggested a discontinuity between autism and schizophrenia, and Kolvin's (1971) systematic comparisons between the two groups showed many differences. In 1972, I argued that the overarching generic concept of 'childhood schizophrenia' should be abandoned (Rutter, 1972). Autism and

■57

schizophrenia constituted disparate conditions requiring separate classification. It was also noted that there might be a possible third group of disintegrative disorders, involving a profound regression and behavioural disintegration after an initial period of apparently normal development – a clinical picture first described by Heller (1930) much earlier in the century, but one subjected to almost no systematic research. About this time, clinicians began to abandon the notion of autism as a psychosis, replacing it with the concept that it might constitute a neurodevelopmental disorder with the need, therefore, to approach treatment with developmental considerations in mind.

Interventions

During the 1960s, educational and behavioural approaches to the treatment of children with autism began to come to the fore. This was the time when the first special schools and classes for such children were established (Bartak & Rutter, 1971) through the initiatives of pioneer teachers such as Sibel Elgar (Elgar & Wing, 1969) with the support of parents and the establishment of self-help organisations such as the National Autistic Society, founded in 1962 (Wing, 1972) in the UK, which brought together parents and professionals to work for a common cause. Parent groups stimulated, fostered and supported the development of educational provision. During the 1960s there were the first reports of the application of operant learning principles to the modification of the behaviour of children with autism (Ferster & DeMyer, 1961; Lovaas, 1967). The positive side of these early reports was the demonstration that experimental methods could be applied to the study of children with autism. They were also important in showing that careful functional analysis of children's behaviour and the appropriate use of reinforcement principles could lead to worthwhile changes in behaviour. Clinicians were, nevertheless, reluctant to move uncritically in the direction urged by these early behavioural enthusiasts. Four concerns predominated. First, behaviourists used their findings to argue that there was no need to postulate any kind of neurodevelopmental disorder, and this seemed to run counter to other evidence. Second, although the immediate changes in behaviour were striking, they had been brought about in rather artificial circumstances in the laboratory, and the long-term gains in the natural environment remained unknown. Third, there was distaste over the use of punitive techniques, such as the employment of electric cattle prods in order to shape social behaviour (Lovaas et al, 1965). Fourth, the use of material reinforcers, such as sweets or chocolates (Lovaas et al, 1966), seemed to carry the danger that the children's behaviour would become reliant on artificial rewards.

As clinicians gained experience in the application of behavioural and educational approaches in the treatment of children with autism, the need for some modifications in treatment method became apparent. Up to that time, it had been thought desirable to provide treatment on an in-patient basis because that enabled a higher intensity of therapeutic input. It soon became evident that, although behavioural methods did indeed result in symptomatic gains, the benefits tended to dissipate either on return home or on moving to a different setting within the residential facility (Lovaas et al, 1973). It was necessary to consider what steps should be taken to ensure that behavioural gains generalised. It was concluded that it was likely to be helpful to engage the participation of parents as co-therapists (Schopler et al, 1980, 1986) and to seek to introduce the educational and behavioural modifications in the children's natural environments of home and school. Various forms of community interventions were developed, including working with parents in their own homes (Rutter, 1973).

The other therapeutic shift arose in part from clinical experience and in part from an appreciation that if autism constituted an abnormality of development (rather than a psychosis), it was important to plan treatment with developmental goals in mind and also in the light of considerations of the principles of psychological development and of how the basic deficits of children with autism might be impeding that development (Rutter & Sussenwein, 1971). Thus, there was a need to consider how to foster more normal social development, how to facilitate language development and communicative skills and how to reduce abnormal stereotyped patterns of behaviour. It was decided that the clinical and cognitive research findings suggested that the social problem lay in the difficulties children with autism faced in engaging in social interaction, rather than in their withdrawing from social encounters. Attention came to be paid to how to intrude on the child in order deliberately to engage him or her in interaction that was meaningful and pleasurable. Similarly, behavioural attempts to modify language came to focus more on communicative skills than on the acquisition of words as such. By the end of the 1960s, a quite radical change in the therapeutic approaches to autism was beginning to be established.

Aetiology

This first phase included relatively little research into causes. However, there was the beginning of a series of reports that autism was sometimes associated with one or other of a mixed bag of medical conditions that had in common the presence of organic brain pathology. The 1971 study by Chess *et al* of children with congenital rubella provides a good example of just such a systematic study. At first, the importance seemed to lie simply in the demonstration that autism might arise on the basis of some defined medical condition (and hence the implication that such conditions should be searched for). Questions also began to be asked on what these medical aetiologies might have in common and what brain mechanisms might underlie the development of autism.

The answers to these questions, however, had to await a much later phase of research, as the next 15 years saw a concentration on the diagnosis and delineation of autism.

Phase 2: the 1970s to mid-1980s

Diagnosis and syndrome delineation

■ 59

The 1970s into the mid-1980s were associated with two main trends in diagnostic studies. As a degree of consensus on diagnosis came to be achieved, it was appreciated that it would be hugely advantageous for both research and clinical practice to develop standardised assessments (Parks, 1983). At first, a range of questionnaires were produced but, although they have their value, they did not prove to be satisfactory for individual diagnosis. Rather, it seemed preferable to develop standardised interviews and methods of observation. Once more, various methods were tried (see Schopler & Mesibov, 1988), with Wing & Gould's (1978) Schedule of Handicaps, Behaviors and Skills and Schopler's Childhood Autism Rating Scale (CARS; Schopler *et al*, 1980, 1986) leading the way. But, over time, the Autism Diagnostic Interview (ADI; Le Couteur *et al*, 1989) and the Autism Diagnostic Observation Schedule (ADOS; Lord *et al*, 1989) came to be the tools that were most widely adopted. The ADI, as the interview came to be called, provides an interesting bringing-together of clinical and research approaches. Clinical researchers who developed it were aware that although many of the problems associated with autism were severe, they were also quite subtle and specific in terms of the aspects of social reciprocity and communicative deviance that needed to be tapped. Accordingly, the interview was designed to obtain detailed descriptions of actual behaviour (rather than yes/no answers to structured questions) and behavioural codings made by the investigator on the basis of an operationalisation of diagnostic concepts. The interview is well standardised and has been shown to be reliable and have discriminative validity, but its style and qualities approximate closely to the ways in which most clinicians approach the task of differential diagnosis. The ADOS, the observation method, also had the particular quality of using a series of social tasks and situations to provide a 'press' for social interactions. As with the interview, although systematically standardised and operationalised, the style of observation required considerable clinical skills and appropriate training in the use of the observational tasks.

The second trend during the 1970s and early 1980s involved the growing appreciation of the heterogeneity of autism, together with the increasing awareness of the need to consider where to draw the boundaries of autism and how to differentiate it from other pervasive developmental disorders that seemed similar in many respects yet different in others. Five areas of inquiry warrant particular mention.

First, Rett (1966) described a hitherto unrecognised syndrome in which girls plateaued or regressed in their early development, showing a loss of purposive movements, a failure of head growth and social deficits that seemed somewhat autistic-like in their pattern. His initial paper did not get much recognition at first, but when Hagberg *et al*

(1983) picked up the importance of the observation and reported a series of cases, Rett's syndrome was rapidly put on the map. Some child psychiatrists emphasised the high frequency with which girls with Rett's syndrome had been diagnosed as having autism (Witt-Engerström & Gillberg, 1987), but a more careful study of the children's behaviour indicated important differences (Olsson & Rett, 1987, 1990).

Second, there were numerous reports of autistic-like abnormalities shown by children with the newly recognised syndrome of the fragile-X anomaly, an unusual form of chromosomal abnormality made manifest by culturing the chromosomes in folate-deficient media. As with Rett's syndrome, however, more detailed studies showed that, although the anomaly could indeed be associated with the characteristic syndrome of autism (Hagerman et al, 1986), a particular form of social anxiety and turning away might be even more characteristic (Cohen et al, 1989; Wolff et al, 1989).

Third, there were several reports of cases showing behavioural disintegration (Corbett et al, 1977; Hill & Rosenbloom, 1986). In a few instances, this pattern was associated with some form of overt acquired brain disease, but in the great majority of cases, medical investigations proved negative. It remained uncertain whether this syndrome was an atypical variety of autism or something different (Volkmar & Cohen, 1989; Kurita et al, 1992). That question remains unanswered today.

Fourth, Wing & Gould's (1979) epidemiological study of individuals with learning disability drew attention to the high frequency with which autistic-like syndromes occurred in children with profound learning disability. Only some of these showed the classical syndrome as described by Kanner, but Wing argued that the syndromes nevertheless represented the same basic condition. The study was important in emphasising the several different ways in which the social deficits of autism might be manifest.

Fifth, there was a resurgence of interest in the concepts first proposed by Asperger and in the manifestations of autistic-like patterns in children of normal intelligence. Wing's (1981) espousal of Asperger's syndrome and Wolff's (Wolff & Chick, 1980; Wolff, 1995) descriptions of what she at that time called schizoid disorder of childhood were particularly important in this connection. Questions were asked about whether these syndromes represented mild autism or some different condition.

Both clinicians and researchers therefore became aware of the need for careful systematic observation that went well beyond general statements about social impairment and social withdrawal. The importance of shrewd clinical observations (as by Rett & Hagberg) were crucial in identification of the clinical heterogeneity, although subsequent research was necessary in order to validate it. The field had moved on dramatically from the undifferentiated concept of childhood schizophrenia.

During the second phase, attention turned to the nature of the language problems associated with autism. Research during the 1960s had made clear that it was not just that speech was slow to develop (or did not develop at all); also, the quality of language was abnormal and so was its communicative usage (Rutter, 1968). Was this, however, because the language deficit was so severe and pervasive in autism, or was the nature of the language problem different in kind from that associated with developmental disorders of language? Bartak, Cantwell and others (Bartak et al, 1975, 1977; Cox et al, 1975; Cantwell et al, 1978) sought to investigate this question by comparing boys of normal non-verbal intelligence with autism and boys of similar cognitive level who showed a developmental disorder of receptive language. The findings showed that the language deficit in children with autism was indeed more severe and more extensive, but the marked differences between the two groups could not be accounted for by the level of language. It was clear that autism involved a quite widespread cognitive deficit that included language but extended much more broadly.

Nature of the disorder

Following the lead provided by Hermelin & O'Connor (1970), studies of the nature of autism during this period continued to focus on gaining a better understanding of its cognitive deficits. The importance of low IQ as a predictor of outcome had been shown, but in itself that finding did not deal with the possibility that the low IQ scores might be secondary to social withdrawal. Several research programmes tackled this question. One research strategy was to determine, through naturalistic follow-ups, whether children's IQ scores varied with changes in their psychiatric state. Findings showed that they did not to any substantial extent (Rutter *et al*, 1967; Rutter, 1979, 1983). The second strategy was to test whether intensive educational and behavioural treatments led to significant IQ gains. The findings showed that they did not (Rutter & Bartak, 1973; Hemsley *et al*, 1978; Howlin & Rutter, 1987). A further strategy was to use a variety of tactics to examine the extent to which motivational factors might influence cognitive performance. Clark & Rutter (1977, 1979) found that the IQ scores of children with autism were largely explicable in terms of cognitive factors, without the need to invoke motivation. Of course, motivational factors influenced the performance just as they did with any other group of children, but they did not account for the low IQ scores shown by many individuals.

The conclusion was clear. Many children with autism had a general cognitive deficit that was not in any way secondary to social withdrawal. On the other hand, it was equally evident that low IQ in itself could not possibly account for autism. To begin with, a substantial minority of children with autism had a normal non-verbal intelligence and there were many children with marked learning disability who did not show autism. Where the low IQ was associated with a particular medical condition, the risk of autism seemed to vary according to the medical diagnosis, as shown by Wing & Gould (1979) among others. Thus, although Down's syndrome and cerebral palsy occasionally co-occurred with autism, the association was much less strong than with, for example, tuberose sclerosis and infantile spasms (Riikonen & Amnell, 1981; Hunt & Dennis, 1987). The implication was that the specific nature of the underlying neuropathology might well be crucially important, although it was not at all apparent which aspects might predispose to autism. In addition, as already noted, the IQ scores of children with autism tended to show an unusual and distinctive pattern (Lockyer & Rutter, 1970; DeMyer *et al*, 1972; DeMyer, 1975; Tymchuk *et al*, 1977). Although a general impairment in intelligence could well be important, there was also a need to search for more specific cognitive deficits.

In this search, researchers and clinicians had become increasingly aware of the need to focus on the possible ways in which a cognitive deficit might lead to the abnormalities in social reciprocity and in social functioning more generally. Tinbergen & Tinbergen (1972) and Richer (1978) had hypothesised that children with autism were motivated to avoid social encounters, but several studies showed that individuals with autism were most likely to respond socially when the social demands on them were increased (McHale *et al*, 1980; Clark & Rutter, 1981). The findings provided no support for the motivational hypothesis, and this view of autism began to fade away.

During both Phase 1 and Phase 2, there was much research in which a range of physiological and psychological functions were examined in children with autism, their responses being compared with those of normal children. This led to claims that autism arose on the basis of perceptual inconstancy (Ornitz & Ritvo, 1968), or of a delay in sensorimotor integration (Ornitz, 1971) or of overselective attention (Lovaas *et al*, 1979). Many of the experiments were elegant and carefully designed. The problem was that there were no controls for mental age, and hence there was an inevitable uncertainty as to whether the findings were a function of low mental age or of autism. The need for appropriate controls was noted in an international symposium held in 1970 (Rutter, 1971) and was underlined by DeMyer in 1975 and Yule in 1978. When the appropriate controls were introduced, as was the case in further studies of overselectivity (see Schover & Newsom, 1976), it became apparent that the level of cognitive impairment was more influential than the diagnosis of autism. Why it took so long for experienced researchers to accept the need for appropriate controls remains a bit of a mystery.

Two new approaches started to come to the fore in the 1980s. First, Hobson (1982, 1983, 1993) put forward the notion that children with autism might lack the ability to experience empathy and that this socio-emotional deficit might constitute the key. The postulate fitted in well with clinical experience and his experimental studies confirmed the reality of the problems experienced by such children in differentiating emotions and some aspects of people.

The second approach focused on mentalising aspects of cognition, rather than emotions as such. Rutter (1983) reported a young adult with autism who complained

61

that he could not "mind-read". The man explained that he thought that other people seemed to have a special sense by which they could read the thoughts of others and thereby anticipate their responses and feelings. By contrast, he was always upsetting people because he did not realise he was doing or saying the wrong thing until *after* the other person had become angry or upset. A breakthrough occurred with the development of experimental methods to test whether there was an understanding of other people's mental states. Wimmer & Perner (1983) devised experimental procedures based on tests of false belief. The paradigm involves a story in which a person (say, Jane) sees an article hidden in one place. Without Jane's knowledge, someone else then moves the object to an entirely different place. The test is provided by finding out whether the subject believes that Jane, in returning to reclaim the object, will look where the object actually is (which would require knowledge not available her) or where she *thinks* it is. Given some form of portrayal of this story, children over the age of 4 anticipated that Jane would look where she *thought* the object was rather than where it actually was. Younger children, on the other hand, could not do that.

Baron-Cohen *et al* (1985) applied this false belief test to individuals with autism and showed that even older children with autism failed it. It was postulated that the social impairments in autism might have arisen on the basis of this lack of appreciation of what other people might be thinking – something that came to be called a lack of a 'theory of mind'. What caught the imagination of the research world with this interesting finding was that, for the first time, it provided a possible means of directly linking a cognitive deficit with the social problem and that it did so in terms of an aspect of cognition known to follow a predictable developmental course. If confirmed, it was clear that this might well have major clinical implications.

Aetiology

The second phase of research saw many studies investigating different possible medical causes of autism (Coleman, 1976; Coleman & Gillberg, 1985; Golden, 1987). Several different strands with lessons for research and for clinical practice may be delineated.

First, there were many reports that autism was associated with some medical condition. Almost all of these were based on single case reports or very small samples. The inferences to be drawn from these reports were problematic for several reasons, as came to be recognised later. The findings were important, nevertheless, in highlighting the possibility that autism could arise on the basis of diagnosable medical conditions. These reaffirmed the need for a careful medical evaluation of all cases of autism.

The second strand is that more detailed studies of proven associations often showed that the autistic syndromes associated with medical conditions were atypical in one way or another. This was noted earlier in relation to Rett's syndrome and the fragile-X anomaly. The follow-up of the congenital rubella sample by Chess (1977) gave the same message.

The final strand to mention is the evidence that genetic factors play an important part in autism. Earlier reviews had concluded that it was unlikely that there was a strong genetic influence, because it was so rare for individuals with autism to be born to parents with the same disorder and because the rate of autism in siblings was so low when considered in absolute terms (estimates at that time suggested it was about 2% – see Rutter, 1967). The situation changed when it was appreciated that these were not the relevant features. Follow-up studies had already shown how extremely rare it was for individuals with autism to marry and have children; accordingly, vertical transmission was not to be expected. Also, the point about the 2% rate was not that it was low in absolute terms, but rather that it was so extremely high relative to the base rate of autism in the general population (estimated at that time at about 4 per 10 000. This led Folstein & Rutter (1977*a,b*) to undertake the first systematic twin study of autism. The sample was small, but the findings were striking in pointing to the likelihood of a strong genetic liability and also in their indication that the liability probably extended beyond the traditional diagnosis of autism to include a broader range of social and communicative deficits in individuals of normal intelligence. Up to that time, most clinicians had tended to see autism as an extreme handicapping condition that was qualitatively distinct from variations within the normal range. Also, the general tendency within psychiatry was to view genetic factors as being likely to apply to the direct inheritance of disorders. Despite its slender empirical base (because of the small sample size), the study was one of the first to raise queries about both assumptions. It seemed that the genetically influenced liability to autism extended somewhat more broadly than had hitherto been appreciated and also that genetic factors might operate within a multi-factorial context, rather than through Mendelian direct inheritance of discrete conditions.

Interventions

The period of the 1970s and early 1980s was marked by the very widespread development of behavioural and educational approaches in the treatment of children with autism and by systematic investigations of their efficacy. At the beginning of the 1970s there were still claims that psychotherapeutic methods were better than educational approaches in the treatment of autism. Accordingly, Bartak & Rutter (1971, 1973; Rutter & Bartak, 1973) undertook systematic comparisons of a psychotherapeutic unit with little emphasis on teaching, a second unit in which regressive techniques and an emphasis on relationships were combined with special educational methods, and a third unit that provided a structured and organised setting with the focus on the teaching of specific skills. The results showed that clinical progress was greatest in the third unit – indicating the value of educational methods. The results were qualified, however, by the indication of the limited generalisation of behavioural gains at school to the home environment, the continuing difficulties in understanding what they had learned shown by many of the children and the marked individual differences in outcome. The problem of generalisation was tackled by a range of programmes explicitly focused on working with parents in relation to the children's behaviour at home.

■63

Schopler and his colleagues (Schopler & Reichler, 1971; Lansing & Schopler, 1978) established the TEACCH programme, in which there was a behaviourally oriented curriculum, using parents as co-therapists, and with the details worked out on an individual basis, taking into account the child's developmental level and the parent's priorities and resources. Somewhat similarly, Hemsley, Howlin and their colleagues (Rutter & Sussenwein, 1971; Howlin *et al*, 1973; Hemsley *et al*, 1978; Rutter, 1985; Howlin & Rutter, 1987) developed a home-based treatment programme. A functional analysis of the children's behaviour was undertaken with the parents to determine when, where, how often and for what apparent reason behaviours occurred. Parents were helped to be consistent in their styles of interaction and handling and were advised to set aside short periods each day to teach the child specific social and communication skills, making the sessions as pleasurable as possible for both child and parents.

Research into the home-based treatment involved four main elements. First, systematic individual case studies were employed to determine whether the benefits demonstrated in laboratory or hospital settings could be replicated in the home, where there was much less control over the environment and with much more limited professional time. Second, studies addressed the question of whether the treatment methods were superior to other approaches, examining longitudinal changes over a 6-month period. Third, the same 6-month comparison was used to determine the efficacy of the methods in altering parental behaviour. Fourth, long-term benefits were assessed by means of an individually matched control group of children seen at the same clinic, but who lived too far away to be involved in the home-based approach, although the same principles were applied in giving the parents advice. The findings showed that the treatment programme brought about quite dramatic changes during the 6 months of intervention and that the long-term gains were both worthwhile and superior to those that followed other methods of treatment. On the other hand, the programme made no difference to IQ levels and the gains in language development were quite modest. The main benefits were seen in relation to the behavioural problems and to overall social functioning. It was also noteworthy that there were huge individual differences in outcome, which were related in the same systematic fashion to the children's IQ and language as found in the earlier follow-up studies of children not treated in the same way.

This same time period was also marked by the beginnings of a series of strong claims on the efficacy of treatment. Thus, the Nobel laureate Tinbergen (Tinbergen & Tinbergen, 1983) stated boldly that "it is becoming clear that many cases of autism can be cured and even prevented by a return to healthier forms of parenting" (p. 214). Similarly,

Welch (1983) asserted that "it is possible to restore an autistic child to normal development by establishing a secure mother–child bond" (p. 334). These various claims that autism could be cured proved controversial but, not surprisingly, they raised expectations among parents and professionals who wished to believe the optimistic message. Unfortunately, none of the claims was supported by controlled, comparative studies, and now, almost 30 years later, such evidence has still to be obtained. The lesson is that we need to pay careful attention to the evidence put forward by researchers and not be overawed by their status or reputation.

Similar issues arose with respect to the unwarranted excitement over the claim (made rather prematurely on the basis of an uncontrolled study of just 3 children) that fenfluramine produced intellectual and behavioural gains in children with autism (Geller *et al*, 1982). The reason why many people got carried away with the promise was because the benefits seemed to reflect what could be an underlying causal biochemical mechanism. It had long been appreciated that about a third of children with autism have raised serotonin levels in the blood (Cook, 1990), and one of the main effects of fenfluramine is to reduce serotonin levels. Many researchers were, nevertheless, sceptical because raised serotonin levels are found in many neuropsychiatric conditions (it is not in the least bit diagnosis-specific) and because there was no evidence in the published report that any benefits were systemically related to changes in serotonin level. The consequence was a mass of further studies with the much needed controls. The findings showed that the benefits were modest indeed and such slight behavioural gains as occurred in some children were unrelated to changes in serotonin levels (Campbell, 1988; Aman & Kern, 1989). Looking back, it is doubtful whether, on the basis of such slender and inadequate evidence, it was justifiable to spend so much money testing the benefits of fenfluramine. In the event, the drug has now been withdrawn from the market because of its possible toxic effects.

The claim was also made that high doses of vitamin B6 led to worthwhile benefits in some children with autism (Rimland *et al*, 1978; Rimland, 1987). There was more substance to this claim, but the results were far from dramatic and, even now, there is uncertainty over the value of this form of treatment. Reviews of the evidence have usually resulted in the conclusion that the regular use of megavitamins is not justified (Sloman, 1991).

Phase 3: the late 1980s and early 1990s

This result brings us to Phase 3 of developments, during the late 1980s and early 1990s.

Aetiology

One of the most important products of the late 1980s and early 1990s was consolidation of the quantitative genetic findings. Both a population-wide twin study in Scandinavia (Steffenberg *et al*, 1989) and a similar nationwide twin study in Britain (Bailey *et al*, 1995) showed a huge difference in the concordance rate for monozygotic and dizygotic pairs (60–90% *v.* less than 5%). These figures translated into a heritability of the underlying liability to autism of about 90%, making it the most strongly genetically influenced of all multi-factorial child psychiatric disorders. Because twins differ from singletons in various respects (for example, a higher level of obstetric complications), it is always necessary to check findings using other research strategies. Family studies of singletons were undertaken during this same period by several different research groups in both Europe and North America (see Rutter *et al*, 1997, 1998*a*). The findings were consistent in showing a rate of autism in siblings of about 2–6%. This represents an increase in rate of some 6- to 10-fold as compared with the base rate of autism in the general population (Fombonne, 1998). The inference from this finding is the same as that from the twin studies. At first, it had been thought that part of the increased risk might stem from obstetric complications, but a more detailed examination of the evidence suggested that these did not account for the increased rate of autism in family members (Bolton *et al*, 1994, 1997).

Non-geneticists sometimes find it puzzling that researchers can conclude from the massive relative increase in risk of autism in the relatives of autistic individuals that genetic factors are powerfully influential, when the absolute rate of autism in relatives is so low. Initial estimates had put the rate in siblings at about 2% (Smalley *et al*, 1988). The more thorough family studies showed that this was probably an underestimate, with the true rate being more like 5%. Nevertheless, that still means that the great majority of siblings do not have autism. One of the main reasons for this apparent paradox is that several genes are involved. Pickles *et al* (1995), using statistical modelling approaches applied to a combination of twin and family data, concluded that the findings suggested that autism was most unlikely to be due to a single gene but that, equally, more than 10 genes were unlikely. What this means is that many family members will have some of the genes that provide the susceptibility to autism, but they will not have all of them. In consequence, if combinations of genes are required for autism to develop, they will escape the handicapping condition.

The first twin study by Folstein & Rutter (1977*a,b*) had suggested that the genetically influenced liability to autism extended beyond the handicapping disorder. The twin and family studies undertaken during the late 1980s and early 1990s have confirmed this (Rutter *et al*, 1997, 1998*a,b*; Bailey *et al*, 1998*a,b*; Szatmari *et al*, 1998). The findings are persuasive that autism extends beyond the traditional handicapping disorder to include a broader range of social and communicative deficits in individuals of normal intelligence. This has come to be termed 'the broader phenotype' of autism. What has proved much more difficult, however, has been the definition of the boundaries of this broader phenotype and, therefore, determination of its frequency in relatives.

In essence, the relevant research strategies sought to tackle this question by determining not just whether there is an increased rate of some problem in relatives, but also whether its distribution in families was associated with other, better-established aspects of the broader phenotype and whether its distribution followed expected patterns and was not due to some other risk factor not representing a genetic liability. On this basis, it has been shown that learning disability, isolated reading and spelling difficulties, and verbal deficits in cognitive functioning are almost certainly not indicators of autism unless they are accompanied by other autistic features – except possibly in the case of autism associated with profound learning disability (Fombonne *et al*, 1997; Pickles *et al*, 1998; Starr *et al*, 2000).

DeLong and his colleagues (DeLong & Dwyer, 1988; DeLong & Nohria, 1994) noted an increased rate of affective disorders in the relatives of autistic individuals, and it has seemed possible that depression or anxiety might, in some circumstances, constitute part of the broader phenotype. In the event, the lack of overlap with other features of the broader phenotype and the lack of an association with the severity of autism, but an association with affective disorder in other relatives, suggest that affective disturbance does not reflect a genetic liability to autism (Bolton *et al*, 1998). On the other hand, an increased rate of affective disorders in relatives seems to be a valid finding and its explanation remains obscure. The empirical evidence also does not support Gillberg's claim (1992) that eating disorders might be part of autism or the Comings' claim (Comings & Comings, 1991) that Tourette's syndrome might also be part of the disorder. Family studies have been consistent in confirming earlier findings that autism was not associated with an increased rate of schizophrenia in relatives. Follow-up studies (Volkmar & Cohen, 1991) have also confirmed that there was no increased likelihood, as compared with the general population, that autistic individuals would develop schizophrenia in adult life. It might well be expected that the broader phenotype would include obsessive-type features, highly circumscribed interests and ritual or repetitive patterns of behaviour. Studies have indeed shown that such features are more common in the relatives of individuals with autism than in the relatives of controls, but the differences have been rather modest and so far it has not proved possible to derive good criteria to determine when such features are, and when they are not, part of the broader phenotype.

Much progress has been made in sorting out which characteristics define the broader phenotype, but many questions remain. So far, the evidence is compatible with a frequency of this broader phenotype in relatives of anything up to 20% or so, and the findings do not, as yet, rule out the possibility that the liability is dimensionally distributed. That is, it always used to be assumed that you either had autism or you did not. That may still be the case, but the possibility that the autistic propensity operates as a continuum, with individuals varying as to how much or how little they have of autism, now needs to be reconsidered.

One clear clinical consequence of these quantitative genetic findings is that it has now become mandatory for clinicians to discuss with families the role of genetic factors in autism. The need for skilled genetic counselling is obvious. This is no straightforward matter, because of the uncertainty over just how autism is inherited. It seems unlikely that it is inherited directly. Several genes are almost certainly involved and there may be an interplay with as yet unidentified environmental risk factors. It is also apparent that the concept of the broader phenotype inevitably raises queries and anxieties in families in relation to the possibility that family members with social oddities or communicative problems may have a mild variety of autism. Clearly, this requires skilled handling. It has become necessary both for child psychiatrists to have a much greater understanding of genetics than has been the case in years gone by, and equally for clinical and medical geneticists offering genetic counselling to have a much better understanding of the ways in which autism may present than will have been offered in their training in the past. The importance of genetic factors in multi-factorial psychiatric disorders is no longer in doubt (Rutter *et al*, 1999*a,b*), but it is clear that there are challenges to both researchers and clinicians in the understanding of how genetic factors operate in these disorders and in developing sensitive and well-informed ways of handling the clinical implications.

The quantitative genetic findings just discussed all apply to autism when it arises in the absence of some associated, and possibly causal, medical condition. Over the same time period, there was a veritable flood of reports, mostly of isolated cases, of associations between autism and either some diagnosable medical condition or some somatic abnormality such as a chromosome anomaly (see Gillberg & Coleman, 1992). It has proved extremely difficult to know how to interpret these findings. They could represent nothing more interesting than coincidence, and very few have been replicated. On the other hand, it is possible that some of the associations do reflect a valid connection and the challenge is to know which is which. It might have been hoped that the associations would give rise to a pattern that would provide clues on the nature of the underlying neural processes. Unfortunately, that has not proved to be the case either. Thus, when last reviewed, there were reports that autism was associated with anomalies in all but three chromosomes (Gillberg, 1998). Similarly, autism has been associated with a mixed bag of metabolic abnormalities and with a range of infections in the prenatal period, and occasionally postnatally (Gillberg & Coleman, 1992). The supposed frequency of the association between autism and a diverse range of medical conditions was used by some to argue that autism was just an administrative category comprising nothing more than a set of non-specific behavioural symptoms mirroring underlying brain dysfunction and, hence, that there was no point in searching for autism-specific causal factors (Coleman, 1990; Gillberg, 1992).

These arguments, although put forward by experienced researchers, were always unjustified and were regarded as such by other researchers at the time (see, e.g., Rutter, 1991; Rutter & Schopler, 1992). The fallacy derived from several different considerations. First, the great majority of the associations were unreplicated and so their validity was not established. Second, the quantitative genetic findings suggested quite a high degree of specificity. Third, as already noted, it was not the case that all the medical causes of organic brain dysfunction greatly increased the likelihood of autism. The existence of differential associations according to the type of medical condition suggests that there may well be some commonality in the basis of different causes of autism, even if the nature of that commonality is at present not known. Finally, the claim that 37% of cases of autism were associated with a diagnosable medical condition (Gillberg, 1992) seems likely to have been a substantial overestimate. Rutter *et al* (1994), putting together the evidence from several studies, concluded that the rate was probably of the order of 10%.

Much the same story of inconsistent findings has applied to a wide range of biological investigations, including brain imaging, metabolic studies and neurophysiological investigations (Gillberg & Coleman, 1992; Bailey *et al*, 1996). By sharp contrast, there has been a relatively high degree of consistency in the neuropsychological findings. It is clear that part of the problem in biological studies has lain in the lack of methodological rigour and a lack of concern that findings be replicated by other investigators under blind conditions. In addition, all too often there has been no attempt to determine whether the abnormalities are specific to autism or would be found in a range of other neurodevelopmental disorders. A further problem, however, is that investigators have often regarded an initial positive finding as providing a 'minimum figure' (e.g. Gillberg & Wahlström, 1985), failing to appreciate the dangers of relying on findings based on small samples (Pocock, 1983; Cohen et al, 1995). The ratio of false to true positives in a small sample is necessarily much greater than in a large sample, and the size of the difference between groups is no guide to the true strength of the association. The point is that to achieve statistical significance, the difference in a small sample is bound to be large and the true difference will almost certainly be very much smaller. This crucial methodological point has been well demonstrated by Cohen et al (1995).

A further clinical implication drawn by some researchers was that a wide range of medical investigations, including lumbar puncture, electroencephalogram (EEG), brain imaging and metabolic studies, should be undertaken as a routine (Elia et al, 1990; Federico et al, 1990; Gillberg, 1990a,b; Gillberg & Coleman, 1996). Most clinicians have resisted this invasive approach to medical investigation. The key question is how often the investigations lead to a diagnosis that cannot be obtained more straightforwardly through clinical history and examination. The answer is that it is rare for the tests to reveal undiagnosed medical conditions; many supposedly abnormal laboratory findings have no unambiguous clinical implications; and the clinical value seems so slight as not to justify the distress inevitably caused to young children if such investigations are routinely undertaken.

Despite the plethora of false dawns and misleading inferences, it would be wrong to dismiss as uninformative all the biological findings during this decade of research. On the contrary, considerable progress was made in clarifying the few associations that do appear to be valid and probably meaningful. First, there is good replicated evidence that tuberose sclerosis is associated with autism. Pooling studies, probably about 25% of individuals with tuberose sclerosis show autism and nearly half show a pattern of behaviour that would meet the broader diagnostic criteria of a pervasive developmental disorder (Smalley et al, 1992; Smalley, 1998). Considered the other way round, the frequency of tuberose sclerosis among individuals with autism is quite low, probably about 1–4%, but this represents a substantial increase over the base rate expectation. It is quite likely that this is particularly so when the autism is associated with epilepsy. It is easy to miss the signs of tuberose sclerosis unless they are specifically looked for, and the clinical implication is that the medical examination should always seek to determine whether it might be present. The one chromosome anomaly that seems to be particularly associated with autism is a partial tetrasomy of chromosome 15 (Gillberg et al, 1991; Baker et al, 1994; Cook et al, 1997a). The meaning of the association with other chromosome anomalies remains obscure but, given that they are not detectable clinically, routine karyotyping is probably desirable. The other chromosome anomaly that needs to be considered is the fragile X. The initial claims of a strong association with autism have not been borne out, but although the true rate of fragile X in autism is probably below 5% (Bailey et al, 1993), that is still high enough to warrant routine screening using DNA methods.

Strong claims had also been made for an association between a lack of development of the posterior cerebellar vermis and autism (Courchesne et al, 1987, 1994), but this has not been confirmed by other investigators (Bailey et al, 1996). It may be that cerebellar abnormalities are occasionally implicated in the causal processes leading to autism, but it now seems implausible that a specific lesion in the cerebellum usually underlies the condition.

Diagnosis and syndrome delineation

To a considerable extent, diagnostic research during this third phase was driven by genetic findings. Thus, an appreciation that the diagnosis extends more widely than originally envisaged has led to a focus on Asperger's syndrome or mild autism occurring in individuals of normal intelligence (see, e.g., Ozonoff et al, 1991a,b; Klin et al, 1995; Happé et al, 1996). Because these milder varieties tend to be diagnosed much later (Howlin & Moore, 1997) there has also been an increasing interest in the diagnosis in adult life. Attention also turned to the other end of the age span, with studies focusing on the very early diagnosis of autism (Baron-Cohen et al, 1993; Lord, 1995; Cox et al, 1999). The standardised interview and observation measures were modified with an eye to making them more suitable for very young children and for older adolescents (Lord *et al*, 1993, 1994, 1998; DiLavore *et al*, 1995). Home videos (Osterling & Dawson, 1994) and health visitor records (Johnson *et al*, 1992) were used to determine whether autism could be diagnosed when the children were very young; screening questionnaires (Dahlgren & Gillberg, 1989) were applied to general populations; and clinical studies (Gillberg *et al*, 1990) were undertaken to answer the same question. The findings showed that, although some children show recognisable features in the first year of life, in most cases it cannot be detected in a reliable and valid fashion until 18 months of age or thereabouts. Moreover, it is clear that the diagnosis is particularly difficult when learning disability means that the child's mental age is below 18 months. The difficulties with respect to diagnosis in adult life, when autism has not been recognised earlier, are also considerable. In the absence of good information on developmental course during the preschool years, it can be quite difficult to sort out which problems in adult life are due to autism and which are due to some other sort of psychiatric disorder. A decade earlier it had seemed that the diagnostic difficulties were becoming resolved, but the extension of the diagnosis to a broader clinical picture emphasised that problems still remained to be tackled.

Both DSM–IV (American Psychiatric Association, 1994) and ICD–10 (World Health Organization, 1992) moved in the same direction in recognising the need to make provision for a range of autistic-like pervasive developmental disorders. There was explicit recognition at the time that the validity of these diagnostic differentiations within the broader group were unestablished in some cases and the need was for more systematic studies to examine the matter more closely. The provisional attempt to subdivide the disorders represented a step forward in the realisation that classification needed systematic research if it was to progress and that this demanded specification of the differentiations that required testing.

Nature of the disorder

This third phase of research involved an explosion of neuropsychological research, initially focused primarily on the theory of mind findings, but then broadening out to examine other significant functions. There can be no doubt that this has been a strong area of research. A range of ingeniously designed tests employed by several independent research groups have made clear that there is indeed a strong association between an impaired ability to understand mental states and autism (Frith, 1989; Baron-Cohen *et al*, 1993; Happé, 1994*a,b*; Baron-Cohen, 1995; Bailey *et al*, 1996; Yirmiya *et al*, 1998). Both the strength of the association and its relative (but not complete – see Yirmiya *et al*, 1998) diagnostic specificity strongly suggest that it is likely to be implicated in the cognitive basis of autism. Five main problems, however, remain to be resolved.

First, if the cognitive deficit constituting the basis for autism (as postulated) is so narrow and highly specific, why is there such a strong association between autism and general learning disability (Rutter & Bailey, 1993)?

Second, if a deficit in theory of mind is responsible, and yet theory of mind itself does not ordinarily develop until the age of 3 or 4 years, why are the manifestations evident as early as 12 to 18 months? It could be that autism arises from cognitive mechanisms that are precursors of the mentalising ability but, so far, it has not been possible unambiguously to demonstrate a causal relationship between a precursor and later theory of mind skills.

Third, the relationship between theory of mind skills and language has not yet been adequately sorted out. The two are associated (Happé, 1995; Yirmiya *et al*, 1998), but the mechanisms involved have yet to be elucidated. Language impairments do not seem sufficient to account for failures on theory of mind tests, because many autistic individuals with high verbal skills nevertheless fail the tests. On the other hand, the association is closer than originally envisaged.

Fourth, some 20% of verbal children with autism pass theory of mind tests. It remains unclear whether they truly have theory of mind skills or whether they use alternative strategies to pass the tests.

Fifth, although it is not difficult to see how an impaired ability to understand other people's mental states might lead to the social and communicative deficits associated with autism, it is by no means so clear how it could give rise to the obsessive-like preoccupations and repetitive patterns of behaviour. It is also not evident how it could give rise to the unusual cognitive talents, or 'idiot-savant' skills, found in a substantial minority of individuals with autism (Hermelin, 2001). Psychological studies during the 1980s and early 1990s extended to include studies of executive planning (Ozonoff, 1994) and of central coherence (Frith, 1989; Frith & Happé, 1994). Empirical findings have shown that many individuals with autism have problems in planning and organisation, in using feedback, in switching to a new cognitive set and in disengaging from perceptually salient stimuli (Bailey et al, 1996). The findings fit in well with clinical observations, but problems in executive planning have been found in a wide range of disorders, and it remains uncertain whether there is a particular type of executive planning deficit that is more specifically associated with autism. Research into central coherence is at a much earlier stage, but the evidence so far does suggest that individuals with autism have a tendency to process information in a piecemeal fashion rather than according to the overall gestalt or meaning. It seems possible that weak central coherence may play a role in the development of idiot-savant skills (Pring et al, 1995) and may predispose to repetitive behaviour patterns. However, that remains to be determined.

The neuropsychological findings undoubtedly carry the potential of providing a means of differentiating social deficits that are part of autism from those that are due to some other kind of problem. This is likely to be particularly important in studying the broader phenotype. That potential has, however, yet to be realised. Clinically, the findings have been crucially important in emphasising the role of cognitive deficits in socialisation and communication, and that has changed concepts of the meaning of the social deficit in autism. Hobson's research (1993) had been crucially important in forcing investigators to seek to understand its origins and in demonstrating that a difficulty in appreciating emotions was part of the problem. On the other hand, the overall pattern of evidence does not seem to support Hobson's notion that an emotional deficit is primary and accounts for the other features (Rutter & Bailey, 1993).

Interventions

Intervention research during this decade provided a consolidation of what was known on the value of developmentally oriented behavioural and educational treatments (Howlin & Rutter, 1987; Howlin, 1998). However, the period was also marked by three areas of controversy. First, Lovaas and his colleagues (Lovaas, 1987, 1996; McEachin et al, 1993) made strong claims that a very intensive (40 hours per week) home-based behavioural programme during the early preschool years can bring about normal functioning in some two-fifths of autistic individuals; and that the findings were inconsistent with the view that autism was due to a neural abnormality. Critics have pointed to limitations in subject selection, research design and most especially in the criteria used to conclude that the children were functioning normally (Schopler et al, 1989; Gresham & MacMillan, 1998). Clinicians have been concerned regarding the emotional, financial and practical costs to families if parents are expected to give up so much to concentrate on the child with autism. Also, the massive improvements that are supposed to follow the intensive treatment seem out of keeping with a broader range of evidence from other interventions (see, e.g., Sheinkopf & Siegel, 1998). What is clearly needed at this point is a systematic comparative study undertaken by independent investigators and that has yet to be done. Lovaas et al's findings cannot be dismissed, but, equally, they cannot be accepted as valid until there has been independent replication.

Second, there have been strong claims on the benefits of a range of specific therapies, including auditory integration and facilitated communication. The latter term was applied to a variety of techniques in which children with autism were supposed to be helped to communicate by a facilitator, who provided physical support to enable the children to point to letters or type or use some other mechanical means of expressing themselves. Quite a range of systematic studies have been undertaken to test these claims and the results have almost always shown that the responses are under the control of the facilitator rather than of the child (Green, 1994; Bebko et al, 1996; Rutter et al, 1998a). Most of the other special interventions have not been adequately evaluated and uncertainty

■ 69

remains on the benefits. What is clear, however, is that the claims currently far outrun the empirical supporting evidence and it seems appropriate for clinicians to be sceptical about what can be achieved by these means.

Third, it has been argued that intervention programmes are much more effective if they can begin when the children are quite young – say, aged 2–4 years. It seems entirely reasonable that treatments should begin early and also it seems desirable to begin interventions before secondary problems develop. Nevertheless, although there is some indication that it pays to start treatment early (see Rogers, 1996), there is still a lack of good evidence on the extent to which really early treatments are more effective than similar methods that begin later. Even so, given that there are no obvious advantages in postponing treatment, it seems reasonable to begin early, while at the same time undertaking studies to test the extent to which this makes a major difference.

Phase 4: the late 1990s

In turning now to the most recent phase of research, the late 1990s, it is inevitable that it is rather too soon to assess the clinical implications and value of the research findings. Nevertheless, a brief survey of the state of play may be useful in indicating the clinical advances to be anticipated.

Aetiology

With respect to aetiology, probably the most exciting development is provided by molecular genetics. A combination of technological and conceptual advances has meant that it is now possible to localise susceptibility genes for psychiatric disorders and therefore, potentially, to identify the precise genes involved and to undertake the necessary research to determine their functional consequences (Rutter & Plomin, 1997; Plomin & Rutter,1998; Rutter et al, 1999a,b). There is no doubt that this quest for susceptibility genes is likely to be successful over the next decade and that it will make a real difference to the power to determine the neural processes involved in the causation of autism. That should make it possible to devise more effective methods of prevention and intervention, although the extent to which this will be possible, and the means by which it will happen, will be hugely dependent on the details of what is found out. Meanwhile, given the unfortunate history of false-positive findings in psychiatric molecular genetics in the past, there needs to be an appropriate combination of enthusiasm for the potential of this research and caution against premature acceptance of positive findings before they are replicated.

Study of the molecular genetics of autism got off to an unfortunate start with the claim of a positive finding in which a non-replication followed within days. Cook et al (1997b), using an association strategy, reported a connection between autism and the promoter region of the serotonin transport gene. Klauck et al (1997), however, not only failed to replicate this finding, but found the reverse (i.e. an excess of the long, rather than the short, variant). Most recently, the International Molecular Genetic Study of Autism Consortium (1998) reported the first positive lod score finding, using an affective sib-pair strategy, in relation to a location on chromosome 7. It remains to be seen whether this finding will hold up on replication in other samples by other groups. Whether or not it does, the existence of several large-scale molecular genetic studies in both North America and Europe (Maestrini et al, 1998) means that replicated findings can certainly be anticipated in the years to come. What will emerge, however, is not *the* gene for autism, but rather several genes that, in combination, give rise to an increased vulnerability to autism. Such findings will revolutionise our ability to define the boundaries of autism and should open the way to understanding the basic neural processes involved. The much needed integration of clinical, genetic, neuropsychological and neurobiological perspectives in autism (Bailey et al, 1996) may at last be on the horizon, but the implementation is still some way off.

Although there had been earlier reports of post-mortem studies (see, e.g., Darby, 1976), it is only during the 1990s that more systematic neuropathological studies have come to the fore. Kemper & Bauman reported findings on six cases in 1993 and 5 years later Bailey et al (1998a) similarly reported six cases. Several of the brains were of unusually large size and abnormalities were found in both the brain stem and the cortex. The findings do not seem compatible with the notion that autism arises on the basis of some localised brain lesion. There is, nevertheless, still a difficulty in knowing how to interpret the findings. Do the abnormalities, for example, index the age when neural development went awry, or do they index the parts of the brain involved in a system-wide malfunction? We do not know.

In his first paper in 1943 Kanner noted in passing that several of the children had unusually large heads. Recent clinical studies have confirmed this observation (Woodhouse et al, 1996), and it may be that this provides a clue to the nature of the neurodevelopmental abnormality. It remains to be determined, however, whether this characteristic is confined to individuals with autism or whether it is a feature that runs in families including members both with and without autism.

Diagnosis and syndrome delineation

In many ways, the most striking recent findings on diagnostic patterns have concerned unexpected groups. Thus, Brown et al (1997) reported autistic-like patterns in children with congenital blindness and Rutter et al (1998b) have done the same in children who had suffered profound privation in institutions in Romania prior to adoption by UK families. In both cases, although the children's behavioural patterns showed many similarities with 'ordinary' autism, there were important atypicalities in both the details of the pattern and its developmental course. These findings emphasise the need for careful clinical attention to the details of children's social and communicative deficits and unusual repetitive behaviour patterns, and raise queries about the diverse ways in which these may develop.

■71

The follow-up into adult life by Mawhood and her colleagues (Rutter et al, 1992; Howlin et al, 2000; Mawhood et al, 2000) of boys with a severe developmental disorder of receptive language also showed a surprisingly high frequency of social deficits. The overall clinical picture was not that of autism, but it was much closer to autism than had been the case when the boys were young. The findings raise again the queries over the interconnections between autism and semantic–pragmatic language disorders (Bishop, 1989; Brook & Bowler, 1992; Eales, 1993).

Twin and family data (Le Couteur et al, 1996; Pickles et al, 1998) have also been used to examine the possibility that variations in symptom pattern may index genetic heterogeneity. The findings so far have emphasised the huge variability in clinical pattern even when the genetic basis must be the same, as is the case within monozygotic pairs. Such pairs have been found to differ by more than 50 IQ points, for example. It is possible that there is a meaningful difference between autism that is associated with a lack of development of spoken language and other varieties (Pickles et al, 1998), and it may be, too, that the association with epilepsy (perhaps particularly when it develops during late adolescence and early adult life) may be a meaningful differentiator, although even those possibilities remain rather uncertain. The history of medical genetics (as well as the findings in autism showing associations with tuberose sclerosis or the fragile-X anomaly) indicate that genetic heterogeneity must be expected but we have yet to determine quite how it can be recognised clinically.

Nature of the disorder

In the field of neuropsychological studies, the development that is likely to make most difference in the years to come is that provided by functional imaging (Rugg, 1997). It provides the means of determining which parts of the brain are active during particular cognitive tasks (Fletcher et al, 1995). Despite occasional assumptions to the contrary, it does not provide direct information on which parts of the brain are abnormal. What it does do, however, is give a means of relating brain function and psychological performance. Thus, for example, it will provide a way of determining whether the minority of individuals with autism who pass theory of mind tests do so using the same part of the brain as that employed by normal individuals in dealing with similar tasks. It remains to be seen just what functional imaging findings will show, but the method is likely to provide psychological studies with the means to span brain and mind in a way that has not been possible satisfactorily up to now.

Interventions

There have been no major therapeutic advances in the past few years, although certainly there have been worthwhile developments. For example, there has been increasing attention to the steps that may help adults with milder varieties of autism to gain and hold down jobs and become more socially independent (Mawhood & Howlin, 1999). Reviews of the findings on pharmacological treatments (Campbell *et al*, 1996; Lewis, 1996) have reaffirmed earlier conclusions that there is no drug that produces major behavioural improvements in most individuals with autism. Several drugs produce modest benefits in some children and their use for symptom reduction in selected cases is well justified. However, there is nothing equivalent to the major improvements in schizophrenia brought about by appropriate neuroleptics or the value of tricyclics and serotonin reuptake inhibitors in the treatment of depression. This is puzzling, because it might have been expected that neurotransmitters would be involved in the brain processes underlying autism and, hence, that one or other of the drugs affecting neurotransmitters would have been helpful. Nevertheless, at least so far, that has not proved to be the case. Whether or not genetic findings will open up more productive new avenues remains to be seen, but that is certainly a possibility.

Conclusions

72 ∎

Clinical practice has changed out of all recognition in the past half century, and research findings have been crucially important in bringing about those changes. It has not, however, been a one-way traffic. Many key advances were prompted by astute clinical observations, and some extravagant research claims were given a more balanced perspective through their interpretation in the light of clinical experience. Many of the advances have come through clinicians and scientists working closely together and through clinician-scientists who combine skills and practice in both areas. Specialist, research-oriented clinics have constituted an important development and are likely to continue to be so in the future. It has been crucially important, too, for researchers to be aware of the potential of advances in other areas of science and of the need to use new concepts and new technologies. The fields of genetics and functional imaging provide examples but so, too, do the contributions from experimental, developmental and cognitive psychology. In many respects, academic psychologists transformed the study of autism at least as much as did clinician-scientists.

We may wonder what Emanuel Miller, were he alive today, would make of the transformation of clinical practice with autism that has taken place. Undoubtedly, he would be pleased at the ways in which interdisciplinary collaboration has been important in both research and clinical developments. Certainly, too, he would obtain great satisfaction from the ways in which research and practice, working together, have led to such worthwhile improvements in what can be done to help individuals with autism and their families, even though it remains a seriously handicapping disorder for which no cure is even remotely on the horizon. Nevertheless, he would, I think, be concerned to ensure that these advances feed through to community services and do not remain confined to tertiary care specialist centres. Doubtless, too, he would be relieved that some of the more mechanical, less humane, experimental treatments have not come to dominate clinical practice. I think he would be troubled by the extent to which evangelists among both researchers and clinicians have sometimes made excessive claims. Perhaps, too, he might be worried lest the market economy emphasis on destructive competition may foster such claims. However, I suspect that, most of all, he would be pleased at the ways in which careful attention to empirical research findings and to their replication and testing in the field has enabled an avoidance of the worst excesses without too much proceeding down blind alleys. He would be delighted by the receptivity to new ideas and I imagine that he would look to the future with a mixture of great hope and enthusiasm, combined with caution and concern to ensure both an appropriate depth of scientific understanding and a continued dedication to meeting the needs of patients and their families. Or am I projecting my own views onto this important pioneer in the establishment of child psychiatry, as Emanuel Miller undoubtedly was? The research and clinical tasks ahead of us are even greater than those in which there has been progress over the past half century, but the means to meet them are there, provided the opportunities are taken and attention is paid to the lessons of the past.

References

Aman, M. & Kern, R. (1989) Review of fenfluramine in the treatment of the developmental disabilities. *Journal of the American Academy of Child and Adolescent Psychiatry*, **28**, 249–565.

American Psychiatric Association (1994) *Diagnostic and Statistical Manual of Mental Disorders* (4th edn) (DSM–IV). Washington, DC: APA.

Bailey, A., Bolton, P., Butler, L., *et al* (1993) Prevalence of the fragile X anomaly amongst autistic twins and singletons. *Journal of Child Psychology and Psychiatry*, **34**, 673–688.

——, Le Couteur, A., Gottesman, I., *et al* (1995) Autism as a strongly genetic disorder: evidence from a British twin study. *Psychological Medicine*, **25**, 63–77.

——, Phillips, W., & Rutter, M. (1996) Autism: towards an integration of clinical, genetic, neuropsychological, and neurobiological perspectives. *Journal of Child Psychology and Psychiatry Annual Research Review*, **37**, 89–126.

——, Luthert, P., Dean, A., *et al* (1998a) A clinicopathological study of autism. *Brain*, **121**, 889–905.

——, Palferman, S., Heavey, L., *et al* (1998b) Autism: the phenotype in relatives. *Journal of Autism and Developmental Disorders*, **28**, 369–392.

Baker, P., Piven, J., Schwartz, S., *et al* (1994) Duplication of chromosome 15q11–13 in two individuals with autistic disorder. *Journal of Autism and Developmental Disorders*, **24**, 529–535.

Baron-Cohen, S. (1995) *Mindblindness: An Essay on Autism and Theory of Mind*. Cambridge, MA: MIT Press.

——, Leslie, A. M. & Frith, U. (1985) Does the autistic child have a 'theory of mind'? *Cognition*, **21**, 37–46.

——, Tager-Flusberg, H. & Cohen, D. (1993) *Understanding Other Minds: Perspectives from Autism*. Oxford: Oxford University Press.

Bartak, L., & Rutter, M. (1971) Educational treatment of autistic children. In *Infantile Autism: Concepts, Characteristics and Treatment* (ed. M. Rutter), pp. 258–280. London: Churchill Livingstone.

——, & —— (1973) Special educational treatment of autistic children: a comparative study. I. Design of study and characteristics of units. *Journal of Child Psychology and Psychiatry*, **14**, 161–179.

——, —— & Cox, A. (1975) A comparative study of infantile autism and specific developmental receptive language disorder. I. The children. *British Journal of Psychiatry*, **126**, 127–145.

——, —— & —— (1977) A comparative study of infantile autism and specific developmental receptive language disorder. III. Discriminant function analysis. *Journal of Autism and Childhood Schizophrenia*, **7**, 383–396.

Bebko, J. M., Perry, A. & Bryson, S. (1996) Multiple method validation study of facilitated communication. II. Individual differences and subgroup results. *Journal of Autism and Developmental Disorders*, **26**, 19–42.

Bettelheim, B. (1967) *The Empty Fortress: Infantile Autism and the Birth of the Self*. London: Collier-Macmillan.

Bishop, D. V. M. (1989) Autism, Asperger's syndrome and semantic-pragmatic disorder: where are the boundaries? *British Journal of Disorders of Communication*, **24**, 107–121.

Bolton, P., Macdonald, H., Pickles, A., *et al* (1994) A case–control family history study of autism. *Journal of Child Psychology and Psychiatry*, **35**, 877–900.

——, Murphy, M., Macdonald, H., *et al* (1997) Obstetric complications in autism: consequences or causes of the condition? *Journal of the American Academy of Child and Adolescent Psychiatry*, **36**, 272–281.

——, Pickles, A., Murphy, M., *et al* (1998) Autism, affective and other psychiatric disorders: patterns of familial aggregation. *Psychological Medicine*, **28**, 385–395.

Brook, S. L. & Bowler, D. M. (1992) Autism by another name? Semantic and pragmatic impairments in children. *Journal of Autism and Developmental Disorders*, **22**, 61–82.

Brown, R., Hobson, R. P. & Lee, A. (1997) Are there autistic-like features in congenitally blind children? *Journal of Child Psychology and Psychiatry*, **38**, 693–704.

Campbell, M. (1988) Fenfluramine treatment of autism. *Journal of Child Psychology and Psychiatry*, **29**, 1–10.

——, Schopler, E., Cueva, J. E., & Hallin, A. (1996) Treatment of autistic disorder. *Journal of the American Academy of Child and Adolescent Psychiatry*, **35**, 134–143.

Cantwell, D., Baker, L. & Rutter, M. (1978) A comparative study of infantile autism and specific developmental receptive language disorder. IV. Syntactical and functional analysis of language. *Journal of Child Psychology and Psychiatry*, **19**, 351–362.

Chess, S. (1977) Follow-up report on autism in congenital rubella. *Journal of Autism and Childhood Schizophrenia*, **7**, 69–81.

——, Kern, S. J. & Fernandez, P. B. (1971) *Psychiatric Disorders of Children with Congenital Rubella*. New York: Brunner/Mazel.

Clark, P., & Rutter, M. (1977) Compliance and resistance in autistic children. *Journal of Autism and Childhood Schizophrenia*, **7**, 33–48.

73

—— & —— (1979) Task difficulty and task performance in autistic children. *Journal of Child Psychology and Psychiatry*, **20**, 271–285.

—— & —— (1981) Autistic children's responses to structure and to interpersonal demands. *Journal of Autism and Developmental Disorders*, **11**, 201–217.

Cohen, I. L., Vietze, P. M., Sudhalter, V., *et al* (1989) Parent–child dyadic gaze patterns in Fragile X males and non-Fragile X males with autistic disorder. *Journal of Child Psychology and Psychiatry*, **30**, 845–856.

Cohen, P., Cohen, J. & Brook, J. S. (1995) Bringing in the sheaves, or just gleaning? A methodological warning. *International Journal of Methods in Psychiatric Research*, **5**, 263–266.

Coleman, M. (1976) *The Autistic Syndromes*. New York: Praeger.

—— (1990) Delineation of the subgroups of the autistic syndrome. *Brain Dysfunction*, **3**, 208–217.

—— & Gillberg, C. (1985) *The Biology of the Autistic Syndromes*. Oxford: Blackwell Scientific.

Comings, D. E. & Comings, B. G. (1991) Clinical and genetic relationships between autism-pervasive developmental disorder and Tourette's syndrome: a study of 19 cases. *American Journal of Medical Genetics*, **39**, 180–191.

Cook, E. H. (1990) Autism: review of neurochemical investigation. *Synapse*, **6**, 292–308.

——, Lindgren, V., Leventhal, B. L. *et al* (1997a) Autism or atypical autism in maternally but not paternally derived proximal 15q duplication. *American Journal of Human Genetics*, **60**, 928–934.

——, Courchesne, R., Lord, C., *et al* (1997b) Evidence of linkage between the serotonin transporter and autistic disorder. *Molecular Psychiatry*, **2**, 247–250.

Corbett, J., Harris, R., Taylor, E., *et al* (1977) Progressive disintegrative psychosis of childhood. *Journal of Child Psychology and Psychiatry*, **18**, 211–219.

Courchesne, E., Hesselink, J. R., Jernigan, T. L., *et al* (1987) Abnormal neuroanatomy in a nonretarded person with autism. *Archives of Neurology*, **44**, 335–341.

——, Townsend, J. & Saitoh, O. (1994) The brain in infantile autism: posterior fossa structures are abnormal. *Neurology*, **44**, 214–223.

Cox, A., Rutter, M., Newman, S., *et al* (1975) A comparative study of infantile autism and specific developmental receptive language disorder. II. Parental characteristics. *British Journal of Psychiatry*, **126**, 146–159.

——, Klein, A., Charman, T., *et al* (1999) Autism spectrum disorders at 20 and 42 months of age: stability of clinical and ADI–R diagnosis. *Journal of Child Psychology and Psychiatry*, **40**, 719–732.

Creak, M. (1961) Schizophrenic syndrome in childhood: progress report of a working party. *Cerebral Palsy Bulletin*, **3**, 501–504.

—— (1963a) Schizophrenia in early childhood. *Acta Paedopsychiatrica*, **30**, 42–47.

—— (1963b) Childhood psychosis: a review of 100 cases. *British Journal of Psychiatry*, **109**, 84–89.

Dahlgren, S. O. & Gillberg, C. (1989) Symptoms in the first two years of life: a preliminary population study of infantile autism. *European Archives of Psychiatric and Neurological Science*, **283**, 169–174.

Darby, J. K. (1976) Neuropathological aspects of psychosis in children. *Journal of Autism and Childhood Schizophrenia*, **6**, 339–352.

DeLong, G. & Dwyer, J. (1988) Correlation of family history with specific autistic subgroups: Asperger's syndrome and bipolar affective disease. *Journal of Autism and Developmental Disorders*, **18**, 593–600.

DeLong, R. & Nohria, C. (1994) Psychiatric family history and neurological disease in autistic spectrum disorders. *Developmental Medicine and Child Neurology*, **36**, 441–448.

DeMyer, M. K. (1975) The nature of the neuropsychological disability in autistic children. *Journal of Autism and Childhood Schizophrenia*, **5**, 109–128.

——, Barton, S. & Norton, J. A. (1972) A comparison of adaptive, verbal, and motor profiles of psychotic and non-psychotic subnormal children. *Journal of Autism and Childhood Schizophrenia*, **2**, 359–377.

DiLavore, P. C., Lord, C. & Rutter, M. (1995) The Pre-Linguistic Autism Diagnostic Observation Schedule. *Journal of Autism and Developmental Disorders*, **25**, 355–379.

Dollery, C. (1978) *The End of an Age of Optimism: Medical Science in Retrospect and Prospect*. London: Nuffield Provincial Hospitals Trust.

Eales, M. J. (1993) Pragmatic impairments in adults with childhood diagnoses of autism or developmental receptive language disorder. *Journal of Autism and Developmental Disorders*, **23**, 593–617.

Eisenberg, L. (1956) The autistic child in adolescence. *American Journal of Psychiatry*, **112**, 607–612.

Elgar, S. & Wing, L. (1969) *Teaching Autistic Children*. London: College of Special Education.

Elia, M., Bergonzi, P., Ferri, R., *et al* (1990) The etiology of autism in a group of mentally retarded subjects. *Brain Dysfunction*, **3**, 228–240.

Federico, A., Battistini, S., De Stefano, N., *et al* (1990) The strategy of investigating autistic syndromes in childhood. *Brain Dysfunction*, **3**, 261–270.

Ferster, C. B. & DeMyer, M. K. (1961) The development of performances in autistic children in an automatically controlled environment. *Journal of Chronic Disorders*, **13**, 312–345.

Fletcher, P., Happé, F., Frith, U., *et al* (1995) Other minds in the brain: a functional imaging study of 'theory of mind' in story comprehension. *Cognition*, **57**, 109–128.

Folstein, S., & Rutter, M. (1977a) Genetic influences and infantile autism. *Nature*, **265**, 726–728.

—— & —— (1977b) Infantile autism: a genetic study of 21 pairs. *Journal of Child Psychology and Psychiatry*, **18**, 297–321.

Fombonne, E. (1998) Epidemiological studies of infantile autism. In *Autism and Developmental Disorders* (ed. F. Volkmar), pp. 32–62. New York: Cambridge University Press.

——, Bolton, P., Prior, J., *et al* (1997) A family study of autism: cognitive patterns and levels in parents and siblings. *Journal of Child Psychology and Psychiatry*, **38**, 667–683.

Frith, U. (1989) *Autism: Explaining the Enigma*. Oxford: Blackwell.

—— (ed) (1991) *Autism and Asperger Syndrome*. Cambridge: Cambridge University Press.

—— & Happé, F. (1994) Autism: beyond 'theory of mind'. *Cognition*, **50**, 115–132.

Geller, E., Ritvo, E., Freeman, B., *et al* (1982) Preliminary observations on the effect of fenfluramine on blood serotonin and symptoms in three autistic boys. *New England Journal of Medicine*, **307**, 165–169.

Gillberg, C. (1990a) Autism and pervasive developmental disorders. *Journal of Child Psychology and Psychiatry*, **31**, 99–119.

—— (1990b) Medical work-up in children with autism and asperger syndrome. *Brain Dysfunction*, **3**, 249–260.

—— (1992) Autism and autism-like conditions: sub-classes among disorders of empathy. *Journal of Child Psychology and Psychiatry*, **33**, 813–842.

—— (1998) Chromosomal disorders and autism. *Journal of Autism and Developmental Disorders*, **28**, 415–425.

—— & Coleman, M. (1992) *The Biology of the Autistic Syndromes* (2nd edn). London: MacKeith Press.

—— & —— (1996) Autism and medical disorders: a review of the literature. *Developmental Medicine and Child Neurology*, **38**, 191–202.

—— & Wahlström, J. (1985) Chromosome abnormalities in infantile autism and other childhood psychoses: a population study of 66 cases. *Developmental Medicine and Child Neurology*, **27**, 293–304.

——, Ehlers, S., Schaumann, H., *et al* (1990) Autism under age 3 years: a clinical study of 28 cases referred for autistic symptoms in infancy. *Journal of Child Psychology and Psychiatry*, **31**, 921–934.

——, Steffenberg, S., Wahlström, J. *et al* (1991) Autism associated with marker chromosome. *Journal of the American Academy of Child and Adolescent Psychiatry*, **30**, 489–494.

Golden, G. S. (1987) Neurological functioning. In *Handbook of Autism and Pervasive Developmental Disorders* (eds D. J. Cohen & A. M. Donnellan), pp. 133–147. New York: John Wiley & Sons.

Goodman, R. (1997) *Child and Adolescent Mental Health Services: Reasoned Advice to Commissioners and Providers*. Maudsley Discussion Paper No.4. London: Bethlem & Maudsley NHS Trust.

Green, G. (1994) The quality of the evidence. In *Facilitated Communication: The Clinical and Social Phenomenon* (ed. H. C. Shane), pp. 156–226. San Diego, CA: Singular Press.

Gresham, F. M. & MacMillan, D. L. (1998) Early intervention project: can its claims be substantiated and its effects replicated? *Journal of Autism and Developmental Disorders*, **28**, 5–13.

Hagberg, B., Aircardi, J., Dias, K., *et al* (1983) A progressive syndrome of autism, dementia, ataxia and loss of purposeful hand use in girls: Rett syndrome; report of 35 cases. *Annals of Neurology*, **14**, 471–479.

Hagerman, R. J., Jackson, A. W., Levitas, A., *et al* (1986) An analysis of autism in 50 males with the fragile X syndrome. *American Journal of Medical Genetics*, **23**, 359–370.

Happé, F. G. E. (1994a) *Autism: An Introduction to Psychological Theory*. London: UCL Press.

—— (1994b) Annotation: current psychological theories of autism: the "theory of mind" account and rival theories. *Journal of Child Psychology and Psychiatry*, **35**, 215–229.

—— (1995) The role of age and verbal ability in the theory of mind task performance of subjects with autism. *Child Development*, **66**, 843–855.

——, Ehlers, S., Fletcher, P., *et al* (1996) 'Theory of mind' in the brain: evidence from a PET scan study of Asperger syndrome. *NeuroReport*, **8**, 197–201.

Heller, T. (1930) Uber dementia infantalis. *Zeitschrift fur Kinderforschung*, **37**, 661–667.

Hemsley, R., Howlin, P., Berger, M., *et al* (1978) Treating autistic children in a family context. In *Autism: A Reappraisal of Concepts and Treatment* (eds M. Rutter & E. Schopler), pp. 379–412. New York: Plenum Press.

Hermelin, B. (2001) *Bright Splinters of the Mind: A Personal Story of Research with Autistic Savants*. London: Jessica Kingsley (in press).

—— & O'Connor, N. (1970) *Psychological Experiments with Autistic Children*. New York: Pergamon Press.

Hill, A. E. & Rosenbloom, L. (1986) Disintegrative psychosis of childhood: teenage follow-up. *Developmental Medicine and Child Neurology*, **28**, 34–40.

Hobson, R. P. (1982) The autistic child's concept of persons. In *Proceedings of the 1981 International Conference on Autism, Boston, USA* (ed. D. Park), pp. 97–102. Washington, DC: National Society for Children and Adults with Autism.

—— (1983) Early childhood autism and the question of egocentrism. *Journal of Autism and Developmental Disorders*, **14**, 85–104.

—— (1993) *Autism and the Development of Mind*. Hillsdale, NJ: Lawrence Erlbaum Associates.

Howlin, P. (1998) Practitioner review: psychological and educational treatments for autism. *Journal of Child Psychology and Psychiatry*, **39**, 307–322.

—— & Moore, A. (1997) Diagnosis in autism: A survey of over 1200 parents. *Autism: International Journal of Research and Practice*, **1**, 135–162.

—— & Rutter, M. (1987) *Treatment of Autistic Children*. Chichester: John Wiley & Sons.

——, Marchant, R., Rutter, M., *et al* (1973) A home-based approach to the treatment of autistic children. *Journal of Autism and Childhood Schizophrenia*, **3**, 308–336.

Howlin, P., Mawhood, L. & Rutter, M. (2000) Autism and developmental receptive language disorder - a follow-up comparison in early adult life. II. Social, behavioural and psychiatric outcomes. *Journal of Child Psychology and Psychiatry*, **41**, 561–578.

Hunt, A. & Dennis, J. (1987) Psychiatric disorder among young children with tuberous sclerosis. *Developmental Medicine and Child Neurology*, **29**, 190–198.

International Molecular Genetic Study of Autism Consortium (1998) A full genome screen for autism with evidence for linkage to a region on chromosome 7q. *Human Molecular Genetics*, **7**, 571–578.

Johnson, M. H., Siddons, F., Frith, U., *et al* (1992) Can autism be predicted on the basis of infant screening tests? *Developmental Medicine and Child Neurology*, **34**, 316–320.

Kanner, L. (1943) Autistic disturbances of affective contact. *Nervous Child*, **2**, 217–250.

—— (1949) Problems of nosology and psychodynamics in early infantile autism. *Human Molecular Genetics*, **19**, 416–426.

—— (1971) Follow-up study of eleven autistic children originally reported in 1943. *Journal of Autism and Childhood Schizophrenia*, **1**, 119–145.

——, Rodriguez, A. & Ashenden, B. (1972) How far can autistic children go in matters of social adaptation? *Journal of Autism and Childhood Schizophrenia*, **2**, 9–33.

Kemper, T. L. & Bauman, M. L. (1993) The contribution of neuropathologic studies to the understanding of autism. *Neurologic Clinics*, **11**, 175–187.

Klauck, S. M., Poustka, F., Benner, A., *et al* (1997) Serotonin transporter (5-HTT) gene variants associated with autism? *Human Molecular Genetics*, **6**, 2233–2238.

Klin, A., Volkmar, F. R., Sparrow, S. S., *et al* (1995) Validity and neuropsychological characterization of Asperger syndrome: convergence with non-verbal learning disabilities syndrome. *Journal of Child Psychology and Psychiatry*, **36**, 1127–1140.

Kolvin, I. (1971) Psychosis in childhood – a comparative study. In *Infantile Autism: Concepts, Characteristics, and Treatment* (ed. M. Rutter), pp. 7–26. Edinburgh: Churchill Livingstone.

Kurita, H., Kita, M. & Miyake, Y. (1992) A comparative study of development and symptoms among disintegrative psychosis and infantile autism with and without speech loss. *Journal of Autism and Developmental Disorders*, **22**, 175–188.

Lansing, M. D. & Schopler, E. (1978) Individualized education: a public school model. In *Autism: A Reappraisal of Concepts and Treatment* (eds M. Rutter & E. Schopler), pp. 439–453. New York: Plenum Press.

Le Couteur, A., Rutter, M., Lord, C., *et al* (1989) Autism Diagnostic Interview: a standardized investigator-based interview. *Journal of Autism and Developmental Disorders*, **19**, 363–387.

——, Bailey, A. J., Goode, S., *et al* (1996) A broader phenotype of autism: the clinical spectrum in twins. *Journal of Child Psychology and Psychiatry*, **37**, 785–801.

Lewis, M. H. (1996) Brief report: psychopharmacology of autism spectrum disorders. *Journal of Autism and Developmental Disorders*, **26**, 231–236.

Lockyer, L., & Rutter, M. (1969) A five- to fifteen-year follow-up study of infantile psychosis. III. Psychological aspects. *British Journal of Psychiatry*, **115**, 865–882.

—— & —— (1970) A five- to fifteen-year follow-up study of infantile psychosis. IV. Patterns of cognitive ability. *British Journal of Social and Clinical Psychology*, **9**, 152–163.

Lord, C. (1995) Follow-up of two-year-olds referred for possible autism. *Journal of Child Psychology and Psychiatry*, **36**, 1365–1382.

——, Rutter, M., Goode, S., *et al* (1989) Autism Diagnostic Observation Schedule: a standardized observation of communicative and social behavior. *Journal of Autism and Developmental Disorders*, **19**, 185–212.

——, Storoschuk, S., Rutter, M., *et al* (1993) Using the ADI–R to diagnose autism in preschool children. *Infant Mental Health*, **14**, 234–252.

76

—, Rutter, M., & Le Couteur, A. (1994) Autism Diagnostic Interview – Revised: a revised version of a diagnostic interview for caregivers of individuals with possible pervasive developmental disorders. *Journal of Autism and Developmental Disorders*, **24**, 659–685.

—, Rutter, M. & DiLavore, P. (2000) Autism Diagnostic Observation Schedule – Generic: a standard.measure of social and communication deficits associated with the spectrum of autism. *Journal of Autism and Developmental Disorders*, **30**, 205–223.

Lotter, V. (1974*a*) Social adjustment and placement of autistic children in Middlesex: a follow-up study. *Journal of Autism and Childhood Schizophrenia*, **4**, 11–32.

—— (1974*b*) Factors related to outcome in autistic children. *Journal of Autism and Childhood Schizophrenia*, **4**, 263–277.

—— (1978) Follow-up studies of autistic children. In *Autism: A Reappraisal of Concepts and Treatment* (eds M. Rutter & E. Schopler), pp. 475–495. New York: Plenum Press.

Lovaas, O. I. (1967) Behavior therapy approach to the treatment of childhood schizophrenics. In *Minnesota Symposia on Child Psychology. Vol. 1* (ed. J. Hill), pp. 108–159. Minneapolis: University of Minneapolis Press.

—— (1987) Behavioral treatment and normal educational and intellectual functioning in young autistic children. *Journal of Consulting and Clinical Psychology*, **55**, 3–9.

—— (1996) The UCLA young autism model of service delivery. In *Behavioral Intervention for Young Children with Autism* (ed. C. Maurice), pp. 241–250. Austin, TX: Pro-Ed.

—, Schaeffer, B., & Simmons, J. Q. (1965) Experimental studies in childhood schizophrenia: Building social behavior in autistic children by use of electric shock. *Journal of Experimental Research on Personality*, **1**, 99–109.

—, Freitag, G., Kinder, M. I., *et al* (1966) Establishment of social reinforcers in two schizophrenic children on the basis of food. *Journal of Experimental Child Psychology*, **4**, 109–125.

—, Koegel, R., Simmons, J. Q., *et al* (1973) Some generalizations and follow-up measures on autistic children in behavior therapy. *Journal of Applied Behavior Analysis*, **6**, 131–166.

—, —— & Schreibman, L. (1979) Stimulus overselectivity in autism: a review of research. *Psychological Bulletin*, **86**, 1236–1254.

Maestrini, E., Marlow, A. J., Weeks, D. E., *et al* (1998) Molecular genetic investigations of autism. *Journal of Autism and Developmental Disorders*, **28**, 427–437.

Makita, K. (1966) The age of onset of childhood schizophrenia. *Folia Psychiatrica et Neurologica Japanica*, **20**, 111–121.

Mawhood, L. & Howlin, P. (1999) The outcome of a supported employment scheme for high functioning adults with autism or Asperger syndrome. *Autism*, **3**, 229–254.

—, —— & Rutter, M. (2000) Autism and developmental receptive language disorder – a follow-up comparison in early adult life. I. Cognitive and language outcomes. *Journal of Child Psychology and Psychiatry*, **41**, 547–559.

McEachin, J. J., Smith, T. & Lovaas, O. I. (1993) Long-term outcome for children with autism who received early intensive behavioral treatment. *American Journal of Mental Retardation*, **97**, 359–372.

McHale, S. M., Simeonsson, R. J., Marcus, L. M., *et al* (1980) The social and symbolic quality of autistic children's communication. *Journal of Autism and Developmental Disorders*, **10**, 299–310.

Medawar, P. (1982) *Pluto's Republic.* Oxford: Oxford University Press.

Miller, E. (1960) A discourse on method in child psychiatry. *Journal of Child Psychology and Psychiatry*, **1**, 3–16.

—— (1968) The problem of classification in psychiatry: some epidemiological considerations. In *Foundations of Child Psychiatry* (ed. E. Miller), pp. 251–269. Oxford: Pergamon Press.

Olsson, B. & Rett, A. (1987) Autism and Rett syndrome: behavioural investigations and differential diagnosis. *Developmental Medicine and Child Neurology*, **29**, 429–441.

—— & —— (1990) A review of the Rett syndrome with a theory of autism. *Brain and Development*, **12**, 11–15.

Ornitz, E. M. (1971) Childhood autism: a disorder of sensorimotor integration. In *Infantile Autism: Concepts, Characteristics and Treatments* (ed. M. Rutter), pp. 50–68. London: Churchill Livingstone.

—— & Ritvo, E. R. (1968) Neurophysiologic mechanisms underlying perceptual inconstancy in autistic and schizophrenic children. *Archives of General Psychiatry*, **19**, 22–27.

Osterling, J. & Dawson, G. (1994) Early recognition of children with autism: a study of first birthday home videotapes. *Journal of Autism and Developmental Disorders*, **24**, 247–259.

Ozonoff, S. (1994) Executive functions in autism. In *Learning and Cognition in Autism* (eds E. Schopler & G. Mesibov), pp. 199–219. New York: Plenum Press.

—, Pennington, B. F. & Rogers, S. J. (1991*a*) Executive function deficits in high-functioning autistic individuals: relationship to theory of mind. *Journal of Child Psychology and Psychiatry*, **32**, 1081–1105.

—, Rogers, S. J. & Pennington, B. F. (1991*b*) Asperger's Syndrome: evidence of an empirical distinction from high-functioning autism. *Journal of Child Psychology and Psychiatry*, **32**, 1107–1122.

■ 77

Parks, S. L. (1983) The assessment of autistic children: a selective review of available instruments. *Journal of Autism and Developmental Disorders*, **13**, 255–267.

Pickles, A., Bolton, P., Macdonald, H., *et al* (1995) Latent class analysis of recurrence risk for complex phenotypes with selection and measurement error: a twin and family history study of autism. *American Journal of Human Genetics*, **57**, 717–726.

Pickles, A., Starr, E., Kazak, S., *et al* (2000) Variable expression of the autism broader phenotype: findings from extended pedigrees. *Journal of Child Psychology and Psychiatry*, **41**, 491–502.

Plomin, R. & Rutter, M. (1998) Child development, molecular genetics and what to do with genes once they are found. *Child Development*, **69**, 1223–1242.

Pocock, S. J. (1983) *Clinical Trials: A Practical Approach*. Chichester: John Wiley & Sons.

Pring, L., Hermelin, B. & Heavey, L. (1995) Savants, segments, art and autism. *Journal of Child Psychology and Psychiatry*, **36**, 1065–1076.

Rett, A. (1966) Uber ein eigenartiges himatrophisches Syndrom bei Hyperammonie in Kindesalter. *Weiner Medizinische Wochenschrift*, **116**, 723–726.

Richer, J. (1978) The partial noncommunication of culture to autistic children – an application of human ethology. In *Autism: A Reappraisal of Concepts and Treatments* (eds M. Rutter & E. Schopler), pp. 47–61. New York: Plenum Press.

Riikonen, R. & Amnell, G. (1981) Psychiatric disorders in children with earlier cognitive spasms. *Developmental Medicine and Child Neurology*, **23**, 747–760.

Rimland, B. (1965) *Infantile Autism*. London: Methuen.

—— (1987) Megavitamin B6 and magnesium in the treatment of autistic children and adults. In *Neurobiological Issues in Autism* (eds E. Schopler & G. B. Mesibov), pp. 389–405. New York: Plenum Press.

——, Callaway, E. & Dreyfuss, P. (1978) The effect of high doses of vitamin B6 on autistic children: a double blind crossover study. *American Journal of Psychiatry*, **135**, 472–475.

Rogers, S. J. (1996) Early intervention in autism (Brief report). *Journal of Autism and Developmental Disorders*, **26**, 243–246.

Rugg, M. D. (ed) (1997) *Cognitive Neuroscience*. Hove, Sussex: Psychology Press.

Rutter, M. (1965) Classification and categorization in child psychiatry. *Journal of Child Psychology and Psychiatry*, **6**, 71–83.

—— (1966) Behavioral and cognitive characteristics of a series of psychotic children. In *Early Childhood Autism: Clinical, Educational and Social Aspects* (ed J. K. Wing), pp. 51–81. Oxford: Pergamon Press.

—— (1967) Psychotic disorders in early childhood. In *Recent Developments in Schizophrenia* (eds A. J. Coppen & A. Walk), pp. 133–158. Ashford, Kent: Headley Bros.

—— (1968) Concepts of autism: a review of research. *Journal of Child Psychology and Psychiatry*, **9**, 1–25.

—— (1970) Autistic children: infancy to adulthood. *Seminars in Psychiatry*, **2**, 435–450.

—— (ed) (1971) *Infantile Autism: Concepts, Characteristics and Treatment*. London: Churchill Livingstone.

—— (1972) Childhood schizophrenia reconsidered. *Journal of Autism and Childhood Schizophrenia*, **2**, 315–337.

—— (1973) The assessment and treatment of pre-school autistic children. *Early Child Development and Care*, **3**, 13–29.

—— (1979) Language, cognition and autism. In *Congenital and Acquired Cognitive Disorders* (ed. R. Katzmann), pp. 247–264. New York: Raven Press.

—— (1983) Cognitive deficits in the pathogenesis of autism. *Journal of Child Psychology and Psychiatry*, **24**, 513–531.

—— (1985) The treatment of autistic children. *Journal of Child Psychology and Psychiatry*, **26**, 193–214.

—— (1990) Interface between research and clinical practice in child psychiatry – some personal reflections (Discussion paper). *Journal of the Royal Society of Medicine*, **83**, 444–447.

—— (1991) Autism: pathways from syndrome definition to pathogenesis. *Comprehensive Mental Health Care*, **1**, 5–26.

—— (1998) Routes from research to clinical practice in child psychiatry: retrospect and prospect. *Journal of Child Psychology and Psychiatry*, **39**, 805–816.

—— (1999) The Emmanuel Miller Memorial Lecture 1998. Autism: two-way interplay between research and clinical work. *Journal of Child Psychology and Psychiatry and Allied Disciplines*, **40**, 169–188.

—— & Bailey, A. (1993) Thinking and relationships: mind and brain (some reflections on theory of mind and autism). In *Understanding Other Minds: Perspectives from Autism* (eds S. Baron-Cohen, H. Tager-Flusberg & D. J. Cohen), pp. 481–504. Oxford: Oxford University Press.

—— & Bartak, L. (1973) Special educational treatment of autistic children: a comparative study. II. Follow-up findings and implications for services. *Journal of Child Psychology and Psychiatry*, **14**, 241–270.

—— & Plomin, R. (1997) Opportunities for psychiatry from genetic findings. *British Journal of Psychiatry*, **171**, 209–219.

—— & Schopler, E. (1992) Classification of pervasive developmental disorders: some concepts and practical considerations. *Journal of Autism and Developmental Disorders*, **22**, 459–482.

—— & Sussenwein, F. (1971) A developmental and behavioral approach to the treatment of pre-school autistic children. *Journal of Autism and Childhood Schizophrenia*, **1**, 376–397.

——, Greenfeld, D. & Lockyer, L. (1967) A five to fifteen year follow-up study of infantile psychosis. II. Social and behavioural outcome. *British Journal of Psychiatry*, **113**, 1183–1199.

——, Tizard, J. & Whitmore, K. (1970) *Education, Health and Behaviour*. London: Longmans.

——, Mawhood, L. & Howlin, P. (1992) Language delay and social development. In *Specific Speech and Language Disorders in Children* (eds P. Fletcher & D. Hall), pp. 63–78. London: Whurr Publishers.

——, Bailey, A., Bolton, P., *et al* (1994) Autism and known medical conditions: myth and substance. *Journal of Child Psychology and Psychiatry*, **35**, 311–322.

——, ——, Simonoff, E., *et al* (1997) Genetic influences and autism. In *Handbook of Autism and Pervasive Developmental Disorders* (eds D. J. Cohen & F. R. Volkmar) (2nd edn), pp. 370–387. New York: John Wiley & Sons.

——, Maughan, B., Pickles, A., *et al* (1998*a*) Retrospective recall recalled In *Methods and Models for Studying the Individual* (eds R. B. Cairns, L. R. Bergman & J. Kagan), pp. 219–242. Thousand Oaks, CA: Sage Publications.

——, Andersen-Wood, L., Beckett, C., *et al* (1998*b*) Quasi-autistic patterns following severe early global privation. English and Romanian Adoptees (ERA) Study Team. *Journal of Child Psychology and Psychiatry*, **40**, 537–549.

——, Silberg, J., O'Connor, T., *et al* (1999*a*) Genetics and child psychiatry. I. Advances in quantitative and molecular genetics. *Journal of Child Psychology and Psychiatry*, **40**, 3–18.

——, ——, ——, *et al* (1999*b*) Genetics and child psychiatry. II. Empirical research findings. *Journal of Child Psychology and Psychiatry*, **40**, 19–55.

Schopler, E., & Mesibov, G. (eds) (1988) *Diagnosis and Assessment in Autism*. New York: Plenum Press.

—— & Reichler, R. J. (1971) Parents as cotherapists in the treatment of psychotic children. *Journal of Autism and Childhood Schizophrenia*, **1**, 87–102.

——, Reichler, R. J., DeVellis, R. F., *et al* (1980) Towards objective classification of childhood autism: Childhood Autism Rating Scale (CARS). *Journal of Autism and Developmental Disorders*, **10**, 91–103.

——, ——, Rochen Renner, B., *et al* (1986) *The Childhood Autism Rating Scale (CARS) for Diagnostic Screening and Classification of Autism*. New York: Irvington Publishers.

——, Short, A. & Mesibov, G. (1989) Relation of behavioral treatment to 'normal functioning': Comment on Lovaas. *Journal of Consulting and Clinical Psychology*, **57**, 162–164.

Schover, L. R. & Newsom, C. D. (1976) Overselectivity, developmental level, and overtraining in autistic and normal children. *Journal of Abnormal Child Psychology*, **4**, 289–298.

Sheinkopf, S. J. & Siegel, B. (1998) Home-based behavioral treatment of young children with autism. *Journal of Autism and Developmental Disorders*, **28**, 15–23.

Sloman, L. (1991) Use of medication in pervasive developmental disorders. *Psychiatric Clinics in North America*, **14**, 165–182.

Smalley, S. (1998) Autism and tuberous sclerosis. *Journal of Autism and Developmental Disorders*, **28**, 407–414.

——, Asarnow, R. & Spence, M. (1988) Autism and genetics: a decade of research. *Archives of General Psychiatry*, **45**, 953–961.

——, Tanguay, P. E., Smith, M., *et al* (1992) Autism and tuberous sclerosis. *Journal of Autism and Developmental Disorders*, **22**, 339–355.

Starr, L, Kazak, S., Tomlins, M., *et al* (2001) Family genetic study of autism accompanied by profound mental retardation. *Journal of Autism and Developmental Disorders*, in press.

Steffenberg, S., Gillberg, C., Helgren, L., *et al* (1989) A twin study of autism in Denmark, Finland, Iceland, Norway, and Sweden. *Journal of Child Psychology and Psychiatry*, **30**, 405–416.

Szatmari, P., Jones, M.B., Zwaigenbaum, L., *et al* (1998) Genetics of autism: overview and new directions. *Journal of Autism and Developmental Disorders*, **28**, 351–368.

Tinbergen, E. A. & Tinbergen, N. (1972) *Early Childhood Autism: An Ethological Approach*. Berlin: Paul Parey.

—— & —— (1983) *'Autistic' Children: New Hope for a Cure*. London: George Allen & Unwin.

Tymchuk, A. J., Simmons, J. Q. & Neafsey, S. (1977) Intellectual characteristics of adolescent childhood psychotics with high verbal ability. *Journal of Mental Deficiency Research*, **21**, 133–138.

Volkmar, F. R. & Cohen, D. J. (1989) Disintegrative disorder or 'late-onset' autism. *Journal of Child Psychology and Psychiatry*, **30**, 717–724.

—— & —— (1991) Comorbid association of autism and schizophrenia. *American Journal of Psychiatry*, **148**, 1704–1707.

■79

Welch, M. G. (1983) Retrieval from autism through mother–child holding therapy. In *'Autistic' Children: New Hope for a Cure* (eds E. A. Tinbergen & N. Tinbergen), pp. 322–336. London: George Allen & Unwin.

Wimmer, H. & Perner, J. (1983) Beliefs about beliefs: representation and constraining function of wrong beliefs in young children's understanding of deception. *Cognition*, **13**, 103–128.

Wing, L. (1972) *Autistic Children*. London: Constable.

—— (1981) Asperger's syndrome: a clinical account. *Psychological Medicine*, **11**, 115–129.

—— & Gould, J. (1978) Systematic recording of behaviors and skills of retarded and psychotic children. *Journal of Autism and Childhood Schizophrenia*, **8**, 79–97.

—— & —— (1979) Severe impairments of social interaction and associated abnormalities in children: epidemiology and classification. *Journal of Autism and Developmental Disorders*, **9**, 11–29.

Witt-Engerström, I. & Gillberg, C. (1987) Rett syndrome in Sweden (Letter). *Journal of Autism and Developmental Disorders*, **17**, 149–150.

Woodhouse, W., Bailey, A., Rutter, M., *et al* (1996) Head circumference and other pervasive developmental disorders. *Journal of Autism and Developmental Disorders*, **37**, 665–671.

Wolff, P. H., Gardner, J., Paccia, J., *et al* (1989) The greeting behavior of fragile X males. *American Journal of Mental Retardation*, **93**, 406–411.

Wolff, S. (1995) *Loners: The Life Path of Unusual Children*. London: Routledge.

—— & Chick, J. (1980) Schizoid personality in childhood: a controlled follow-up study. *Psychological Medicine*, **10**, 85–100.

World Health Organization (1992) *The ICD–10 Classification of Mental and Behavioural Disorders. Clinical Descriptions and Diagnostic Guidelines*. Geneva: WHO.

Yirmiya, N., Erel, O., Shaked, M., *et al* (1998) Meta-analyses comparing theory of mind abilities of individuals with autism, individuals with mental retardation, and normally developing individuals. *Psychological Bulletin*, **124**, 283–307.

Yule, W. (1978) Research methodology: what are the 'correct controls'? In *Autism: A Reappraisal of Concepts and Treatment* (eds M. Rutter & E. Schopler), pp. 155–162. New York: Plenum Press.

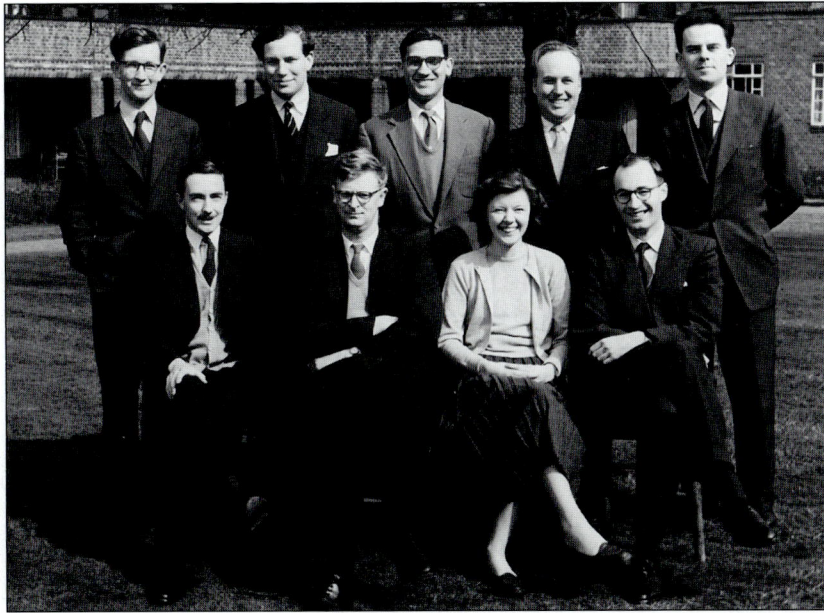

New senior house officers at the Maudsley Hospital, April 1958. Back, l. to r.: Sandy Brown, Hugh Freeman, Larry Sharpe, Clifford Salter, Eddie Kenyon; front, l. to r.: Tony Fairburn, Hyla Holden, Anne Darquier, M.R.

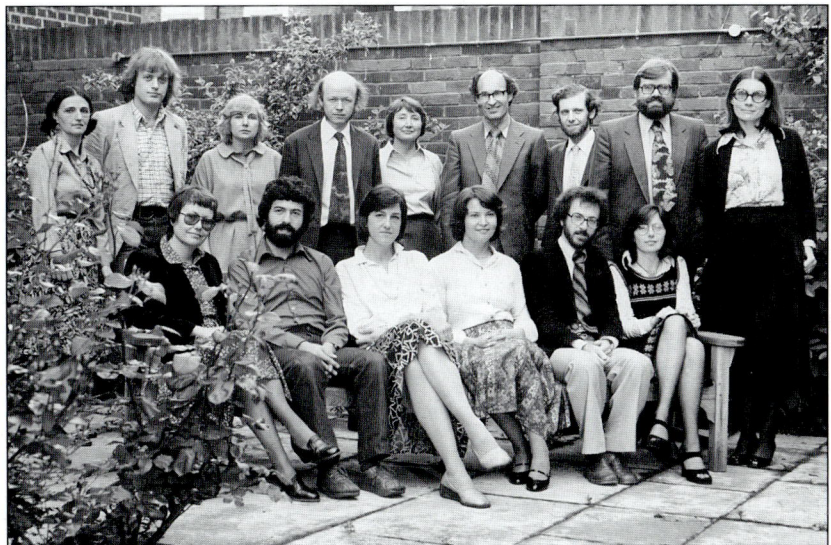

The academic department of child and adolescent psychiatry at the Maudsley Hospital, 1978. Back row, l. to r.: Grace Gray, Peter Clark, Daphne Holbrook, Eric Taylor, Joy Maxwell, M.R., Michael Weiselberg, David Mrazek, Libby Ryan. Front, l. to r.: Janet Ouston, Oliver Chadwick, Barbara Maughan, Christine Liddle, Russell Schachar, Linda Dowdney.

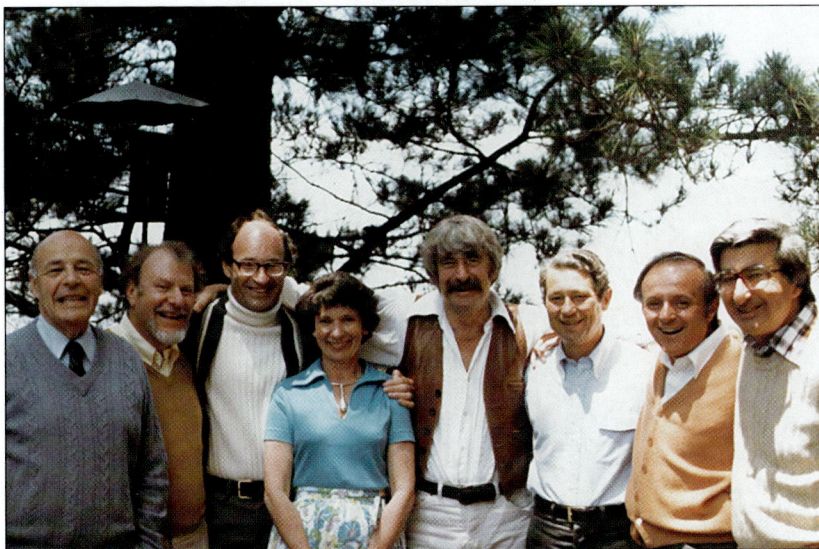

"An important turning point": the Stress, Coping and Development Group at the Centre for Advanced Study in the Behavioral Sciences, Stamford 1980. L. to r.: Norman Garmezy, Herb Leiderman, M.R., Judy Wallerstein, Jerry Patterson, Jerry Kagan, Julius Segal, Lew Lipsitt.

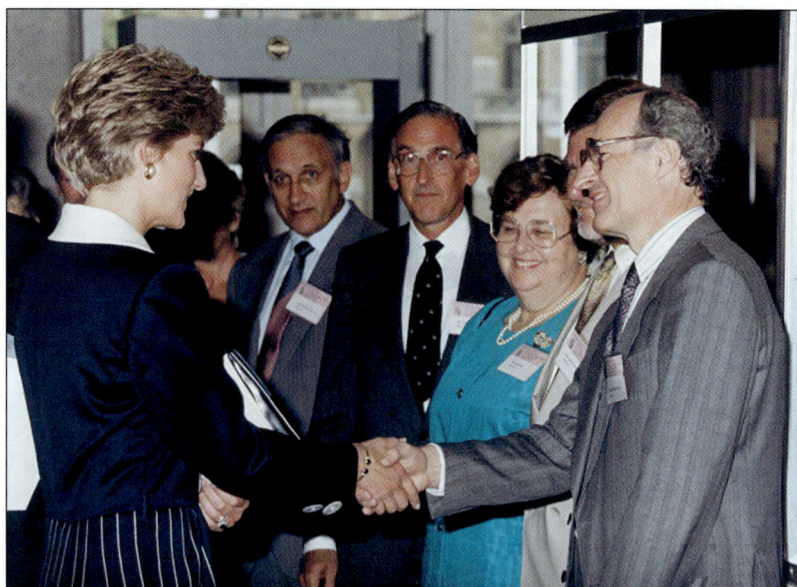

Meeting Diana, Princess
of Wales, with (l. to r.)
Issy Kolvin, Ian Berg,
Dora Black, 1991.
Photo: Monitor Picture
Library.

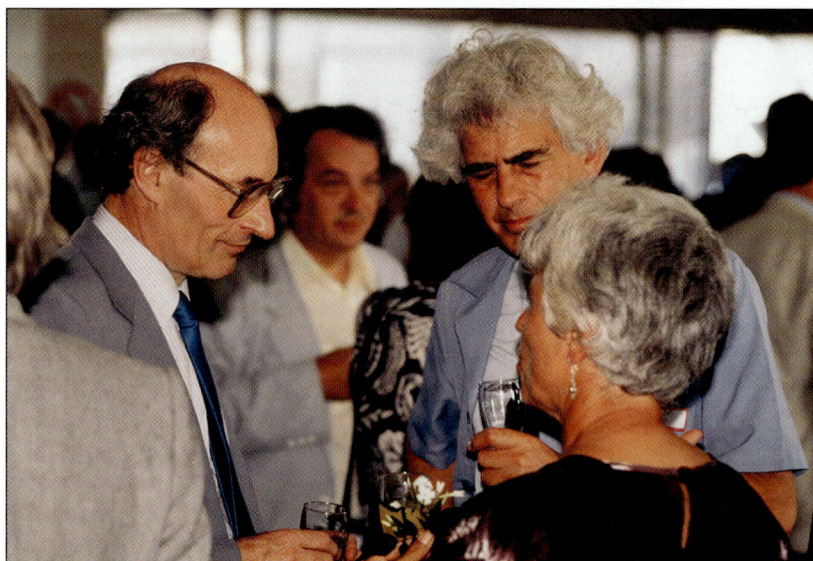

At a party celebrating his
knighthood in 1992:
M.R. with Julian Leff and
Naomi Richardson.

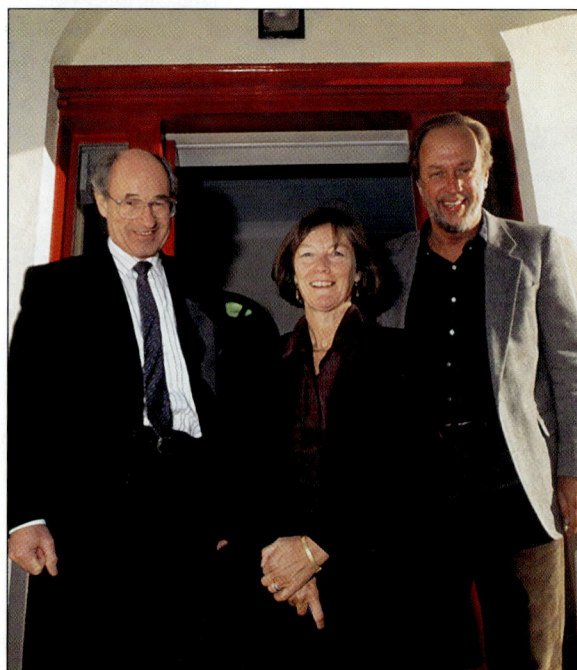

The opening of the Social,
Genetic and
Developmental Psychiatry
Research Centre at the
Institute of Psychiatry,
London 1994:
M.R. with Judy Dunn and
Robert Plomin.

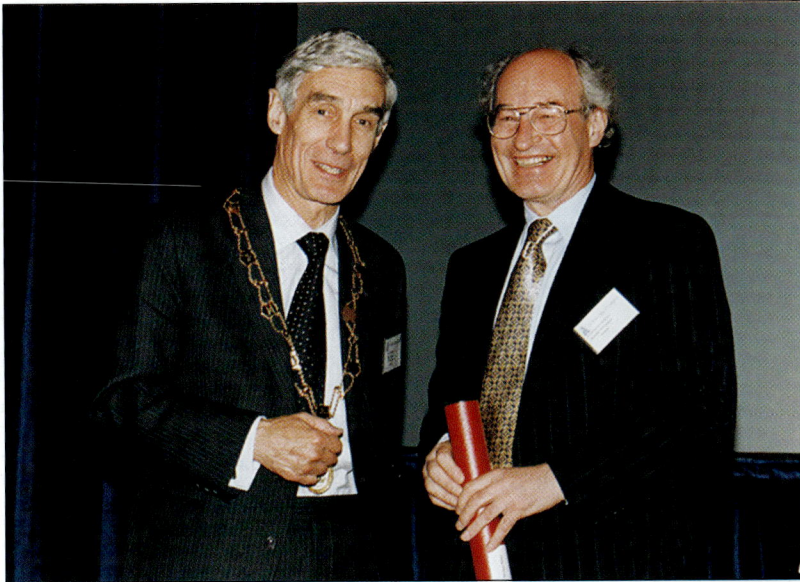

On the occasion of the
conferring of an Honorary
Fellowship of the Royal
College of Psychiatrists,
London 1997: M.R. with
Bob Kendall, then
President of the College.

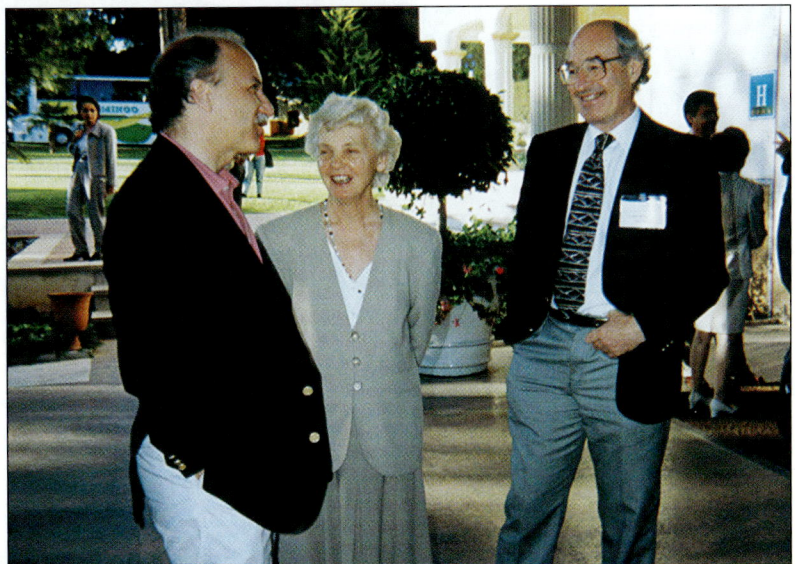

M.R. with Tony Bailey and
Marjorie Rutter at the
Castilla del Pino 1997.

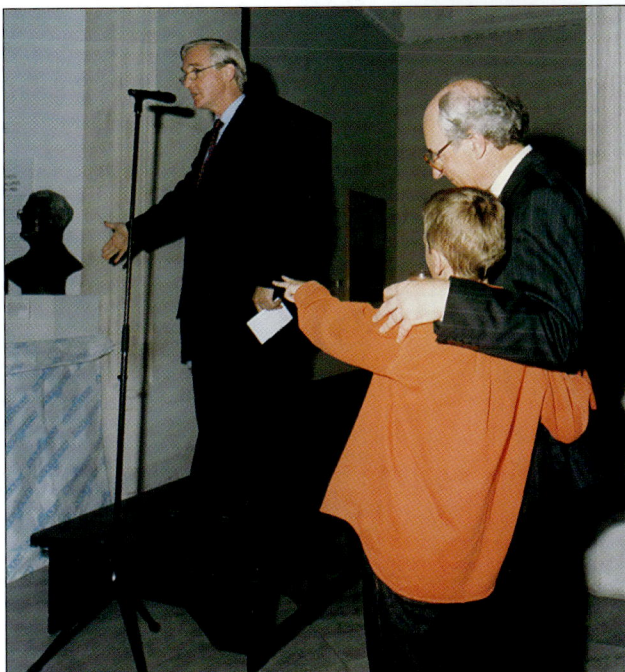

The retirement party at the
National Portrait Gallery,
London 1998: M.R. with
James, his grandson, during
a speech by the Dean, Stuart
Checkley.

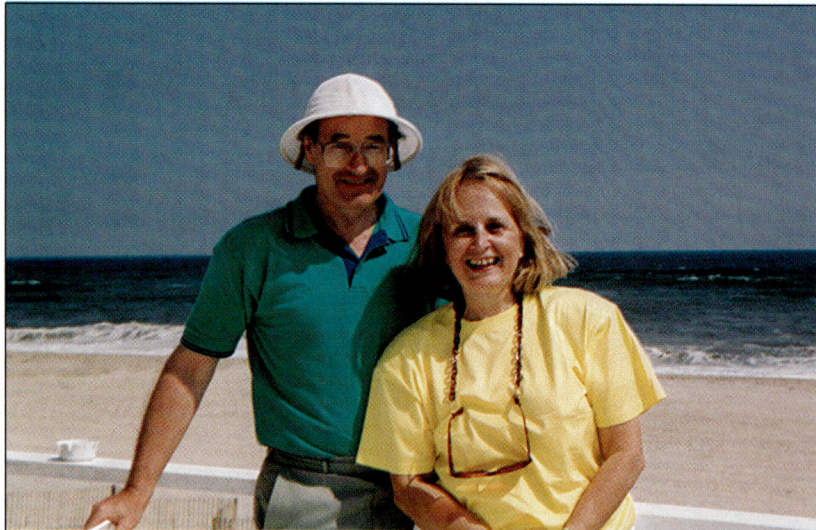

M.R. with Myrna Weissman in relaxed mood on Long Island 1993.

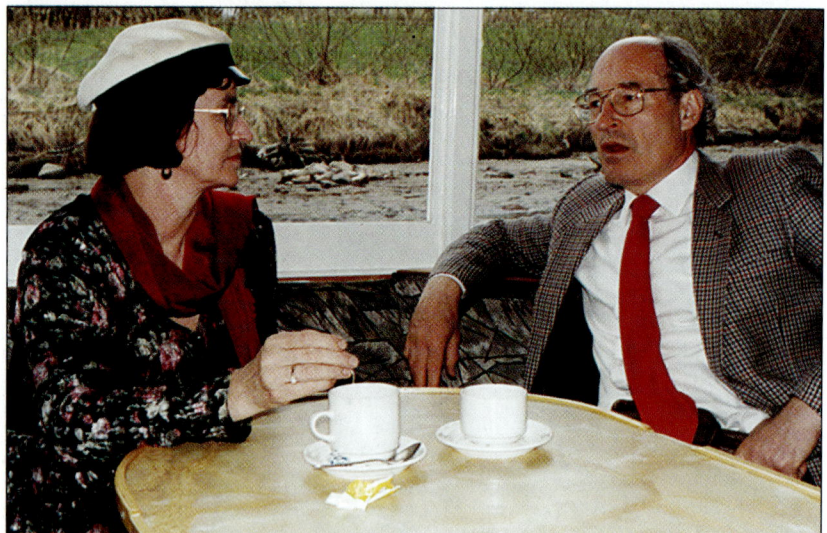

M.R. with Lea Pulkkinen on a boat trip during a visit to Finland in 1997, to receive an honorary degree from the University of Jyväskylä.

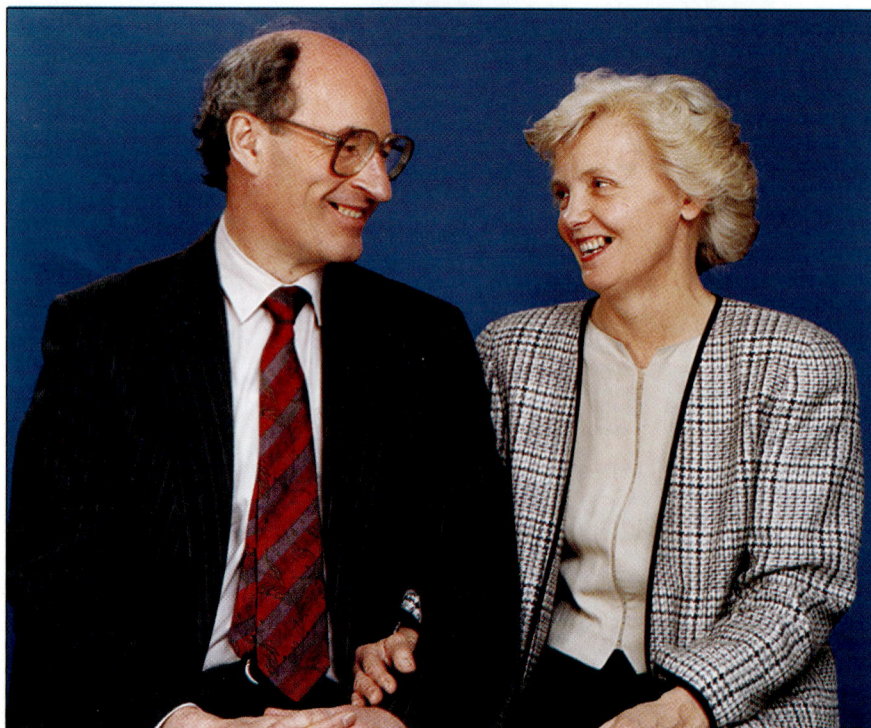

"My most crucial collaborator": M.R. and Marjorie Rutter on the occasion of the publication of their book Developing Minds: Challenge and Continuity Across the Lifespan in 1993.

5 Developmental neuropsychiatry

The foundations

of neuropsychiatry in childhood

Eric Taylor

Michael Rutter brought his programme of sceptical enquiry to neuropsychiatry in the 1970s, a time of high polemic concerning the extent to which children's psychological disturbance could be attributed to brain dysfunction. His epidemiological work cleared the ground and contributed to the central question in this debate, as well as raising a host of issues about the developmental pathways involved that are still energising research.

This chapter begins with a selection of key findings from the early stages of the programme. Its purpose is to consider how they relate to both the current state and the future of developmental neuropsychiatry, which has been called an 'impossible science'. If the brain is the most complicated thing in the universe, then its development is even more complex, and patterns of alteration in this developmental change must baffle the understanding. How, therefore, is it possible to ask useful questions in this area? As is often the case with the Rutter approach, the trick is to make the questions both simple and fundamental.

One of the debates at the time concerned the nature of 'the' brain damage syndrome: what were the clinical features that allowed the clinician to diagnose that a problem was due to deviant development of the brain, rather than to normal reactions to abnormal environments? Posing the question in this way is perhaps evidence of what was going wrong conceptually. The brain is more like a collection of organs than a single one, and to think that the consequences of dysfunction would be a unitary syndrome was an excessive simplification.

With hindsight it is clear that evidence was needed regarding the types of problem actually apparent in children with a damaged brain. Having perceived how crucial it was to approach the question from an epidemiological perspective, Rutter and colleagues set out to provide just that information, publishing their results in *A Neuropsychiatric Study in Childhood* (Rutter *et al*, 1970). This was a remarkable book in many ways.

One of its basic achievements was to establish the rates of prevalence of psychiatric disorders in children with and without brain disease. Figure 5.1, based on results from that survey, shows how much more frequent psychiatric disorder is in children with structural brain disease than in those with physical illness. It is characteristic of Rutter's work in several ways. It is simple, clear, robust and highly persistent. This figure or versions of it still serve as the beginning of many a talk on developmental neuropsychiatry and many a textbook chapter (e.g. Goodman, 1994). How many other scientific results from 30 years ago are quoted as frequently as these?

The diagnostic breakdown of disorders was another of the famous findings (Fig. 5.2). All disorders were more common, and in that sense there was certainly no unitary brain damage syndrome. This helped to kill the notion of minimal brain dysfunction as a distinctive disorder. Nevertheless, some syndromes were disproportionately common

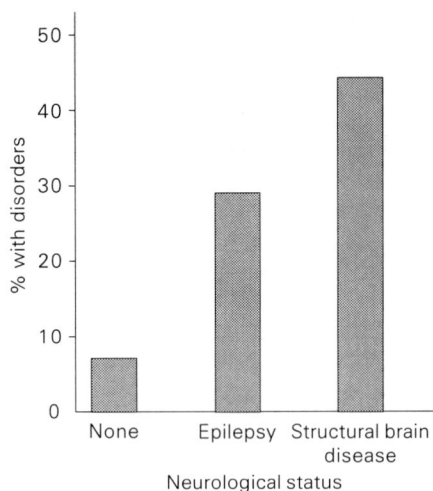

Fig. 5.1 Prevalence of
psychiatric disorder as a
percentage of all children.

82 ■

within the group of children with a dysfunctional brain who had a psychological disorder. Such 'neuropsychiatric' syndromes included hyperkinetic disorder, autism, the spectrum of pervasive developmental disorder, and related behaviours such as repetitive self-injury, stereotypies and pica. The presence of those symptom patterns creates, therefore, some presumption of an associated biological disorder – not an absolute diagnosis but a reason for further enquiry. The presence of autism is, in itself and without other neurological evidence, a strong indicator of physical disorder of the brain. One might now include further syndromes that are disproportionately common in some brain diseases, such as the schizophreniform disorders seen in temporal lobe epilepsy. Conceptually, what had been achieved was an operational meaning for the concept of a neuropsychiatric syndrome using epidemiological association.

Another consequence of this survey was very practical. The high level of psychiatric need in populations with brain disorder was clearly documented, and this has influenced the delivery of services. Many child psychiatrists are now working more closely with populations with neurological impairments than did our predecessors. Child psychiatry expanded to include within itself the special problems of those with impaired brains.

Fig. 5 2 Diagnostic
breakdown of psychiatric
disorders. The prevalence
of each disorder is
expressed as a percentage
of those in each group
who showed any disorder.
PDD, pervasive
developmental disorders.

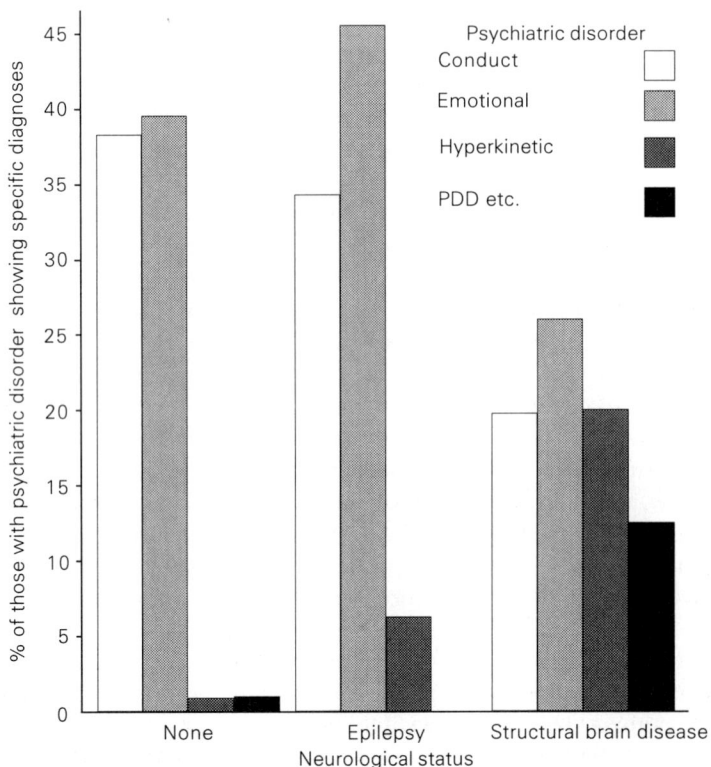

This process is still incomplete, and the meeting of needs of this population is still inadequate in many ways. Surveys in brain-damaged populations still find that needs for physical illnesses are well met, but there is continuing poor recognition of mental health needs (Chadwick *et al*, 1999). One obstacle is the persistence of 'pre-Rutterian' thinking. Some purchasers and professionals in primary care still seem to hold the unstated supposition that the mental illnesses of those with brain damage are an inevitable part of their handicap and that they differ from the mental illnesses of other people. The epidemiological findings about the types of disorder actually found should have dispelled these views, but they evidently still need to be disseminated and acted on.

There has been considerable progress in the sciences basic to child neuropsychiatry since the epidemiological work described above (Harris, 1995). Some of the themes need to be drawn out here, because they create new possibilities of thinking about how brain disorder causes psychopathology.

Recent advances in developmental neuroscience

Genetic factors

There has been a greatly increased appreciation of the strength of genetic contributions to the developmental neuropsychiatric disorders. For many of them – hyperkinetic disorders, autism, Tourette disorder – a strong genetic component has been identified, and molecular genetic investigations are in full cry after the genes that convey susceptibility. Much of this work is reviewed elsewhere in this volume, so is not repeated here. It has already changed the way that clinicians make their formulations and holds promise of further elucidating the developmental processes that are involved.

■83

Developmental neurobiology

Neuroanatomy has contributed a substantial amount to studies of the different phases of brain development and an appreciation of how much development happens postnatally. Early researchers tended to think of the brain's formation as shaped essentially by the prenatal phases of neuronal proliferation and migration, and therefore thought of environmental influences as being primarily those that had an effect in embryonic life and around the time of birth. It is now apparent that the anatomical structure of the brain is not fully established until adult biological maturity.

In the first stages of brain development, during the first 120 days of embryonic life, the neural plate invaginates to form a neural tube, and a rapidly proliferating epithelium generates the cells that will become neurons (Rakic, 1988). The cortical layer to which a cell will belong is determined at this stage of cell formation – before the cells have migrated to their eventual positions (McConnell & Kaznowski, 1991).

A migration of neurons then takes place, the first-formed neurons settling into an inner layer near the surface of the ventricle, and later-formed neurons moving past them to outer, more superficial layers of cortex. This migration is an interactive process: it is influenced by the expression of neurotransmitters and neuromodulators (Rakic, 1988; Komuro & Rakic, 1993) and by contact with the surfaces of neighbouring cells (Rakic, 1990). Abnormalities at this stage of development are likely to give rise to widespread abnormalities of brain function.

The neurons then differentiate into various types that will come to make use of various neurotransmitters. This seems to be determined after cell migration and is influenced by the connections made with other cells and by circulating levels of hormones (Patterson & Nawa, 1993). Abnormalities in the early stages of development have been proposed as causes of major mental disorders, including learning disability and schizophrenia. Nowakowski (1991) summarised a considerable variety of single autosomal recessive gene mutations that cause anatomical abnormalities of the hippocampus in mice. In one such abnormality (Hippocampus Lamination Defect mutant), the migration of nerve cells begins correctly, but is arrested before the cells have reached their normal destination. In another (Dreher mutant) there is an abnormality at a stage of proliferation of the pyramidal cells of the hippocampus, so that the cyto-architecture is marked not only by misplaced neurons, but also by abnormal cell numbers.

One must be cautious about extrapolating from animal models to human disease, but the ectopias and other brain abnormalities seen in these mutant mice do bear a similarity to the types of neuropathology that have been described in post-mortem studies of schizophrenia (Nowakowski, 1991). The general point is that many different genetic alterations of brain development are probable. We do not yet know the extent to which each brain disorder has a specific neuropsychiatric expression, or whether each gives rise to a non-specific vulnerability with similar eventual results.

The migration and differentiation of neurons is followed by an extensive period of cell death. This is controlled by afferent connections and influences from the cells' synaptic targets (Oppenheim, 1991). Throughout development, and even into adult life, a neuron's survival is dependent on the afferent and efferent connections that it makes. The neurological process of selective cell death is succeeded by a similar process at the level of the synapse: early proliferation is followed by massive and selective culling in postnatal life in interaction with the organism's experience.

This neural pruning is a controlled and regulated process. Genetic factors are involved, and there is also a process of natural selection for synaptic connections that have been established by use (Keshavan *et al*, 1994). Failures of the process can be responsible for localised neuropathology and consequent brain dysfunction. It is also possible that there could be widespread failures in the selective pruning of synapses, so that large areas of the brain could show a dysfunctional overconnectedness. Advances in functional neuroimaging make this, in principle, detectable. At the level of speculation, some aspects of childhood psychopathology could be seen as reflecting an indiscriminately overconnected pattern of brain organisation. Unselectiveness of attention, failure to inhibit irrelevant responses, and overflow of motor movements could all be viewed as the random activation of neural circuits that are unnecessary to the task at hand.

Major neurodevelopmental changes continue throughout early childhood. The number of synapses diminishes dramatically, and the volume of white matter increases, due to further myelination of those axonal connections that survive regressive elimination. This reorganisation can be expected both to modify the expression of pre-existing abnormalities and to create new kinds of vulnerability to the operation of genetic and environmental risk factors.

During later childhood, psychological functions may be taken over by higher cortical centres, as the latter mature. Further function becomes more molecular – the amount of cortex dealing with any given task becomes smaller and more specialised. Advances in neuroimaging technology mean that the site and extent of cortex devoted to any particular function can, in principle, be measured. Deviations from the normal course of development can therefore be detected, and their significance for psychopathology should become clearer. Later childhood and adolescence are also marked by an increase in neurotransmitter receptors, while dopamine receptors in the frontal lobes may not reach their full numbers until adult life. There is an accelerated cull of synapses in adolescence, which may eliminate dysfunctional connections and create an opportunity for psychological problems to diminish in severity or change in form during young adulthood.

The immediate clinical significance of these postnatal developmental changes in the brain is that they help us to understand the otherwise puzzling developmental changes in disorders over the life span. For example:

(a) autism sometimes appears rather late in development, at about age 2 years, and atypical syndromes may begin even later;

(b) during adolescence there appears to be an evolution from the impulsions with which obsessive–compulsive disorder presents in children to the resisted compulsions of the adult illness;

(c) adolescent changes in schizophrenia often bring the onset of first-rank symptoms in people who previously have had only the neurocognitive deficits that predispose to it;

(d) the presentation of hyperkinetic disorders may change, with a waning of hyperactivity and an evolution of antisocial problems in later childhood and adolescent development.

All of these changes in disorder have eluded clear explanations, and may be better understood from the perspective of the child's brain as developing in structure as well as in function.

Molecular neuroscience has also contributed, but has perhaps not yet fulfilled its promise. The accidental discovery of the antihyperkinetic effect of sympathomimetic central nervous stimulants remains the main pharmacological contribution to treating childhood disorders. The neurochemical basis of their action is still not worked out. There are some important puzzles that invite investigation, for example, the apparent lack of effect of tricyclic antidepressants on the depressive disorders of childhood despite the efficacy of serotonin reuptake inhibitors for obsessional disorder, in which the mode of action is usually thought of as similar. Promisingly, pharmaceutical companies have appreciated that some of their products have high potential relevance for child psychiatric disorders. There are now screening programmes in place in which developmental animal models are used to examine the effects of many candidate drugs. One result should be a deeper understanding of the chemical pathways through which psychotropic drugs act on the immature brain.

Animal neuropharmacological models have been explored, but usually there is much doubt at the level of behavioural analysis. There are, for instance, so many animal models for attention-deficit hyperactivity disorder (ADHD) that no single one has carried great credibility. A knock-out gene mouse model of deficient dopamine transporter has been well analysed for the differing effects of stimulants, by comparison with neurochemical actions in ordinary mice. But it is still unclear whether this gene knock-out is a good model for ADHD. The experimental mice are overactive, especially in novel situations; humans with ADHD are overactive, but often *not* in novel situations. Should this invalidate the model? No clear answer is possible. Other animal models carry similar problems of interpretation. However, it is worth noting Sagvolden's model – applying to both rats and humans – of a rapid decay of reward effectiveness with time (Sagvolden & Sergeant, 1998). This is a process by which some animals and some people lose interest and motivation. The model has shown that it can make surprising and interesting predictions about the operant conditioning behaviour of children with impulse control disorders.

Advances in measurement

Advances in measurement are now driving progress in both research and clinical issues. Child psychopathology has long been denied the advances of biological psychiatry because of practical and ethical constraints on biological measurement. This is now changing, especially because of developments in imaging, such as functional magnetic resonance imaging (fMRI), that make it feasible to identify neurophysiological alterations that could be part of the pathogenesis of disorder.

One important application to clinical problems has already appeared: the investigation of the significance of perinatal abnormalities. As considered below, there has been a pendulum-like swing in the views of experts about the extent to which early environmental adversity can cause lasting abnormalities of psychological function. The advent of non-invasive methods of imaging such as ultrasound allowed their routine use in intensive neonatal care, and it swiftly became apparent that the presence of physical lesions was a crucial predictor of neuropsychological dysfunction (Taylor, 1991).

Developmental mechanisms

The complexity of pathogenic mechanisms has become much better appreciated: genetic susceptibility interacts with environmental factors; the expression of a risk from genetic constitution or early brain damage is modified by qualities of the environment; and there are a variety of developmental tracks, with symptom patterns that remain constant, problems that wane and problems that appear late in development.

Psychological assessment over extended time periods has also shown that different sorts of cerebral pathology may give rise to different types of developmental course: for example, the falling IQ of children with Down's syndrome and fragile-X syndrome, by contrast with the stable or rising IQ of children with learning disability associated with cerebral palsy (Burack *et al*, 1988).

One of the constant themes in Rutter's contributions to developmental neuropsychiatry has been an emphasis on process and mechanism, studying the routes

■85

through which brain dysfunction is expressed, and asking whether it is a direct expression of brain function or the result of more complex pathways and interacting mechanisms. In different circumstances both theories may well hold true, and the question becomes that of when and under what circumstances these different routes apply. The study of how genes and environments interact has become crucial.

There is a sense in which all genetic disorders involve gene–environment interactions: genes can express themselves only through a relationship with the environment. Indeed, genetic and environmental influences are both important in most disorders. But this is only the beginning of the developmental enquiry: how do these influences work, and how might they be modified?

The most widely recognised influences are additive, with both genetic and environmental contributions acting independently. True gene–environment interactions involve a genetic control of sensitivity to the environment and environmental control of gene expression. Gene–environment correlations are present when the exposure to environmental experiences is determined by genetic propensities.

One way forward is the possibility that describing different types of DNA change will lead to the finding that an apparently weak environmental influence is in fact of great importance in a specifically vulnerable group. For example, Seeger has reported preliminary findings of a strong association between ADHD and season of birth – but only in a subgroup characterised by a variant form of the gene coding for the D4 dopamine receptor (further details available from E.T. upon request). By the same token, other genetic risk factors may operate through creating a sensitivity to foetal toxins such as nicotine.

Another possibility arises from the finding that the transition of ADHD into conduct disorder may be predicted by the critical expressed emotion of the families in which children live (Rutter *et al*, 1997). On the one hand, the genetic constitution of the child is altering the environment: their genes for hyperactivity are evoking criticism from their parents. (This route is likely, because of the finding that when children's hyperactivity is treated, the critical expressed emotion from their parents tends to fall.) On the other hand, the parents' criticism and volatility may be an expression of their own hyperactivity. This would be an example of a correlation between the genetic constitution of the parents and the environment that they are producing for the child. The unteasing of these various and complex pathways is likely to dominate much future research and to be crucial for clinical applications.

Revisiting the conclusions of developmental neuropsychiatry

In the light of these scientific advances, do the conclusions from Rutter's early epidemiological surveys require modification? On the whole, they have been robust. 'Minimal brain dysfunction' has not risen from the ashes. The factors modifying the expression of brain damage are still considered as important as the brain damage itself. Nevertheless, the ability to make finer discriminations and investigate more closely what brain dysfunction is present has opened the way to finding more examples of specific links between brain and behaviour.

It is probably not very useful to ask in a global way whether the consequences of brain dysfunction are specific or non-specific. In some situations there may be very direct and specific behavioural manifestations of a neurological disorder. A mouse with a 5HT-1B receptor knock-out changes predictably as a direct result of the lesion, and every mouse who has had this procedure shows marked impulsiveness. In humans, too, some inherited disorders (such as Prader–Willi and Angelmann syndromes) show a rather constant form of disorder that is determined by the details of the DNA constitution of the child, rather than by what has happened after birth. In other inherited disorders, there is a wider range of presentations. The pedigrees of people with a specific neurodevelopmental disability often include a wide range of other neurodevelopmental problems (Elbert & Seale, 1988). In yet other disorders, such as the fragile-X chromosome constitution, the presentation is sometimes typical, but more often falls short of being a distinct phenotype (Bregman *et al*, 1988). Individual children may show a wide range of intellectual and behavioural changes, but there remain striking similarities between affected children (such as that of the rhythm of their speech). In still other situations – such as the range of problems that may follow severe closed-head injuries – the consequences may include virtually any kind of child psychopathology.

There is, in other words, no single 'brain dysfunction' about which one can generalise. Different types of pathology need separate consideration. I will mention here those that carry implications for clarifying the mechanisms of expression, such as anatomically lateralised brain lesions and their accompanying psychological syndromes; the consequences of metabolic disorder, in which the reversibility of chemical changes allows natural experiments; and the effects of brain trauma, where there is usually clear knowledge about the time of onset and the localisation of lesions.

Lateralisation

The lateralised syndromes have aroused much interest as a royal road to understanding the specifics of brain–behaviour relationships. The hemispheres specialise early, especially for language. Auditory evoked potential responses to speech sounds are more prominent on the left side than the right, even in neonates (Molfese & Molfese, 1980). Sounds presented to the right ear – and therefore to the left hemisphere – have a greater effect on physiological measures of response (such as heart rate changes) than those presented to the left ear (Best *et al*, 1982).

Nevertheless, and despite this early specialisation, language survives early local lesions. A left-sided vascular lesion (as in congenital hemiplegia) or injury to the head during early childhood does not have the same specific effects on language as would be seen had the injury occurred in adult life. Normal language development can follow even complete destruction (e.g. by excision) of the left hemisphere in early childhood (Goodman, 1987). The most characteristic result of an early hemiplegia, whichever side of the brain is damaged, is an impairment in visuospatial abilities. There may still be some subtle aspects of language that are impaired by having to be dealt with by the right hemisphere, and the age at which the lesion is sustained is a determinant of how much transfer takes place (Taylor, 1991).

Does this contradict the conclusion of early specialisation? No: rather, it emphasises the plasticity of the immature brain and the preservation of language even at the expense of other abilities.

The effect of lateralised lesions on behaviour patterns has not yet been subjected to definitive study. Comparisons of children with left- and right-sided hemiplegias do not suggest that the type of behaviour abnormality is determined by the side of the lesion (Goodman,1987). This is in keeping with the general conclusion that the results of early lesions are diffuse rather than localised, and heavily determined by the processes of compensation – which are not always benign.

However, some accounts of children with minor coordination problems of the right side of the body, or electroencephalogram findings suggestive that the left side of the brain is compromised, have emphasised specific consequences in the understanding of social relationships. A 'right-hemisphere syndrome' of social and attentional impairment has been highlighted by Weintraub & Mesulam (1983). This is hard to square with the above results of children selected by the side of their abnormality, rather than by their psychiatric presentation. It may therefore be that an ascertainment bias in the reporting of this syndrome is responsible for the apparent effects. Alternatively, the time of onset of an abnormality may be crucial. I have suggested elsewhere (Taylor, 1991) that genetically determined lesions of very early onset may not stimulate the processes of compensation and may therefore have more specific consequences than acquired lesions. Lesions acquired in later childhood may carry the same localising sequelae as they would in adult life, by contrast with the diffuse effects of lesions in early childhood.

Psychological phenotypes

The presentations of single-gene disorders and chromosomal anomalies are sometimes so characteristic that the genetic abnormality can be predicted with some reliability from the psychological pattern. Such 'behavioural phenotypes' (O'Brien & Yule, 1996) are of particular promise for tracking how DNA changes may lead to brain dysfunction. In Turner's syndrome, for example, the neuropsychological functioning of the affected children is determined by the subtle changes in the DNA that are associated with a maternal as opposed to a paternal transmission (Skuse *et al*, 1997).

■87

Associations such as these seem to imply that genetic change can be closely and directly causative to intellectual function. It is even possible that behavioural changes can be analysed in the same terms. For example, the characteristic pattern of self-mutilation in Lesch–Nyhan syndrome – with destructive biting of lips and fingers – is very seldom seen in other self-injurious disorders. As another example, the behavioural problems of Smith–Magenis syndrome are often linked to sleep disturbance and appear on falling asleep or on waking. Many of the affected children have abnormalities of sleep, sometimes a specific deficiency of rapid-eye-movement (REM) sleep. Pathogenetic mechanisms are most likely to be found when both the cause and the presentation of the syndrome are known and constantly related.

Another lesson that we can learn from these phenotypes concerns which types of dysfunction are related. In Williams' syndrome the capacity for the recognition of faces is relatively preserved when compared with general problems in visuospatial perception; this indicates that different brain systems may be involved (Udwin *et al*, 1987). It emphasises the need to survey a wide range of abilities in assessing children with developmental disorders.

Metabolic disorders

Phenylketonuria (PKU) is usually due to a recessively inherited deficiency of phenylalanine hydroxylase: screening of neonates and dietary treatments (by restriction of phenylalanine) prevent the worst of the structural brain damage that is common in untreated cases. The severity of the disorder is therefore a function chiefly of the adequacy of treatment (Berry *et al*, 1979). Subtle qualities of the treatment may make a great difference to outcome.

If the diet is relaxed after childhood, the level of phenylalanine in the blood predicts poor performance on tests of vigilance, task persistence and reaction time. During treatment in childhood, high phenylalanine levels are associated with a reduction of IQ of about 1 standard deviation (Smith *et al*, 1990). A collaborative perinatal study (Williamson *et al*, 1981) revealed a 6-point difference in mean IQ at age 4 years between a group with treated PKU and a group of their siblings, matched for age and gender; futhermore, the extent to which the parents were able to ensure that the children with PKU kept to the diet was a predictor of IQ at age 6 in a multiple-regression analysis. When treated children were switched back to an unrestricted diet in later childhood or adolescence, they showed a 6-point fall in IQ as phenylalanine levels rose (Smith *et al*, 1978). The decline characterised the early- rather than the late-treated children. Behaviour also shows some abnormality by comparison with the general population when rating scales are applied to children with treated PKU (Smith & Beasley, 1989): behavioural deviance, as rated by teachers, is doubled (Stevenson *et al*, 1979).

The course of PKU therefore suggests a rather close dependence of psychological changes on relatively small changes in the physical substrate of the disorder. However, this is not necessarily reflected in a specific behavioural phenotype. Widespread and diffuse changes are to be expected in a chemical alteration affecting the whole of the brain. Phenylalanine excess reduces the concentration of tyrosine and tryptophan in the brain, and correspondingly inhibits the production of dopamine and serotonin (McKean, 1972). It is likely that some of the psychiatric effects of PKU result from reversible effects on neurotransmitters, as well as from structural effects on myelination of the brain during early childhood. The relationship between the neurochemical changes and psychiatric disturbance can now be addressed.

Although direct physical effects of the PKU on the brain are powerful, it is clear that there are also other influences on disorder. Maternal IQ, for example, is quite strongly associated with children's IQ (Williamson *et al*, 1981), and social class is a strong predictor of IQ in children with PKU, independent of dietary control (Smith *et al*, 1990). The restrictions, frustrations and cognitive blunting imposed by the disease all have powerful effects on behaviour, and relationships may be distorted by the attitudes of others. These too should be addressed in comprehensive treatment

Congenital hypothyroidism, like PKU, has been greatly reduced in its impact by the successful introduction of neonatal screening and effective therapy with replacement thyroxine. As in PKU, more recent study has indicated that the mean IQ score for treated patients is still less than that in the general population. The initial severity of the condition – measured by blood thyroxine levels when the condition is first diagnosed – predicts the degree of reduction of IQ at the ages of 3 and 5 years (Fuggle & Graham, 1991). Again, the psychological presentation is partly determined by subtle aspects of the physical insult to the brain.

Brain trauma

'Birth trauma' used to play a very strong part in aetiological formulations. Its perceived importance declined greatly with the realisation that most obstetric suboptimality was not a direct cause of psychological abnormalities, but reflected psychosocial adversity and abnormalities of foetal development (Goodman, 1988; Hall, 1989; Gaffney et al, 1994). More recently, birth trauma_has again become a focus for study for at least two reasons.

First, imaging of brain structures has revealed marked brain changes in children who survive a very low birth weight but sustain neurological damage (Stewart et al, 1999). Second, a large Danish cohort indicated an association between minor obstetric complications and violent crime (Raine et al, 1996). These Danish results, however, essentially repeat the known association without excluding possible reasons for it, for example, that there is a prior association between abnormalities of foetal development and psychosocial adversity or that obstetric complications result from an abnormal foetus.

Other findings have argued that perinatal influences can be strong. The extent of hypoglycaemia in the first days of life is quite a good predictor of developmental delays later (Lucas et al, 1988). This is very likely to be a causal influence, because the subsequent delays are prevented by better feeding. The low threshold for injury by hypoglycaemia is in contrast to the apparently high thresholds for injury by hypoxia and mechanical damage. The developmental question shifts from the protection of the immature brain to the differing circumstances in which it can be either very vulnerable or highly resilient. The influence of perinatal adversity also needs to be reconsidered, because we can now directly detect the small number of cases in which adversity has indeed overcome the brain's defences and caused damage – for example, the frontal malacia that has been linked to hyperactive behaviour in later childhood (Casaer, 1991).

Postnatal injury

Follow-up research by Rutter and his collaborators on the consequences of head injury in children showed very persuasively a causal path from severe head injuries to cognitive problems – but a probable non-causal association between cognitive problems and minor head injuries (Rutter et al, 1983). In the latter case the cognitive problems were more likely to contribute to the probability of having the accident in the first place. The threshold for psychological disturbance after trauma is therefore relatively high, and clinicians should not give too much emphasis to the possibility of head injury in a child with a psychiatric disorder who does not have a clear history of severe brain trauma.

The course of development after the brain is damaged is influenced by neurological and non-neurological factors. The brain lesions themselves may persist, or wane (as they do in many children who encounter neonatal adversity or later head trauma), or intensify (when, for instance, uncontrolled seizures bring about further deterioration of brain function), or be complicated by other lesions (as when structural defects due to PKU's effects on myelination are compounded by its effects on neurotransmitter metabolism). The lesions may have a variety of effects on the rest of the brain. Other parts of the brain may take over the function of a damaged area, either through the same strategies as were used by the original part or through the substitution of a different strategy for achieving the same end. The neurons involved by damage may – depending on their developmental stage – regenerate new terminals, and connecting neurons may produce new ones. This process of growth within the central nervous system may be both harmful and helpful, because anomalous connections may impair the processing of information (Goodman, 1994). A brain that has suffered damage does not just display a deficit: it has adapted to the abnormality in a variety of ways.

89

The future of child neuropsychiatry

It is impossible to foresee the future of any science. The most one can do is to extrapolate from current trends, and to guess that the investment of research time will produce much more satisfactory knowledge about the causes and course of disorders and that the working out of pathogenetic mechanisms will suggest rational therapies, more productive targets for therapy and better means of monitoring the course and auditing the results of a service.

Neuroimaging

When new techniques appear, they have a way of advancing conceptual understanding. The development of neuroimaging was quite unforeseen 30 years ago, but it has now reached a stage at which we can envisage detailed knowledge of the anatomical and chemical localisation of dysfunctions in the neurodevelopmental disorders.

It is already possible to get reasonable pictures that localise cognitive function in children. For example, my colleagues and I have applied fMRI to children and adults performing a 'stop' test, and have described the activation of a neural network including right-hemispheric mesial frontal cortex, and inferior frontal and caudate nucleus (Rubia *et al*, 1998). We have also used the combination of fMRI with an inhibitory task to test a hypothesis that frontal and striate structures involved in inhibiting responses are underfunctioning in people with ADHD (Rubia *et al*, 1999). We found that adolescents with ADHD showed a significant global reduction in functional neuroactivation. The decrease in signal intensity was found mainly in frontal and striatal brain regions, indicating localised underfunctioning.

For all imaging studies one must ask *what* one has 'understood' in understanding where something is happening; whether it matters; and whether it is a surplus explanation (a kind of phrenology). To take the example of the above ADHD study, is it not obvious that children with ADHD have poor attention, that frontal circuits control attention and therefore that these children have underactive frontal circuits?

Such implied criticism underestimates the range of issues that current imaging techniques can address. We can on occasion infer not only where but also how certain processing takes place. The above findings, for instance, argue against non-localised abnormalities. They refute some of the possible formulations about the nature of impulsiveness – for example, that it reflects a hippocampal dysfunction or an abnormality of reward mechanisms. Indeed, the findings included an excessive activation of other areas of cortex, notably the insula, suggesting that the task of suppressing responses is done in a different way and follows a different strategy in children with ADHD. The imaging results support a particular kind of pathology, excluding some hypotheses and accepting others, and open up possibilities for more precise aetiological research. How far that will lead to the analysis of individual children remains a question for the future.

Clinical implications

The purpose of research into developmental neuropsychiatry is to improve clinical practice. One benefit of research is a fuller understanding of the factors that act to create vulnerability and protection within the groups of children who are at risk because of neurological illness, handicap or injury. In epilepsy, for example, we know a good deal about the factors that influence rates of mental disorder (Table 5.1). These findings provide a kind of map for clinicians: they indicate key features to assess in each case, and therefore how to intervene and what targets to select.

Table 5.1 Predictors of psychiatric disorder in children with epilepsy

Associated neurological abnormalities
Seizure type and frequency
Age at onset
Medication: polytherapy, folate level
Cognitive impairments
Rejection and stigmatisation
Family discord, hostility, divorce

Improved detection using neuropsychology and neuroimaging may also increase the range of what is possible for compensated disorders. Obviously, it is much easier to recognise a disability when there is serious impairment of function. Sometimes a child may in large part be overcoming a handicap and showing minimal impairment because of a great effort of compensation. It may be just as important for that child's well-being that such 'compensated problems' are diagnosed.

The likely impact of molecular genetics is not yet clear and deserves careful consideration at all stages of advance in knowledge. New ethical and clinical choices will arise. The likeliest advances will not be in 'genetic engineering', but in defining high-risk groups. For instance, if we know that a child has a very rapid delay of reward gradient, it might be feasible to develop a preventive programme to bypass the problem. Genetic knowledge may alter our classification schemes: disorders may dissolve into components and reasons for comorbidity may become clearer. Knowledge of pharmacogenetics may allow us to test individual children to determine what drug to give, and therefore to speed up the process of therapy in conditions (such as complicated epilepsy) where multiple drug changes and even confusion of regimes are at present all too common. The range of effective drugs can also be expected to advance rapidly when knowledge of the neurochemical actions that are desired allows the pharmaceutical industry to apply powerful techniques of screening.

Conclusions

General conclusions about the psychological sequelae of brain damage or impairment are dangerous. Knowledge has advanced greatly, but is still at the level where much has to be done in the basic charting of the psychological development of children with different types of abnormal brain function.

Too many investigations in the past have relied on using convenient populations, rather than seeking a representative series; too many have sought the consequences of brain damage in a static deficit, modified only in degree by later recovery and experience. This simple view clearly does scant justice to the complexity of neurological and psychological development.

Michael Rutter's enduring contribution will go beyond his influential findings and his commitment to drawing practical lessons. His emphasis on the importance of elucidating the steps in complex chains of pathogenesis should continue to stimulate a truly developmental neuropsychiatry. Within a very complicated situation he has provided a fine model of what is a soluble question. In a sense we are all Rutterians now: our thinking about developmental neuropsychiatry is based firmly on his.

■91

References

Berry, H. K., O'Grady, D. J., Perlmutter, L. J., *et al* (1979) Intellectual development and academic achievement of children treated early for phenylketonuria. *Developmental Medicine and Child Neurology*, **21**, 311–320.

Best, C. T., Hoffman, H. & Glanville, B. B. (1982) Development of infant ear asymmetries for speech and music. *Perception and Psychophysics*, **31**, 75–85.

Bregman, J. D., Leckman, J. F. & Ort, S. I. (1988) Fragile X syndrome: genetic predisposition to psychopathology. *Journal of Autism and Developmental Disorders*, **18**, 343–354.

Burack, J. A., Hodapp., R. M., & Zigler, E. (1988) Issues in the classification of mental retardation: differentiating among organic etiologies. *Journal of Child Psychology and Psychiatry*, **29**, 765–779.

Casaer, P., de Vries, L., & Marlow, N. (1991) Prenatal and perinatal risk factors for psychosocial development. In *Biological Risk Factors for Psychosocial Disorders* (eds M. Rutter & P. Casaer), pp. 139–174. Cambridge: Cambridge University Press.

Chadwick, O. Taylor, E. & Bernard, S. (1999) *The Prevention of Disorders in Children with Severe Learning Disability*. Report to NHS R & D Executive. London: Institute of Psychiatry.

Elbert, J. C. & Seale, T. W. (1988) Complexity of the cognitive phenotype of an inherited form of learning disability. *Developmental Medicine and Child Neurology*, **30**, 181–189.

Fuggle, P. & Graham, P. (1991) Metabolic and endocrine disorders: biological aspects of continuous or discontinuous psychological functioning during childhood and adolescence. In *Biological Risk Factors for Psychosocial Disorders* (eds M. Rutter & P. Casaer). Cambridge: Cambridge University Press.

Gaffney, G., Sellers, S., Flavell, V., *et al* (1994) Case–control study of intrapartum care, cerebral palsy, and perinatal death. *British Medical Journal*, **308**, 743–750.

Goodman, R. (1987) The developmental neurobiology of language. In *Language Development and Disorders* (eds W. Yule & M. Rutter), pp. 129–145. London: MacKeith Press.

—— (1988) Are complications of pregnancy and birth causes of schizophrenia? *Developmental Medicine and Child Neurology*, **30**, 391–395.

—— (1994) Brain disorders. In *Child and Adolescent Psychiatry: Modern Approaches* (eds. M. Rutter, E. Taylor & L. Hersov), 3rd edn, pp. 172–190. Oxford: Blackwell Scientific.

Hall, D. (1989) Birth asphyxia and cerebral palsy. *British Medical Journal*, **299**, 279–282.

Harris, J. C. (1995) *Developmental Neuropsychiatry*. New York: Oxford University Press.

Keshavan, M. S., Anderson, S., & Pettegrew, J. W. (1994) Is schizophrenia due to excessive synaptic pruning in the prefrontal cortex? The Feinberg Hypothesis revisited. *Journal of Psychiatric Research*, **28**, 239–265.

Komuro, H. & Rakic, P. (1993) Modulation of neuronal migration by NMDA receptors. *Science*, **260**, 95–97.

Lucas, A., Morley, R. & Cole, T. J. (1988) Adverse neurodevelopmental outcome of moderate neonatal hypoglycaemia. *British Medical Journal*, **297**, 1304–1308.

McConnell, S. K. & Kaznowski, C. E. (1991) Cell cycle dependence of laminar determination in developing neocortex. *Science*, **254**, 282–285.

McKean, C. M. (1972) The effects of high phenylalanine concentrations on serotonin and catecholamine metabolism in the human brain. *Brain Research*, **47**, 469–476.

Molfese, D. R. & Molfese, V. J. (1980) Cortical responses of preterm infants to phonetic and nonphonetic speech stimuli. *Developmental Psychology*, **16**, 574–581.

Nowakowski, R. S. (1991) Neuronal migration and differentiation during normal and genetically perturbed development of the hippocampal formation. In *Developmental Neuropathology of Schizophrenia* (eds S. A. Mednick, T. D. Cannon, C. E. Barr, *et al*), pp. 29–60. New York: Plenum Press.

O'Brien, G. & Yule, W. (eds) (1996) *Behavioural Phenotypes*. Cambridge: Cambridge University Press.

Oppenheim, R. W. (1991) Cell death during development of the nervous system. *Annual Review of Neuroscience*, **14**, 453–501.

Patterson, P. H. & Nawa, H. (1993) Neuronal differentiation factors/cytokines and synaptic plasticity. *Cell*, **10**, 123–137.

Raine, A., Brennan, P., Mednick, B., *et al* (1996) High rates of violence, crime, academic problems, and behavioral problems in males with both early neuromotor deficits and unstable family environments. *Archives of General Psychiatry*, **53**, 544–549.

Rakic, P. (1988) Specification of cerebral cortical areas. *Science*, **241**, 170–176.

—— (1990) Principles of neural cell migration. *Experientia*, **46**, 882–891.

Rubia K., Overmeyer S., Taylor E., *et al* (1998) Prefrontal involvement in 'temporal bridging' and timing movement. *Neuropsychologia*, **36**, 1283–1293.

——, ——, ——, *et al* (1999) Hypofrontality in Attention Deficit Hyperactivity Disorder during higher-order motor control: a study with fMRI. *American Journal of Psychiatry*, **156**, 891–896.

Rutter, M., Graham, P. & Yule, W. (1970) *A Neuropsychiatric Study in Childhood*. London: SIMP/Heinemann.

——, Chadwick, O. & Shaffer, D. (1983) Head injury. In *Developmental Neuropsychiatry* (ed. M. Rutter), pp. 83–111. New York: Guilford.

——, Maughan, B., Meyer, J., *et al* (1997) Heterogeneity of antisocial behaviour: causes, continuities, and consequences, *Nebraska Symposium on Motivation*, **44**, 45–118.

Sagvolden, T. & Sergeant, J. A. (1998) Attention deficit/hyperactivity disorder – from brain dysfunctions to behaviour. *Behavioral Brain Research*, **94**, 1–10.

Skuse, D. H, James, R. S, Bishop, D. V., *et al* (1997) Evidence from Turner's syndrome of an imprinted X-linked locus affecting cognitive function, *Nature*, **387**, 705–708.

Smith, I. & Beasley, M. G. (1989) Intelligence and behaviour in children with early treated phenylketonuria. *European Journal of Pediatrics*, **43**, 1–5.

——, Lobascher, M., Stevenson, J. E., *et al* (1978) Effect of stopping low phenylalanine diet on intellectual progress of children with phenylketonuria. *British Medical Journal*, **2**, 723–726.

——, Beasley, M. & Ades, A. (1990) Intelligence and quality of treatment in phenylketonuria. *Archives of Disease in Childhood*, **65**, 472–478.

Stevenson, J. E., Hawcroft, J., Lobascher, M., *et al* (1979) Behavioural deviance in children with early treated phenylketonuria. *Archives of Diseases in Childhood*, **54**, 14–18.

Stewart, A. L., Rifkin, L., Amess, P. N., *et al* (1999) Brain structure and neurocognitive and behavioural function in adolescents who were born very preterm. *Lancet*, **353**, 1653–1657.

Taylor, E. (1991) Developmental neuropsychiatry. *Annual Research Review, Journal of Child Psychology and Psychiatry*, **32**, 3–47.

Udwin, O., Yule, W. & Martin, N. (1987) Cognitive abilities and behavioural characteristics of children with idiopathic infantile hypercalcaemia. *Journal of Child Psychology and Psychiatry*, **28**, 297–309.

Weintraub, S. & Mesulam, M.-M. (1983) Developmental learning disabilities of the right hemisphere: emotional, interpersonal and cognitive components. *Archives of Neurology*, **40**, 463–468.

Williamson, M. L., Koch, R., Azen, C., *et al* (1981) Correlates of intelligence test results in treated phenylketonuric children. *Pediatrics*, **68**, 161–170.

6 Five decades of research on autism

Progress and promise

Fred R. Volkmar

In the 50 years since its first scientific description by Leo Kanner (1943) the syndrome of autism has posed scientific challenges to theories of developmental psychology and neurobiology, as well as to therapy and education. Almost every theory of child development has been used in the attempt to understand the enigmatic impairments and competencies of individuals with this condition. Michael Rutter's contributions have been, and continue to be, seminal in essentially all aspects of research on this interesting and perplexing condition – notably in the areas of nosology and diagnosis, treatment and follow-up studies, and genetics. In addition, his publications and work as an editor have stimulated research.

It is a tribute to Rutter and to the field that the task of providing an exhaustive survey of the subject is no longer possible. Several thousand research publications, numerous books and several journals devoted to autism are a testament to its productivity. The present chapter focuses selectively on progress in several areas: diagnosis and classification; neurobiology; treatment and outcome; and, more briefly, behavioural research and developmental issues.

Diagnosis and classification

Unlike many conditions in child psychiatry, autism does not seem to 'shade off' into normality in the usual sense. Although issues of syndrome boundaries and the balance between broader *v.* narrower definitions are a perennial source of debate (Rutter & Schopler, 1992), autism represents one of the more robust categorical 'disorders' in child psychiatry (Volkmar *et al*, 1997b). The paired processes of diagnosis and classification have been fundamental to both research and clinical service, as Rutter so eloquently demonstrates in his Emmanuel Miller lecture (Rutter, 1998; see also Chapter 4). These issues are also central to the recent convergence, in their definitions of autism and related conditions, of the two major diagnostic systems: the 4th edition of the *Diagnostic and Statistical Manual* (DSM–IV) (American Psychiatric Association, 1994) and the 10th edition of the International Classification of Diseases (ICD–10) (World Health Organization, 1994). Although different in important ways in their overall organisation, and indeed sometimes very different for other classes of disturbance, for autism and related disorders these two diagnostic systems are now much more alike than different (Volkmar *et al*, 1994). This achievement has, in turn, allowed the development of diagnostic assessments that are more rigorously related to these guidelines (Lord *et al*, 1994). At present, autism is probably the disorder with the best empirically based, cross-national diagnostic criteria.

■93

Based on a paper presented at the Annual Residential Meeting of the Child and Adolescent Faculty of the Royal College of Psychiatrists, Bristol, 24 September 1998.

Kanner's (1943) astute clinical description of 11 children with "autistic disturbances of affective contact" proved to be remarkably enduring, but also provided some false leads for research – some of which took several decades to clarify. Early controversies focused on his use of the word 'autism', which suggested to many a possible continuity with schizophrenia, and on some of his other initial speculations, such as associations with 'mental retardation' (learning disability) and with other medical conditions. The severity of autism and rather broad notions of 'psychosis' and 'schizophrenia' led to a widespread presumption during the 1950s and 1960s that autism was the earliest form of schizophrenia (Bender, 1947; Creak, 1963). In many ways this was not dissimilar from the rather broad notions of schizophrenia then employed in work with adults (see Werry, 1996, for a discussion). Indeed, in DSM–I and DSM–II (American Psychiatric Association, 1952, 1968), only the term 'childhood schizophrenia' was officially available to describe children with autism. This proved, of course, very problematic; today, reports from that era are often uninterpretable.

Rigorous clinical studies conducted in the UK by Kolvin (1971), Rutter (1972) and others suggested that autism and schizophrenia were unrelated. In 1978, Rutter synthesised Kanner's original report and subsequent research in a highly influential definition of autism that remained near to the clinical phenomena encountered in the disorder. He noted that the social and communication impairments in autism were distinctive and could not be accounted for solely as a result of associated learning disability, and that the condition was of very early onset and associated with a specific group of unusual behaviours subsumed under the term 'resistance to change' or 'insistence on sameness' (Rutter, 1978). This synthesis proved particularly influential in DSM–III (American Psychiatric Association, 1980) because it was descriptive and remained conceptually close to Kanner's original description.

Although it had many shortcomings, DSM–III was a landmark in the development of psychiatric taxonomy. It emphasised research findings rather than theory in the attempt to produce valid, reliable descriptions of complex clinical phenomena. Autism was included as an 'official' diagnosis for the first time in a new class of disorder – the 'pervasive developmental disorders' (PDDs). This newly coined category clearly differentiated autism from childhood schizophrenia and achieved broad acceptance, and although subsequently debated (e.g. Gillberg, 1991; Volkmar & Cohen, 1991; Rutter & Schopler, 1992), it has been broadly accepted in the field and now seems here to stay.

The recognition of autism in DSM–III represented a major advance in the classification, but had various shortcomings (Rutter & Shaffer, 1980). It lacked a developmental orientation, and even the term 'infantile autism' indicated that the definition was most applicable to younger children and individuals with greater impairment. A category was included for 'residual' infantile autism, but this term was unsatisfactory because the problems of older children, adolescents and adults were quite apparent and not particularly residual. An attempt was made to deal with this problem in DSM–III–R (American Psychiatric Association, 1987), which provided a much more developmentally oriented definition with more detailed diagnostic criteria intended to cover the entire range of syndrome expression in autism – over both age and developmental level. Somewhat oddly, the DSM–III–R system avoided the issue of development and history, rather than current status, in making a diagnosis, and as a result early onset was no longer a necessary diagnostic feature. The changes introduced in DSM–III–R severely complicated the interpretation of studies done with the earlier diagnostic criteria and also presented a major problem relative to the then pending changes in the classification of autism and similar conditions in ICD–10 (World Health Organization, 1994). Discrepancies between the two systems included aspects of both the definition of autism and the inclusion of other 'new' disorders within the PDD class (Rutter & Schopler, 1992; Szatmari, 1992). Various changes were considered at the time DSM–IV was in preparation and as ICD–10 was being completed.

The preparation of DSM–IV was rather more extensive than any of its predecessors, including literature reviews, data reanalyses and a large international field trial (Volkmar et al, 1994). The latter included nearly 1000 cases provided by a range of sites and clinicians who submitted diagnostic information relevant not only to DSM–IV but also to ICD–10. It became clear that the draft ICD–10 definition had reasonable convergence with the diagnosis of experienced clinicians and tended to converge with DSM–III diagnoses as well. The large sample size enabled rapid identification of the shortcomings of the DSM–III–R diagnostic system, by which the false-positive rate for a diagnosis of autism was inversely related to IQ, so that nearly 60% of cases with the most severe mental handicap appeared to receive a diagnosis of autism incorrectly. Changes were made to ICD–10 criteria in terms of both wording and reduced number, and some 'new' conditions were included so that convergence between DSM and ICD was possible.

It is appropriate here to note an important continuing diagnostic tension. To some extent this represents a particularly American problem, since there is, unfortunately, a tendency in the USA to organise services around diagnoses rather than individuals: a diagnosis acts as a 'ticket' for services (Rutter & Schopler, 1992). However, this issue is also part of a broader diagnostic tension. While this tension might be seen as that between research and clinical practice ('service'), it is more appropriately conceptualised as the question of what type of diagnostic error is preferable, i.e., whether false-positive or false-negative cases are of greater concern. If the major concern has to do with securing services for all individuals who might benefit from them, then, of course, the tendency will be to err on the side of overinclusiveness; a disadvantage of this approach is that there is also then potential for diluting available services. However, if the concern is really about identifying cases for research, the impact of false positives looms large. In other words, there is a continuing and appropriate tension between those who lump and those who split. At the moment the splitters tend to dominate, but this may reflect the fact that with an approach somewhat narrower than that employed in DSM–III–R, meaningful distinctions may be drawn in the group of cases who do not seem to exhibit 'classical' autism.

These issues were probably most acute regarding the inclusion of Asperger's syndrome (Asperger, 1944). The relationship of Asperger's syndrome to autism has yet to be clarified, but the disorder is of interest because it may establish areas of continuity between autism and other disorders, while some research suggests important potential differences from autism as well (e.g., in terms of clinical features and increased rates of the disorder in families; Klin & Volkmar, 1997). While there is little controversy that there is indeed a broader PDD phenotype, the question of how Asperger's disorder may best be conceptualised is an open one. It is not uncommon today for researchers and clinicians to use the term in very different ways, e.g., to refer to atypical or sub-threshold autism (PDD–NOS (not otherwise specified)), to adults with autism, to more cognitively able individuals with autism, or to a disorder different from autism. From the point of view of nomenclature it is the last of these views that is most important, but definitive data are lacking.

Similar issues arose with regard to inclusion of Rett's syndrome and 'childhood disintegrative disorders'. There were few concerns about the validity of Rett's syndrome: the issue was whether it should be included as a psychiatric disorder or as a neurological condition (Rutter, 1996). Although there were different views (see Gillberg, 1994; Rutter, 1994), it was clearly important that it be included somewhere. The condition now termed childhood disintegrative disorder (previously termed disintegrative psychosis or Heller's syndrome; Volkmar *et al*, 1997c) was not included in DSM–III or DSM–IV, but had, under a slightly different name, been included in ICD–9. This disorder, first described nearly 100 years ago, is characterised by a marked regression and the development of an 'autistic-like' picture, but only after several years of normal development. The presumption in DSM–III and DSM–III–R was that children with this condition suffered from an identifiable neurological or other progressive process accounting for the deterioration. However, the available literature did not support this view, as such disorders were identified in only a minority of cases. This condition is of interest not because of its frequency, indeed it fortunately is probably rare (Volkmar & Rutter, 1995); rather, the very unusual pattern of onset and distinctive course suggest a potential homogeneity of aetiology, which merits further study and which may have implications for more typical autism.

The area of the broader PDD phenotype is relevant both to service provision and to an understanding of potential genetic mechanisms. As a result of the various genetic studies now underway this issue has assumed greater prominence. It is clear, for example, from Wing & Gould's (1979) epidemiological research that high levels of autistic-like behaviours occur among most individuals with mental handicaps. However, the relationship of these cases to more strictly diagnosed autism remains unclear, because it is in just this group that issues of diagnosis are most complicated and that medical factors are more likely to be aetiologically involved. At the other end of the PDD spectrum there has appropriately been more interest in attempting to disentangle subgroups: in addition to Asperger's disorder, concepts such as

■95

multiplex disorder (Cohen *et al*, 1986), deficits in attention, motor control and perception (DAMP; Hellgren *et al*, 1994) and multiple complex developmental disorder (McKenna *et al*, 1994) have been proposed. Again definitive data are needed.

While considerable advances have been made in this field, and although many aspects of diagnosis and classification are largely settled, some areas of controversy remain. Issues of syndrome boundaries and relationships to basic genetic mechanisms have yet to be clarified. Paradoxically, it may well be that the tendency of the field to move towards more carefully drawn definitions of autism has stimulated interest in conditions that fall just outside it. The advent of assessment tools such as the Autism Diagnostic Interview – Revised (ADI–R; Lord *et al*, 1994) and Autism Diagnostic Observation Schedule – Generic (ADOS–G; DiLavore *et al*, 1995), which are keyed to diagnostic criteria, has also helped increase diagnostic consistency – an issue particularly important for the more ambitious multi-site studies that are now underway at various centres.

Neurobiology

During the 1960s and 1970s a growing body of evidence supported the primacy of biological rather than experiential factors in the pathogenesis of autism. This included the high rates of persistence of primitive reflexes, the delayed development of hand dominance and of so-called 'soft' neurological signs and, as individuals with autism were followed over time, the high rates of emerging seizure disorder, particularly in adolescence (Rutter, 1970; Minshew *et al*, 1997). As the role of organic factors became more clear, attempts were made to associate autism with a host of other medical conditions. The extent and nature of associations has been somewhat controversial. There are claims for very high rates of medical and neurobiological features associated with autism; Gillberg (1992), for example, has argued that more than one-third of cases of autism are associated with such conditions. However, the tendency to publish positive single-case reports, small sample sizes in other studies, issues in ascertainment bias, complexities in making autism diagnoses and ambiguities regarding causal medical conditions may have contributed to these high estimates: careful studies now suggest that, at most, about 10% of cases exhibit such associations (Rutter *et al*, 1994). The two conditions most strongly associated with autism – fragile-X syndrome (Hagerman, 1990) and tuberose sclerosis (Bolton & Griffiths, 1997) – have strong genetic components, and it is this area that appears at present to be of the greatest research interest.

Genetics

In his original description of autism, Kanner (1943) suggested that the syndrome was congenital in nature. Despite this speculation, remarkably little attention was paid to the role of possible genetic factors for many years. In part this reflected the diversion of the field onto issues of diagnosis and early speculations regarding psychogenetic aetiology (Volkmar *et al*, 1997*b*). Furthermore, the condition was rather rare and individuals with autism often did not reproduce. Interest in genetic mechanisms increased as it became clear, following the original Folstein & Rutter (1977*a,b*) twin study, that there was an increased concordance of autism in identical, as opposed to same-gender fraternal, twins. This observation has been replicated in subsequent studies (e.g., Steffenburg *et al*, 1989; Bailey *et al*, 1995), which have consistently revealed higher concordance rates in monozygotic twins. However, although high, the concordance rates were not 100%, which suggested a role for some other factors in pathogenesis. The nature of such a factor or factors is less clear, since the available data do not seem consistently or generally to implicate a role for factors such as obstetric or other complications (Rutter *et al*, 1997).

The role of genetic factors is also suggested by the small but significant increase in rates of autism in non-twin siblings (Rutter *et al*, 1997): at least 2–3% of siblings of a child diagnosed with autism also exhibit the disorder, and a slightly larger number exhibit a broader variety of developmental problems. These rates, compared to the base rate frequency of autism in the population, suggest that the frequency of autism in siblings is increased 50- to 100-fold.

Despite the strong evidence implicating genetic factors, the nature of the underlying predisposition to autism has yet be identified clearly, since it appears that a broad range of difficulties may be seen in other family members. On balance, these difficulties are certainly suggestive of those found, albeit in a much more severe form, in autism. However, while these difficulties are indeed much less overt, they do appear to persist over time and are strong evidence for a broader phenotype (Bolton *et al*, 1994). Important issues of the boundaries of such a broader phenotype remain to be addressed.

Study of the genetics of other conditions within the PDD class are much less advanced than that of autism, but particular interest centres on Asperger's syndrome, given Asperger's observation (1944) that the condition appeared to run in families. The relationship of Asperger's syndrome to autism and the broader phenotype of PDD remains an important topic for research. The most convincing studies are those in which the frequency of Asperger's syndrome is assessed in family members relative to an appropriate comparison group. Preliminary work from our centre (Volkmar *et al*, 1998) using family self-report data has revealed that in a sample of 99 families there was a positive family history of the disorder or something very similar to it in 46% of first-degree relatives. Furthermore, consistent with Asperger's original report, males were affected more frequently than females (19% of fathers *v.* 4% of mothers). The relationship to autism was also highlighted in this study, since 3.5% of siblings were reported to have autism. Data from the study were consistent with the hypothesis that there is a broader phenotype of social and developmental difficulties in family members, but given the preliminary nature of these results the clinical impression of higher rates of the conditions must be regarded as an interesting hypothesis that awaits additional verification.

The nature of the underlying mode of inheritance in autism and related conditions is a topic of much interest. An early study by Ritvo *et al* (1985) seemed to suggest a pattern of autosomal recessive inheritance rather than a more complicated, multi-factorial model. However, more recent work suggests that it is more likely that multiple interacting genes are involved (see Rutter *et al*, 1997). At present, several international studies are addressing these issues using various approaches. Rigorous assessment of the proband and family members is an important aspect of this work and builds on Rutter's earlier studies of diagnosis and classification. Results of these studies should have important implications for both research and clinical work.

■97

The range of methods used to study the non-genetic aspects of autism and related conditions is impressive, but unfortunately the results obtained, at least to date, have been rather less so. There has been a tendency to begin a project with a method or theory without necessarily having a well-formulated research question. As a result, findings often have been inconsistent, unreplicated or sometimes even contradictory (Bailey *et al*, 1996). Considerable interest has centred on both traditional and newer methods of studying the brain and brain–behaviour relations.

Other neurobiological research

Studies using neuroimaging have the potential to clarify both structural and functional aspects of the brain in relation to autism. Unfortunately, results of neuroimaging studies have often been inconsistent. Any of several factors may be responsible. First, of course, it is possible that the brain abnormality in autism is characterised by a diffuse process rather than a localised one, or that present techniques are simply incapable of detecting it. Second, various methodological issues relating to the interpretation of the available results arise because subjects have not always been well characterised, samples have been small and the usual problem intrinsic to false-positive reports arises. Thus, while a few studies have reported focal lesions, these have not been consistent and are therefore probably unrelated to the autistic symptoms (Filipek, 1998).

Given the potential role of the limbic system, it is surprising that to date neuroimaging studies have not identified gross abnormalities in this area (Filipek, 1996). Some findings do appear to be of more consistency and greater interest. Several studies have documented increased head circumference in autism (e.g., Bolton *et al*, 1994; Bailey *et al*, 1998). Others have noted larger cerebral volume, particularly in the temporal, parietal and occipital regions; these appear to be due to increases in white matter (Filipek *et al*, 1992; Piven *et al*, 1995, 1996). It is not yet clear whether increased head size is present at birth or emerges over time (Filipek, 1998).

Various malformations related to disrupted cortical migration have been reported, including polymicrogyria and macrogyria, although these difficulties are not specific with regard to location (Piven *et al*, 1990; Berthier, 1994; Volkmar *et al*, 1996). One of the more intriguing, but still controversial, findings has been the claim for changes reported by Courchesne *et al* (Courchesne *et al*, 1988) in the cerebellum in vermal lobules VI and VII. In general, other groups have not been able to replicate this result (for a discussion see Filipek, 1998, and Piven & Arndt, 1995).

Functional neuroimaging studies are of growing interest in autism, given the opportunities they provide for clarifying relationships between areas of brain activity in response to different tasks (e.g., Chugani *et al*, 1997; Haznedar *et al*, 1997). As Bailey *et al* (1996) noted, it is especially important that results of neuroimaging studies be related to carefully quantified measures of function/dysfunction in autism. Early positron emission tomography (PET) studies have now given way to increasingly sophisticated approaches such as functional magnetic resonance imaging (fMRI). Advances in technology may offer improved methods for clarifying relationships. For example, our group (Schultz *et al*, 2000) has reported abnormalities in areas of cortical activity in higher-functioning individuals with autism or Asperger's syndrome compared with typically developing persons on a facial discrimination task. It should be noted that advances in experimental psychology are no less important here; for example, one would use experimental tasks that are as purely social as possible. This is easier said than done, since paradigms such as 'theory of mind' clearly rely on multiple aspects of the central nervous system, in terms of motor output, verbal mediation and so forth (Happé *et al*, 1996). The difficulties here are, however, not specific to autism – indeed, our understanding of the neurobiological bases of social interaction in normal development remains rather limited (Brothers, 1989; Brothers & Ring, 1992).

Given the severity of the disturbance in autism it might be hoped that abnormalities would be apparent on neuropathological examination. Only a few neuropathological studies have been completed, and it is clear that more are needed. However, given the results of the neuroimaging studies, it is probably not surprising that in general gross neuroanatomy appears normal. Consistent with the reports of larger head circumference, brain weight has been reported to be increased in three of five adults with autism (Bailey *et al*, 1993, 1998). This result differs from that reported by Bauman & Kemper (1997), who did, however, note some neuronal differences and what appeared to be a developmental difference between children and adults with autism. Changes in the forebrain–limbic system, with reduced neuronal size and increased density of neurons, have also been reported (Bauman & Kemper, 1997; Minshew *et al*, 1997), as have neuroanatomical differences in the cerebellum (e.g., Bauman & Kemper, 1994).

Various other neurobiological methods and systems have been studied. Although animal models have been proposed, their practical development is very problematic, given the centrality of social and communicative deficits in the definition and pathophysiology of autism. Probably one of the better animal models relates to the experimental induction of stereotyped movements following administration of stimulant medications that increase levels of the neurotransmitter dopamine, with subsequent administration of dopamine-blocking agents (such as haloperidol), which reduces the movements (Anderson & Hoshino, 1997). Unfortunately this model is, at best, minimally relevant, as studies of dopamine and its metabolites in children with autism have been limited and few systematic differences have been observed (Anderson & Hoshino, 1997). One of the best-replicated neurobiological findings in autism, the high peripheral serotonin level commonly observed (Anderson & Hoshino, 1997), has, to date, lacked meaningful developmental or behavioural correlates.

Treatment

The provision of effective treatments remains of great concern to parents, clinicians and researchers alike. In the first decades of work on autism the mainstay of treatment tended to be relatively unstructured psychotherapy. As children were followed over time and systematic evaluation studies of treatment became available it became evident that structured programmes were much more effective (Lockyer & Rutter, 1969, 1970). The available data continue to indicate that this is the case (Rogers, 1996). Indeed, probably the greatest commonality among treatment programmes that appear to have some degree of efficacy is their reliance on structure and attempts appropriately to focus the child's attention (Rogers, 1996). Behavioural and educational methods remain the major components of treatment (Schreibman, 1997). One of the relative weaknesses in the available literature has been the dearth of more ambitious longer-term studies: those conducted have tended to be of short duration and focused on only one or a small number of interventions. Issues of developmental changes in syndrome expression need to be more carefully considered in intervention research. From the longitudinal studies that are available (Howlin, 1998) it is clear that a small number of individuals with autism did well even before our current armamentarium of treatments was available. This observation also emphasises the importance of systematic and controlled research, past the level of case reports, in interpreting the many claims for cures and dramatic improvement. Thus, the appropriate question is whether a treatment can be systematically applied to a group of individuals in a controlled fashion and be demonstrated to be superior to another intervention or no specific intervention.

In the absence of a definite cause, much less a cure, it is not surprising that claims for dramatic cures continue to appear – seemingly at the rate of about one every 6 months. Few of these are ever systematically evaluated, but some persist none the less, quite independent of any empirical research findings. A distinction needs to be drawn between those treatments that are probably not particularly efficacious but pose little danger to the child and those that may endanger the child's physical well-being or the child's availability for appropriate educational programming. In some cases there may also be a danger for the parents and family in complying with an unusual or demanding treatment programme. While some of the proposed treatments are patently either ridiculous or dangerous, others may be more beguiling. For example, Dr Stanley Greenspan, one proponent of a specific form of therapeutic intervention in the USA, suggests that the parents attempt to follow the child's lead in the intervention programme. While few of us would probably disagree with the importance of using the child's motivation in treatment, the attempt to rely on the child's interests as the mainstay of treatment seems fundamentally wrong. The attempt by the American Academy of Child Psychiatry to provide treatment guidelines for clinicians on the basis of solid, empirical work is a welcome development (Volkmar *et al*, 1999).

A different problem presents itself with regard to the issue of integration of the child with autism into mainstream educational programmes. The battle lines on this issue are poorly drawn, since some argue that all children should be in mainstream settings on a philosophical basis, while others see the question as an empirical one to be guided by the needs of the specific child (Harris & Handleman, 1997). As Rutter has noted (1996), what we need are data that could guide the question of what is right for the individual child.

Although pharmacological interventions can be of benefit for selected target symptoms in autism, they do not seem to address the more fundamental problems of social interaction, communication and cognition. Problem behaviours such as hyperactivity and stereotyped and self-injurious behaviours, and possibly some of the repetitive behaviours more suggestive of obsessive–compulsive disorder, can be effectively treated with medications (McDougle, 1997). Although considerable media attention is focused on the occasional report of a single case or small number of cases, most controlled studies have focused on the major tranquillisers such as haloperidol, or, more recently, the atypical neuroleptics such as risperidone (McDougle, 1997). Important developmental issues remain to be addressed. For example, it appears that there may be differences between children and adults with respect to the efficacy of the selective serotonin reuptake inhibitors. Issues of diagnosis, particularly at the extreme ends of the age and IQ distribution, are a complication for the interpretation of drug and other treatment studies. The issue of pharmacological intervention also raises another topic of current controversy – the approach to comorbidity.

We know that in general comorbidity of psychiatric disorders in children and adolescents is the rule rather than the exception (Angold *et al*, 1999). In autism it is clear that learning disability is a frequently associated condition; it is less clear how and whether other conditions are significantly increased (Ghaziuddin *et al*, 1992). For example, for Asperger's syndrome there have been many reports of associations with numerous other conditions such as schizophrenia and other psychoses, affective disorders, Tourette's syndrome and violent behaviour (Kerbeshian & Burd, 1986; Fujikawa *et al*, 1987; Baron-Cohen, 1988; Ghaziuddin *et al*, 1991). Unfortunately, definitive data that might address this problem are not available, and the reported associations remain impressions rather than established fact. Ultimately, this issue is important for both clinical practice

■99

and research. To some extent, however, particularly in parts of the USA, there is vogue for identifying, and often medicating, many conditions associated with autism. It is clear that the diagnosis of some, if not much, of this alleged comorbidity is fundamentally wrong-headed and mistakes the presence of non-specific symptoms implying the existence of additional syndromes. An important issue here is to clarify these relationships more adequately on the basis of family history and sound epidemiological and other data.

Behavioural and psychological research

In their review of behavioural research in autism Sigman *et al* (1997) has rightly pointed out that the history of the field has essentially paralleled that of developmental psychopathology. Issues of diagnosis complicated early studies. As it became clear that autism was a valid category, behavioural research was helpful in clarifying important issues. For example, some of the apparently highly deviant behaviours of autism, such as echolalia, might have adaptive functions (Prizant *et al*, 1997), and poor performance on tests of intelligence is not due simply to negativism on the part of the child (Klin *et al*, 1997). Investigators turned their attention to the identification of the 'core' deficit in autism – over the years such core deficits have been postulated in a diverse array of psychological functions, including arousal, perception, cognition and language, and, more recently, in social functions as well. It became clear that issues of experiment design were particularly important in the interpretation of this research; for example, as the potential confounders presented by associated learning disability could be disentangled only by use of appropriate comparison groups.

Over the past decade or so, the focus of research has tended to shift more towards the study of social and affective development. Methods and theories from cognitive psychology, such as theory of mind (Baron-Cohen, 1989), executive functioning (Ozonoff *et al*, 1991) and central coherence theory (Happé, 1996), have been used in the attempt to understand the social deficit in autism. Although we have yet to understand this deficit fully, several things have been established. First, the social deficit is evident very early in life, and theories that attempt to account for it must extend back to that time (Volkmar *et al*, 1997a). Second, such theories must account for its persistence over time and across the entire spectrum of dysfunction. Perhaps the study of very young children with autism would present the best opportunity for understanding these phenomena, but unfortunately they are difficult to identify, except in the study of high-risk samples such as siblings of children with autism (Baron-Cohen *et al*, 1996). It is also the case that we do not yet understand all the developmental consequences of the early social deficit and its continuities/discontinuities over time. In my work with individuals who are the most cognitively able, I am impressed both with the persistence and severity of the social deficit and the attempt, on the part of the individual, to make use of whatever skills he or she does have to overcome it.

Summary

A disorder that affects the core of human experience, autism has posed scientific and clinical challenges for theories of developmental psychology and neurobiology as well as for therapy and education. Every conceivable theory of child development has been applied to understanding the enigmatic impairments and competencies of individuals with autism. Autism serves as a paradigmatic disorder for theory testing and research on a wealth of topics: the essential preconditions of normal social development; the expression and recognition of emotions; intersubjectivity; sharing a focus of joint attention; the use and meaning of language; attachments; empathy; and apprehending the minds of others. As we use increasingly sophisticated methods to understand the condition, it is becoming clear that all aspects of the research enterprise are fundamentally interdependent. For example, methods developed to study social behaviour may be useful in the attempt, through neuroimaging, to clarify basic mechanisms of central nervous system functioning; and the identification of different patterns of familial aggregation of conditions other than autism within the families of individuals with autism may provide important clues about more basic relationships between disorders.

As Rutter's work emphasises, it is important that we continue to pay careful attention to both biology and psychology, as well as to the patterns of adaptation that individuals use in an attempt to compensate for their difficulties. Explicating the interaction between genetic and environmental factors in the course of autism will, in the end, bring us back with answers to questions posed by Kanner in his first report of this condition.

American Psychiatric Association (1952) *Diagnostic and Statistical Manual of Mental Disorders* (1st edn) (DSM–I). Washington, DC: APA.

—— (1968) *Diagnostic and Statistical Manual of Mental Disorders* (2nd edn) (DSM–II). Washington, DC: APA.

—— (1980) *Diagnostic and Statistical Manual of Mental Disorders* (3rd edn) (DSM–III). Washington, DC: APA.

—— (1987) *Diagnostic and Statistical Manual of Mental Disorders* (3rd edn, revised) (DSM–III–R). Washington, DC: APA.

—— (1994) *Diagnostic and Statistical Manual of Mental Disorders* (4th edn) (DSM–IV). Washington, DC: APA.

Anderson, G. M. & Hoshino, Y. (1997) Neurochemical studies of autism. In *Handbook of Autism and Pervasive Developmental Disorders* (eds D. J. Cohen & F. R. Volkmar) (2nd edn), pp. 325–343. New York: John Wiley & Sons.

Angold, A., Costello, E. J. & Erkanli, A., (1999) Comorbidity. *Journal of Child Psychology and Psychiatry*, **40**, 57–88.

Asperger, H. (1944) Die 'autistichen Psychopathen' im Kindersalter. *Archive fur Psychiatrie und Nervenkrankheiten*, **117**, 76–136.

Bailey, A., Luthert, P., Bolton, P., *et al* (1993) Autism and megalencephaly. *Lancet*, **341**, 1225–1226.

—— , Le Couteur, A., Gottesman, I., *et al* (1995) Autism as a strongly genetic disorder: evidence from a British twin study. *Psychological Medicine*, **25**, 63–77.

——, Phillips, W. & Rutter, M. (1996) Autism: towards an integration of clinical, genetic, neuropsychological, and neurobiological perspectives (review). *Journal of Child Psychology and Psychiatry*, **37**, 89–126.

—— , Luthert, P., Dean, A., *et al* (1998) A clinicopathological study of autism. *Brain*, **121**, 899–905.

Baron-Cohen, S. (1988) An assessment of violence in a young man with Asperger's syndrome. *Journal of Child Psychology and Psychiatry and Allied Disciplines*, **29**, 351–360.

—— (1989) The theory of mind hypothesis of autism: a reply to Boucher (special issue: Autism). *British Journal of Disorders of Communication*, **24**, 199–200.

—— , Cox, A., Baird, G., *et al* (1996) Psychological markers in the detection of autism in infancy in a large population. *British Journal of Psychiatry*, **168**, 158–163.

Bauman, M. L. & Kemper, T. L. (1994) Neuroanatomic observations of the brain in autism. In *The Neurobiology of Autism* (eds M. L. Bauman & T. L. Kemper), pp. 119–145. Baltimore: Johns Hopkins University Press.

—— & —— (1997) Is autism a progressive process? (abstract). *Neurology*, **48** (suppl.), A285.

Bender, L. (1947) Childhood schizophrenia. *American Journal of Orthopsychiatry*, **17**, 40–56.

Berthier, M. L. (1994) Corticocallosal anomalies in Asperger's syndrome (letter). *American Journal of Roentgenology*, **162**, 236–237.

Bolton, P., Macdonald, H., Pickles, A., *et al* (1994) A case–control family history study of autism. *Journal of Child Psychology and Psychiatry and Allied Disciplines*, **35**, 877–900.

Bolton, P. F. & Griffiths, P. D. (1997) Association of tuberous sclerosis of temporal lobes with autism and atypical autism. *Lancet*, **349**, 392–395.

Brothers, L. (1989) A biological perspective on empathy. *American Journal of Psychiatry*, **146**, 10–19.

—— & Ring, B. (1992) A neuroethological framework for the representation of minds. *Journal of Cognitive Neuroscience*, **4**, 107–118.

Chugani, D. C., Muzik, O., Rothermel, R., *et al* (1997) Altered serotonin synthesis in the dentatothalamocortical pathway in autistic boys. *Annals of Neurology*, **42**, 666–669.

Cohen, D. J., Paul, R. & Volkmar, F. R. (1986) Issues in the classification of pervasive and other developmental disorders: toward DSM–IV. *Journal of the American Academy of Child Psychiatry*, **25**, 213–220.

Courchesne, E., Yeung-Courchesne, R., Press, G. A., *et al* (1988) Hypoplasia of cerebellar vermal lobules VI and VII in autism. *New England Journal of Medicine*, **318**, 1349–1354.

Creak, E. M. (1963) Childhood psychosis: a review of 100 cases. *British Journal of Psychiatry*, **109**, 84–89.

DiLavore, P. C., Lord, C. & Rutter, M. (1995) The pre-linguistic autism diagnostic observation schedule. *Journal of Autism and Developmental Disorders*, **25**, 355–379.

Filipek, P. A. (1996) Structural variations in measures of developmental disorders. In *Developmental Neuroimaging: Mapping the Development of Brain and Behavior* (eds R. W. Thatcher, G. R. Lyon, J. Rumsey, *et al*), pp. 169–186. San Diego, CA: Academic Press.

—— (1999) Neuroimaging in the developmental disorders: the state of the science. *Journal of Child Psychology and Psychiatry and Allied Disciplines*, **40**, 113–128.

——, Richelme, C., Kennedy, D. N., *et al* (1992) Morphometric analysis of the brain in developmental language disorders and autism (abstract). *Annals of Neurology*, **32**, 475.

Folstein, S. & Rutter, M. (1977a) Infantile autism: a genetic study of 21 twin pairs. *Journal of Child Psychology and Psychiatry*, **18**, 297–321.

—— & —— (1977b) Genetic influences and infantile autism. *Nature*, **265**, 726–728.

Fujikawa, H., Kobayashi, R., Koga, Y., *et al* (1987) A case of Asperger's syndrome in a nineteen-year-old who showed psychotic breakdown with depressive state and attempted suicide after entering university. *Japanese Journal of Child and Adolescent Psychiatry*, **28**, 217–225.

■ 101

Ghaziuddin, M., Tsai, L. Y. & Ghaziuddin, N. (1991) Brief report: violence in Asperger syndrome. A critique. *Journal of Autism and Developmental Disorders*, **21**, 349–354.

—, — & — (1992) Comorbidity of autistic disorder in children and adolescents. *European Child and Adolescent Psychiatry*, **1**, 209–213.

Gillberg, C. (1991) Debate and argument: is autism a pervasive developmental disorder? *Journal of Child Psychology and Psychiatry and Allied Disciplines*, **32**, 1169–1170.

— (1994) Debate and argument: having Rett syndrome in the ICD–10 PDD category does not make sense. *Journal of Child Psychology and Psychiatry and Allied Disciplines*, **35**, 377–378.

Gillberg, C. L. (1992) Subgroups in autism: are there behavioural phenotypes typical of underlying medical conditions? *Journal of Intellectual Disability Research*, **36**, 201–214.

Hagerman, R. J. (1990) The association between autism and fragile X syndrome. *Brain Dysfunction*, **3**, 218–227.

Happé, F. G. (1996) Studying weak central coherence at low levels: children with autism do not succumb to visual illusions. A research note. *Journal of Child Psychology and Psychiatry*, **37**, 873–877.

—, Ehlers, S., Fletcher, P., *et al* (1996) 'Theory of mind' in the brain. Evidence from a PET scan study of Asperger syndrome. *Neuroreport*, **8**, 197–201.

Harris, S. L. & Handleman, J. S. (1997) Helping children with autism enter the mainstream. In *Handbook of Autism and Pervasive Developmental Disorders* (eds D. J. Cohen & F. R. Volkmar) (2nd edn), pp. 665–675. New York: John Wiley & Sons.

Haznedar, M. M., Buchsbaum, M. S., Metzger, M., *et al* (1997) Anterior cingulate gyrus volume and glucose metabolism in autistic disorder. *American Journal of Psychiatry*, **154**, 1047–1050.

Hellgren, L., Gillberg, C. & Gillberg, I. C. (1994) Children with deficits in attention, motor control and perception (damp) almost grown up: the contribution of various backgrounds to outcome at age 16 years. *European Child and Adolescent Psychiatry*, **3**, 1–15.

Howlin, P. (2000) Outcome in adult life for more able individuals with autism or Asperger syndrome. *Autism*, **4**, 63–83.

Kanner, L. (1943) Autistic disturbances of affective contact. *Nervous Child*, **2**, 217–250.

Kerbeshian, J. & Burd, L. (1986) Asperger's syndrome and Tourette syndrome: the case of the pinball wizard. *British Journal of Psychiatry*, **148**, 731–736.

Klin, A. & Volkmar, F. R. (1997) Asperger syndrome. In *Handbook of Autism and Pervasive Developmental Disorders* (eds D. J. Cohen & F. R. Volkmar) (2nd edn), pp. 94–122. New York: John Wiley & Sons.

—, Carter, A., Volkmar, F. R., *et al* (1997) Assessment issues in children with autism. In *Handbook of Autism and Pervasive Developmental Disorders* (eds D. J. Cohen & F. R. Volkmar) (2nd edn), pp. 411–418. New York: John Wiley & Sons.

Kolvin, I. (1971) Studies in the childhood psychoses. I. Diagnostic criteria and classification. *British Journal of Psychiatry*, **118**, 381–384 .

Lockyer, L. & Rutter, M. (1969) A five- to fifteen-year follow-up study of infantile psychosis. III. Psychological aspects. *British Journal of Psychiatry*, **115**, 865–882.

— & — (1970) A five to fifteen-year follow-up study of infantile psychosis. IV. Patterns of cognitive ability. *British Journal of Social and Clinical Psychology*, **9**, 152–163.

Lord, C., Rutter, M. & Le Couteur, A. (1994) Autism Diagnostic Interview–Revised: a revised version of a diagnostic interview for caregivers of individuals with possible pervasive developmental disorders. *Journal of Autism and Developmental Disorders*, **24**, 659–685.

McDougle, C. J. (1997) Psychopharmacology. In *Handbook of Autism and Pervasive Developmental Disorders* (eds D. J. Cohen & F. R. Volkmar) (2nd edn), pp. 707–729. New York: John Wiley & Sons.

McKenna, K., Gordon, C. T. & Rapoport, J. L. (1994) Childhood-onset schizophrenia: timely neurobiological research. *Journal of the American Academy of Child and Adolescent Psychiatry*, **33**, 771–781.

Minshew, N. J., Sweeney, J. A. & Bauman, M. L. (1997) Neurological aspects of autism. In *Handbook of Autism and Pervasive Developmental Disorders* (eds D. J. Cohen & F. R. Volkmar) (2nd edn), pp. 344–369. New York: John Wiley & Sons.

Ozonoff, S., Pennington, B. F. & Rogers, S. J. (1991) Executive function deficits in high-functioning autistic individuals: relationship to theory of mind. *Journal of Child Psychology and Psychiatry and Allied Disciplines*, **32**, 1081–1105.

Piven, J. & Arndt, S. (1995) The cerebellum and autism (letter). *Neurology*, **45**, 398–399.

—, Berthier, M. L., Starkstein, *et al* (1990) Magnetic resonance imaging evidence for a defect of cerebral cortical development in autism. *American Journal of Psychiatry*, **147**, 734–739.

—, Arndt, S., Bailey, J., *et al* (1995) An MRI study of brain size in autism. *American Journal of Psychiatry*, **152**, 1145–1149.

—, —, —, *et al* (1996) Regional brain enlargement in autism: a magnetic resonance imaging study. *Journal of the American Academy of Child and Adolescent Psychiatry*, **35**, 530–536.

Prizant, B. M., Schuller, A. L., Wetherby, A. M., *et al* (1997) Enhancing language and communication development: language approaches. In *Handbook of Autism and Pervasive Developmental Disorders* (eds D. J. Cohen & F. R. Volkmar) (2nd edn), pp. 572–605. New York: John Wiley & Sons.

Ritvo, E. R., Spence, M. A., Freeman, B. J., *et al* (1985) Evidence for autosomal recessive inheritance in 46 families with multiple incidences of autism. *American Journal of Psychiatry*, **142**, 187–192.

Rogers, S. J. (1966) Brief report: early intervention in autism. *Journal of Autism and Developmental Disorders*, **26**, 243–246.

Rutter, M. (1970) Autistic children: infancy to adulthood. *Seminars in Psychiatry*, **2**, 435–450.

—— (1972) Childhood schizophrenia reconsidered. *Journal of Autism and Childhood Schizophrenia*, **2**, 315–337.

—— (1978) Diagnosis and definitions of childhood autism. *Journal of Autism and Developmental Disorders*, **8**, 139–161.

—— (1994) Debate and argument: there are connections between brain and mind and it is important that Rett syndrome be classified somewhere. *Journal of Child Psychology and Psychiatry and Allied Disciplines*, **35**, 379–381.

—— (1996) Autism research: prospects and priorities (review). *Journal of Autism and Developmental Disorders*, **26**, 257–275.

—— (1998) The Emmanuel Miller Memorial Lecture 1988. Autism: two-way interplay between research and clincial work. *Journal of Child Psychology and Psychiatry and Allied Disciplines*, **409**, 169–188.

—— & Schopler, E. (1992) Classification of pervasive developmental disorders: some concepts and practical considerations (special issue: Classification and diagnosis). *Journal of Autism and Developmental Disorders*, **22**, 459–482.

—— & Shaffer, D. (1980) DSM–III: a step forward or back in terms of the classification of child psychiatric disorders? *Journal of the American Academy of Child Psychiatry*, **19**, 371–394.

——, Bailey, A., Bolton, P., *et al* (1994) Autism and known medical conditions: myth and substance (review). *Journal of Child Psychology and Psychiatry*, **35**, 311–322.

——, ——, Simonoff, E., *et al* (1997) Genetic influences in autism. In *Handbook of Autism and Pervasive Developmental Disorders* (eds D. J. Cohen & F. R. Volkmar) (2nd edn), pp. 370–387. New York: John Wiley & Sons.

Schreibman, L. (1997) Theoretical perspectives on behvaioural intervention for individuals with autism. In *Handbook of Autism and Pervasive Developmental Disorders* (eds D. Cohen & F. Volkmar), pp. 920–933. New York: John Wiley & Sons.

Schultz, R. T., Gauthier, I., Volkmar, F., *et al* (2000) Abnormal ventral temporal cortical activity during face discrimination among individuals with autism and Asperger syndrome [see comments]. *Archives of General Psychiatry*, **57**, 331–340.

Sigman, M., Dissanayake, C., Arbelle, S., *et al* (1997) Cognition and emotion in children and adolescents with autism. In *Handbook of Autism and Pervasive Developmental Disorders* (eds D. J. Cohen & F. R. Volkmar) (2nd edn), pp. 248–265. New York: John Wiley & Sons.

Steffenburg, S., Gillberg, C., Helgren, L., *et al* (1989) A twin study of autism in Denmark, Finland, Iceland, Norway, and Sweden. *Journal of Child Psychology and Psychiatry*, **30**, 405–416.

Szatmari, P. (1992) A review of the DSM–III–R criteria for autistic disorder (special issue: Classification and diagnosis). *Journal of Autism and Developmental Disorders*, **22**, 507–523.

Volkmar, F. R. & Cohen, D. J. (1991) Debate and argument: the utility of the term pervasive developmental disorder. *Journal of Child Psychology and Psychiatry and Allied Disciplines*, **32**, 1171–1172.

—— & Rutter, M. (1995) Childhood disintegrative disorder: results of the DSM–IV autism field trial. *Journal of the American Academy of Child and Adolescent Psychiatry*, **34**, 1092–1095.

——, Klin, A., Siegel, B., *et al* (1994) Field trial for autistic disorder in DSM–IV. *American Journal of Psychiatry*, **151**, 1361–1367.

——, ——, Schultz, R., *et al* (1996) Asperger's syndrome (clinical conference). *Journal of the American Academy of Child and Adolescent Psychiatry*, **35**, 118–123.

——, Carter, A., Grossman, J., *et al* (1997*a*) Social development in autism. In *Handbook of Autism and Pervasive Developmental Disorders* (eds D. J. Cohen & F. R. Volkmar) (2nd edn), pp. 173–194. New York: John Wiley & Sons.

——, Klin, A. & Cohen, D. J. (1997*b*) Diagnosis and classificiation of autism and related conditions: consensus and issues. In *Handbook of Autism and Pervasive Developmental Disorders* (eds D. J. Cohen & F. R. Volkmar) (2nd edn), pp. 5–40. New York: John Wiley & Sons.

——, ——, Marans, W., *et al* (1997*c*) Childhood disintegrative disorder. In *Handbook of Autism and Pervasive Developmental Disorders* (eds D. J. Cohen & F. R. Volkmar) (2nd edn), pp. 47–59. New York: John Wiley & Sons.

——, ——, Pauls, D. (1998) Nosological and genetic aspects of Asperger syndrome. *Journal of Autism and Developmental Disorders*, **28**, 457–463.

——, Cook, E., Pomeroy, J. , *et al* (1999) Practice parameters for the assessment and treatment of children, adolescents, and adults with autism and other pervasive developmental disorders. *Journal of the American Academy of Child and Adolescent Psychiatry*, **38** (suppl. 12), 32S–54S.

Werry, J. (1996) Childhoood schizophrenia. In *Psychoses and Pervasive Developmental Disorders in Childhood and Adolescence* (ed. F. R. Volkmar). Washington, D.C.: American Psychiatric Press.

Wing, L. & Gould, J. (1979) Severe impairments of social interaction and associated abnormalities. *Journal of Autism and Developmental Disorders*, **9**, 11–29.

World Health Organization (1994) *Diagnostic Criteria for Research* (10th edn) (ICD–10). Geneva: WHO.

7 Classification and categorisation revisited

David Shaffer

In 1965 Michael Rutter published his paper 'Classification and categorisation in child psychiatry" (Rutter, 1965). I would like to use this occasion to review that very important paper and to highlight Rutter's really extraordinary contribution to psychiatric nosology.

Classical beginings

Throughout the history of medical classification there has been a tension between scientists and naturalists who have simply listed what they see and philosophers and theoreticians who have sought to fit their observations to some grander organising principle. This is not to say that the inventories or lists of the observers are without order, but the order is usually based on apparent similarities and differences, rather than on any purported underlying mechanism. This tension between simple nomenclature and grand classification can be traced back to early Greece. Hippocrates – very much a list-maker – is quoted as saying,

> "Whoever having undertaken to speak or write on Medicine, have assumed for themselves some hypothesis to their argument, such as hot, or cold, or moist, or dry, or whatever else they choose (thus reducing their subject within a narrow compass, and supposing only one or two original causes of death among mankind), are manifestly in error in many of their novelties." (Longrigg, 1998: p. 51)

Hippocrates' nomenclature was simple and descriptive, no more than a list, uninformed by any of the theory-based systems that would, in later years, do so much to obscure rather than clarify understanding. His list included symptoms such as spitting of blood, as well as conditions like asthma and epilepsy. The psychiatric conditions were also simple comparisons, symptoms such as 'frightful dreams', or more comprehensive but no less observable phenomena such as 'madness' and 'melancholy'. Aristotle, who authored the first hierarchical classification of living things, was a child when Hippocrates died. He was clearly more imaginative, possibly more self-important than the venerable physician (Pellegrin, 1987), for whom he had limited admiration: "Hippocrates is an excellent geometer but a complete fool in everyday affairs" (Aristotle, edn 1981). In *Topics*, Aristotle outlines the principles of classification, believing that "perfect description and definition is the summit of human knowledge in every part of science". The debate between simple descriptive nomenclature and theory-based, hierarchical classifications had started. It continues to this day.

In the mid-18th century, Boissier de Sauvages (1760) published his *Nosologia Methodica*, which followed hierarchical rules, with orders being subdivided into sections, classes, genera, species and varieties. De Sauvage's classification included 10 classes of disease (giving salient features such as wasting, fever, weakness and pain), 44 orders, 350 genera and a great many more species and varieties. In 1769, William Cullen, the Scottish physician and the first person to use the word 'neurosis' (Knoff, 1970), published his *Synopsis and Nosology*, which was informed by ideas of nervous energy (Cullen, 1792). In 1796, Erasmus Darwin, Charles Darwin's physician grandfather, introduced his own classification, also influenced by ideas of nervous forces, with only four classes: diseases of irritation, sensation, volition and association (Darwin 1809).

These early hierarchical classifications were examples of how unproven theses informed the whole system. They were based at worst on assumed aetiological or physiological relationships and at best on descriptive groups whose similarities concealed considerable differences. These classification systems could and did influence practice. Cullen, in an oration to the Royal College of Medicine, stated,

> "The distinction of the genera of diseases, the distinction of the species of each, and often that of the varieties, I hold to be a necessary foundation of every plan of physic whether medical or empirical." (Gouley, 1888: p. 75)

Cullen was clearly aware of the limitations of these approaches and warned:

> "The structure of genera is an effect of the human mind, which till the species are well known and understood must be fallacious and uncertain." (Gouley, 1888: p. 181)

He also cautioned against classifying different levels of severity as different diseases, a lesson that might be relevant to the way that we differentiate between oppositional-defiant disorder and conduct disorder, and autism and Asperger's syndrome. Dr Parr, author of the *London Medical Dictionary* (1819), objected to prevailing classifications on more pragmatic grounds:

> "An order is an association of genera; but orders are usually too comprehensive, including too great a number of genera; and to facilitate investigation, these are often divided into separate groups which is a proof of imperfection in arrangement." (Gouley, 1888: p. 187)

In a voice that would have been welcomed by the early critics of DSM–III and ICD–9, Parr said, "it is said that nature created only species: it is not true; for she has created only individuals" (Gouley, 1888: p. 185). A strong environmentalist, he concluded that,

> "Individuals differ as a result of circumstances arising from accident … from soil and climate … from constitution … from local varieties … and … when circumstances are changed return to the species from which they started." (Gouley, 1888: pp. 185–186)

Grand schemes continued to issue forth, and many included disorders of the mind. In 1822, Good, considered one of the greatest of 19th-century nosologists, published a system with a class of 'neurotica' (diseases of nervous function) (Fig. 7.1). Good (1824) had a particular penchant for combined categories, including priapism with wry neck, as his preferred solution to the nosological problem of how to deal with the co-occurrence of different conditions.

Classical nosology did not prosper during the latter half of the 19th century, perhaps because scientific discoveries challenged their theoretic assumptions, or perhaps because no particular system of classification had been officially endorsed by the profession. There was also a good deal of healthy scepticism over the pretensions of classificatory models. In 1864, Sir William Aitken, in *Science and Practice of Medicine*, cynically pointed to the various dimensions that had at one time or another been the basis of classification, i.e., aetiology, the nature of the pathological process, the structural effect of the disorder, the functional effect of the disorder and the disease's anatomical location.

```
┌─────────────────────────────────────────────┐
│           GOOD'S TABLE OF CLASSIFICATION.     │
│                                               │
│              CLASS. IV. NEUROTICA,            │
│           Diseases of the nervous function.   │
│                                               │
│                ORD. I. PHRENICA,              │
│              Affecting the intellect.         │
│                                               │
│               Gen. I. Ecphronia,              │
│               Insanity, Craziness.            │
│          Spec.1. E. Melancholia, (Melancholy.)│
│           Spec. 2. E. Mania, (Madness.)       │
│                                               │
│               Gen. II. Empathema,             │
│              Ungovernable passion.            │
│     Spec. 1. E. Entonicum, (Empassioned excitement.) │
│     Spec. 2. E. Atonicum, (Empassioned depression.)  │
│       Spec. 3. E. Inane, (Hare-brained passion.)     │
│                                               │
│                Gen. III. Alusia,              │
│             Illusion, Hallucination.          │
│   Spec. 1. A. Elation, (Sentimentalism, Mental extravagence.) │
│   Spec. 2. A. Hypochondrias (Hypochondrism, Low spirits.)     │
│                                               │
│               Gen. IV. Aphelxia,              │
│                     Revery.                   │
│       Spec. 1. A. Socors, (Absence of mind.)  │
│       Spec. 2. A. Intenta, (Abstraction of mind.) │
│         Spec. 3. A. Otiosa, (Brown-study.)    │
│                                               │
│               Gen. V. Paroniria,              │
│               Sleep-disturbance.              │
│       Spec. 1. P. Ambulans, (Sleep-walking.)  │
│       Spec. 2. P. Loquens, (Sleep-talking.)   │
│       Spec. 3. P. Salax, (Night-pollution.)   │
│                                               │
│                Gen. VI. Moria,                │
│                    Fatuity.                   │
│       Spec. 1. M. Imbecillis, (Imbecility.)   │
│       Spec. 2. M. Demens, (Irrationality.)    │
└─────────────────────────────────────────────┘
```

Fig. 7.1 Good's classification of disorders of the mind (Gouley, 1888).

Stripped of any theoretical underpinnings, British nomenclatures were presented to the Statistical Congresses of the European Nations in Paris (1855) and Vienna (1857) and were favourably received. In 1859, the Royal College of Physicians of London appointed William Farr, Registrar General and founder of modern epidemiology, to preside over an endeavour that would take 10 years and produce a nomenclature of 1146 diseases (Royal College of Physicians of London, 1869). Farr, a practical man, commented that, despite the great academic interest in classification, nomenclatures were rarely consulted by practising physicians. In the best tradition of English common sense, he proposed a simple listing that would not disguise its imperfections. His classification was translated into six languages and remained influential 50 years later (Royal College of Physicians of London, 1918).

The Royal College's nomenclature was seized on eagerly by others. The United States Marine Hospital Service adopted it in 1879, and the New York State Board of Health shortly thereafter (State Board of Health of New York, 1883). A home-grown version was prepared in 1872 by the American Medical Association (AMA; unpublished), but it was extensively criticised and as a result the AMA resolved to meet jointly with the Royal College in London. In this last show of imperial influence, the College lent its imprimatur to a revised edition that met with American approval.

John Gouley, surgeon to Bellevue Hospital, acknowledging his debt to botanists and mineralogists, despaired of contemporary classification systems, complaining that,

"the words, groups, sections, classes, orders ... are so loosely and carelessly employed that it is difficult to understand the meaning these terms are intended to convey". (Gouley, 1888: p. 215)

In a last ditch effort to bring back 'true classifications', Gouley proposed his own system, *Diseases of Man* (1888). This was prefaced with aphorisms such as "to think is to classify and to classify is to think" (p. 2) and "the perfection of a science depends, in no inconsiderable degree, from the perfection of its language; and the perfection of every language upon its simplicity and precision" (p. 2). Alas, his attempt found little favour.

The 20th century

A British proposal to establish an International List of Causes of Death was passed at the International Statistical Institute meeting in Chicago (1893) and was subsequently accepted at a meeting convened by the government of France in Paris. By 1907 this nomenclature had been adopted by most developed countries (International Commission, 1909). Despite their role in its creation, insular Britain, and with it the British Empire, held out until 1909, preferring a derivation of William Farr's original Royal College of Physicians classification system (Royal College of Physicians of London, 1918). The *International List of Causes of Death* (ILCD) was a great success perhaps because it made no pretension of being a proper classification of diseases; it was a simple working nomenclature. The ILCD contained little of psychiatric interest, for mental illness was rarely an immediate cause of death.

Despite the momentous contributions to classification of psychiatric disorders by Kraepelin (1883), Bleuler (1911) and Jaspers (1913), psychiatric, and indeed medical, nosology was, for most physicians at the turn of the 19th century, a parochial matter. Psychiatric training took place in large hospitals and asylums, and each of these had its own method of naming and ordering disorders for statistical purposes. Because they attended mainly to in-patients, these lists overrepresented psychotic conditions and 'mental retardation' (learning disability). The *Terminology of Disease* for the Vanderbilt Clinic of Columbia University (Lambert & Martin, 1910) included a section of 'diseases of the mind' that was confined to various forms of mental retardation, mania, melancholia, paranoia and insanity. The *Bellevue Hospital Nomenclature* (Bellevue, 1911) emerged as the most influential of the North American systems, ultimately becoming the basis of the *Nomenclature of Diseases and Conditions* distributed by the US Public Health Service (1916). These hospital-based nomenclatures were provided to trainees, who in due course disseminated them when they moved out to new practices or hospitals. This process often resulted in minor changes and adaptations so that over time even related systems became inconsistent (Raines, 1951). To address the lack of a uniform nomenclature in psychiatry, the American Psychiatric Association (APA) developed a standard reporting nomenclature in 1917.

In 1929, a conference of expert statisticians was held in Berlin under the auspices of the League of Nations. It resolved that member nations should develop a list of terms, diseases and pathological conditions to help identify disparate prevalences of disease from countries and to facilitate international good health (Emerson & Baehr, 1933). In the USA, at the invitation of the New York Academy of Medicine, a national conference on the nomenclature of disease was held in 1928, with the participation of leading professional associations and physicians drawn from the main teaching hospitals in the country. The president of the conference noted,

> "Hospitals, health organizations, and insurance companies have been obliged to devise their own nomenclatures or, having borrowed an existing one, have promptly proceeded to modify it beyond recognition. A confusing multiplicity of effort has been due to the absence of any central guiding influence … [T]he terminology employed has represented the personal choice of the author and has, therefore, been open to individual criticism and continuous alteration. In none of the existing nomenclatures has a logical plan been followed consistently throughout. If an anatomical arrangement was adopted so as to satisfy the needs of some of the specialists, the original plan was forsaken in places for purely etiological function, epidemiological or less important considerations." (Emerson & Baehr, 1933: p. xi)

In a laudably democratic style, the draft nomenclature – which was to be the forerunner of the International Classification of Diseases – was distributed to the leading

■107

hospitals in the USA and Canada, and feedback was solicited from the users. The psychobiological section of the system inferred subconscious mechanisms for most of the disorders, and the section on neurotic traits included sleep walking, stammering, overactivity and fears. The nomenclature was eventually endorsed by a host of different associations and, with support from the Commonwealth Fund and the New York Academy of Medicine, was widely distributed (National Conference on Nomenclature of Disease, 1933; Standard Nomenclature of Disease, 1933, 1935; American Medical Association, 1942). However, the new system was still primarily oriented to in-patients, and categories such as 'psychopathic personality' or 'psychoneurosis' became overused and lost their value.

The DSM and ICD systems

In 1950, the American Psychiatric Association and Morton Kramer, chief of the biometrics branch of the recently formed National Institute for Mental Health (NIMH), formed a committee of psychiatrists to develop the first Diagnostic and Statistical Manual, DSM–I (American Psychiatric Association, 1952). Following the precedent established by the earlier Standard Nomenclature, it was sent out for review to a representative sample of psychiatrists before being adopted. DSM–I was aetiologically based, delegating psychogenicity to disorders 'without clearly defined physical cause'. Reflecting the weight of psychodynamic influences at the time, both 'mental retardation' and enuresis were grouped as 'adjustment reactions', but in general DSM acknowledged the lack of evidence for the causes of many disorders.

In 1966, the Group for the Advancement of Psychiatry prepared a classification system for child and adolescent psychiatry. Although it was more extensive than DSM–I or –II (American Psychiatric Association, 1968), it was conceptually unsystematic, using both aetiological and descriptive behavioural categories, and included arcane groups such as lymphemic disorders ('disorders of the lymph system that might give rise to psychiatric disorders'). The classification never gained widespread acceptance.

In 1968, the eighth version of the International Classification of Diseases (ICD–8; World Health Organization, 1968) appeared, with only a single category for child psychiatric disorders, lucidly entitled 'psychiatric disorders of childhood'. This extremely reliable, but completely uninformative category signalled to the rest of the world that the disorders of children and adolescents had not been sufficiently explored to merit classification.

Some of Rutter's greatest papers have been those that brought clarity to an area rife with conflicting opinions and concepts. It was clear that the field of classification was in such a state when, in 1965, he published his paper 'Classification and categorisation in child psychiatry' in the *Journal of Child Psychology and Psychiatry* (Rutter, 1965). This classic paper in child psychiatry is as relevant now as when it was written, and it remains, unfortunately, ahead of its time. Its opening paragraph made a persuasive case for classification, and the justification he offered went beyond the uncontroversial goal of facilitating communication. It added an argument that had not previously been voiced, that is the heuristic value of a nomenclature:

> "Until a disorder can be identified and characterised, it cannot be adequately studied. This means that we cannot wait for more information to become available before we develop a classification. Indeed, if we do wait, such information is not likely to be forthcoming." (Rutter, 1965: p. 71)

He seems to be calling for an approach that falls between the creative but overauthoritative approach of 18th-century classifications and the cautious, conservative list-making that followed and prevailed up to and including ICD–8, with its single parsimonious and uninformative category. It heralded a period in which psychiatric classification, equipped with adequately defined entities in carefully constructed glossaries, provided the energy for new discoveries. The disorders defined in the new classifications not only reflect past research; they have become the focus of research that, in some cases, results in confirmation and, in others, in refutation. It is unlikely that this focused cycle of research, change in criteria and then further research would have taken place without the heuristic engine of ICD–9 and –10 and DSM–III and –IV.

Table 7.1 Rutter's classification of childhood psychiatric disorders (Rutter, 1965)

No.	Classification
1	Neurotic disorders
2	Antisocial or conduct disorders
3	Mixed group
4	Developmental disorders
5	The hyperkinetic syndrome
6	Child psychosis
7	Psychosis developing at or after puberty
8	Mental subnormality
9	Educational retardation as a primary problem
10	Depression
11	Adult-type neurotic illnesses
12	Normal variation

Rutter's early classification system was fairly simple (Table 7.1). It included two valuable categories that have been ignored by the subsequent systems. The first is a coding for 'normal variation', which allows the user to assign a neutral code. This reduces the likelihood of coding an inaccurate category or of not assigning any category. The second is 'manifestation of mental subnormality only', which allows learning disability ('mental retardation') and its manifestations to be coded separately from psychiatric disorder.

After the publication of this paper, Rutter worked closely with the World Health Organization to ensure that ICD–9 would venture beyond ICD–8. In the meantime, American investigators had been developing techniques, such as the Research Diagnostic Criteria (RDC; Spitzer *et al*, 1977), to select homogeneous populations to participate in multi-site studies. The RDC became the model of a criterion-based, operationally defined nomenclature on which the APA's DSM–III would be based. The process, begun in 1974 under the leadership of Robert Spitzer, culminated in 1979 with the introduction of DSM–III (American Psychiatric Association, 1980). In the short term, this event had an arguably greater effect on American psychiatry than even the introduction of the more important types of psychotropic medication. It stimulated an explosion of diagnosis-specific treatment and natural-history research, but, more important, it also contributed to the decline of highly speculative, often unprovable aetiological formulations.

It is interesting to see how DSM–III followed the precepts outlined in Rutter's paper of 15 years earlier. DSM–III was proudly atheoretical. Spitzer had decided that there was insufficient knowledge to resolve disputes about aetiology and the basic causes of most mental illnesses, and so aetiological concepts were to be avoided, except in the case of adjustment disorder and disorders due to a pre-existing medical condition. Other innovations that surprised clinicians were the inclusion of operationally defined criteria with specific severity and frequency thresholds, a very detailed and authoritative text and glossary, the statement that this was a classification of disorders and not of people, and the field studies that were carried out before the system was introduced.

When DSM–III was introduced in the USA it provoked a certain indignation, if not outrage. Psychologists claimed that the DSM promoted a 'medical' model, because it was a product of a psychiatric organisation, and that it ignored the contributions of psychologists. This was untrue. There were many psychologists on the editorial board, and they had played a key role in formulating new definitions. There was widespread concern that a DSM–III diagnosis would label people and that, if the label carried a bad prognosis, it would make it difficult for patients to gain access to treatment or educational or employment opportunities. Psychodynamically oriented clinicians criticised it for promoting a simplistic or reductive approach to diagnostic formulation and treatment, while academics reproached it for its overauthoritative style.

Paradoxically, some of the most persuasive rebuttals to these objections could have been found in Rutter's 'Classification and categorisation in child psychiatry' (1965). To claims that the DSM enriched or enhanced a medical model of psychiatric disorder Spitzer, quoting Rutter (1965), might have replied: "Classification in no way implies the existence of disease entities" (p. 71), giving as an example, "Continuities of personality characteristics or temperament or maturational level may be classified just as

■ 109

illness can" (pp. 72–73). To those who complained that the system reduced the complexity and diversity of individual patients to a set of common criteria:

> "It would be a retrograde step to regard every patient as entirely individual ... A diagnostic classification should be able to convey important and relevant information about the patient, but one should not expect it to say all that is relevant or important. Classification is not the same as a diagnostic formulation... The aim is to classify disorders, not to classify children." (pp. 72–73)

To those who expressed concern about operational criteria:

> "If the classification is to be acceptable, it must be based on fact, not concepts. It must be defined in operational terms." (p. 73)

One might have thought that Rutter would have welcomed DSM–III, and I think that in many ways he did. But his style is gentlemanly and diffident, and there was a brash, overconfident quality to DSM–III that both he and I found disturbing. He suggested we write a paper (Rutter & Shaffer, 1980). We pointed out that the DSM included many categories that had never been validated; that its precision on matters of frequency, severity and duration – which were never presented as heuristic, only as authoritative – was pseudoscientific; and that the various thresholds proposed were arbitrary and had no empirical basis. We stated that the manual's overauthoritative tone would promote its use as a definitive textbook. Given our special interest in multi-axial approaches to classification (Rutter *et al*, 1975), we expressed disappointment at the way that multiple axes were being permitted but not required.

In retrospect, my judgement is that Rutter's 1965 paper was closer to being correct and that some of the concerns about the arbitrariness of the categories, criteria and thresholds were the very things that enhanced the value of DSM–III. Less precisely defined criteria would have been insufficient to confirm or disprove the proposed disorders and would have strengthened the hand of inarticulate clinicians who would rely on subjective and intuitive feelings. Paradoxically, DSM–III's arbitrary precision became one of its greatest strengths.

Preparing for DSM–IV

The criticisms made in our paper and by many others were taken seriously. Together, the response to DSM–III influenced the development of DSM–IV (American Psychiatric Association, 1994; Shaffer 1996).

It had been said that DSM–III was written by a few people around a table, with little input from the wider mental health community. There may have been some truth in this. I remember being invited to a DSM–III–R meeting. I had the dubious distinction of being the only psychiatrist in the USA who had an interest in enuresis and was called in to give an opinion on the elimination-disorder categories. I entered the meeting while another disorder was being discussed. The atmosphere was heated, closer to my idea of a tobacco auction then to a scholarly debate. Bob Spitzer, the auctioneer, stood at the head of a long table, crowded with experts, as if looking for bids. Janet Williams sat at his side, with what was then considered a portable computer, the size of a large suitcase, busily recording the proceedings. Spitzer would put forward a suggestion or a question and would wait for the bids to come in. At the end of the day, he and Williams would repair to their office and rewrite the text and criteria in the spirit of whatever gestalt his formidable intelligence had taken from the meeting. This process was sound but not systematic. A consensus of some kind had emerged, and Spitzer did his best to capture it. The process also resulted in a uniform style and approach and avoided the pain of writing by committee.

However, concerns about the lack of 'democratic process' led the APA to approach DSM–IV differently. The DSM–IV committees were told to obtain wide consultation before making their recommendations. Magda Campbell and I were appointed co-chairs of the child and adolescent committee, and we established an intricate system of expert subcommittees for each disorder (see American Psychiatric Association, 1997, 1998).

We travelled around the country to various professional meetings, speaking not only to child psychiatrists, but also to psychologists and paediatricians, describing the committee's proposals and the thinking behind them. The APA published an excellent options book (American Psychiatric Association, 1991) that listed different solutions for classifying different disorders; we distributed it widely and invited comments and criticisms. Although the options book was a fine idea, it elicited very little feedback, at least in the child psychiatry field. Over the course of the 5-year process, we received only about a dozen letters, nearly all from professionals interested in dissociative disorders, who would probably have approved a step back to ICD–8 with the difference that the sole category would be 'dissociative disorders of childhood'. Our own group was also, of course, vulnerable to the usual group processes. Some committee members were more sensitive than others or appeared to have a vested interest in certain diagnostic formulations. They were dismissive of data that conflicted with their views and when few data were available would hold sway. Some distinguished members had forceful personalities and with a withering look or sarcastic comment could effectively curtail discussion. Finally, a certain amount of rewriting took place by the lead editors. This was most often useful, but could sometimes lead to errors, as happened in the 'pervasive developmental disorders' (PDD) category.

The APA also responded to the protests about the short interval between the appearance of the DSM–III and DSM–III–R, and the impact of frequent changes to the systems. There were unfair and untrue allegations that it had been introduced simply to sell more books and make more money, and that the changes had been arbitrary and poorly substantiated. There were to be no changes from DSM–III–R unless they were well grounded in science and well substantiated in the literature. To that end, a series of diagnostics-based reviews were commissioned that would be the basis of every change (American Psychiatric Association, 1997, 1998). In practice, the reviews were of mixed quality; the worst uncritically gave equal weight to papers of poor methodological quality and those that were sound.

The DSM–IV field trials (e.g., Lahey *et al,* 1994; Volkmar *et al,* 1994) were used as a basis for fine-tuning certain criteria. Although helpful, the field trials suffered from certain limitations. They were designed to examine how criteria drawn up in committee mapped onto real patients. Subjects were recruited from different speciality clinics that regularly saw children with disruptive or PDD-related disorders, i.e., clinical convenience samples. Patients and their parents were interviewed to see whether they met old or new criteria and their clinical diagnoses were noted. They were then re-interviewed for the purpose of measuring the test–retest reliability of different criteria. The impact of the new criteria formulations on prevalence was noted. The samples used presented the greatest limitations. For example, patients were recruited from disruptive-disorder clinics to examine the new formulations of attention-deficit hyperactivity disorder, conduct disorder and oppositional defiant disorder (respectively, ADHD, CD and ODD). But these same patients were those used to provide data on, for example, anxiety and mood disorders, resulting in overselection for comorbidity with disruptive disorder and providing no information on normal base rates, false-positive rates, or how many unimpaired youth in the community would meet symptomatic criteria. When population-based studies were eventually carried out, substantial numbers of children were found who met symptomatic criteria for disorders (Shaffer *et al,* 1996) but functioned well at school, within their families and with their peers. Concern about this phenomenon led, at the last minute, to the inclusion of impairment criteria for every diagnosis. Although this might be clinically valuable, it undermines risk-factor and genetic research. It would be unheard of to not diagnose cancer or hypertension until they caused symptoms. This call for impairment criteria is perhaps a reflection of the degree of uncertainty that we still feel about our diagnostic systems.

DSM–IV was far better received than DSM–III. I doubt whether this was because of our attempts to consult widely and arrive at decisions openly. I suspect that the real reason for the lack of protest was that the protesters had been worn out or ground down or were simply less interested than they had been in the early 1980s.

One of the real accomplishments of DSM–IV was that the WHO and ICD–10, represented by Rutter, played an active role in the formulation of diagnoses and in ensuring that there were only slight differences between the two systems for the more

■ 111

important disorders. A 10-year process of coordinating the DSM–IV and ICD–10 revisions was initiated by the late Gerald Klerman and Norman Sartorius in 1980, followed by multiple joint-revision conferences founded by the Alcohol, Drug Abuse, and Mental Health Administration (ADAMHA) and coordinated by Darrel Regier of NIMH (Sartorius *et al,* 1990). Among the remaining differences between the two systems, ICD–10 retained compound categories like mixed anxiety and depressive disorder and mixed conduct and depressive disorder; but these do occur somewhat more commonly than priapism and wry neck. The DSM takes the view that compound diagnoses imply that there is some essential element about two diagnoses combined that is different from the sum of the two considered separately. It does recognise that some 'comorbidity' is artefactual, either for structural reasons (e.g., because similar criteria contribute to more than one diagnosis), or because the criteria for one diagnosis (e.g., separation anxiety), are also 'epiphenomena' of another (e.g., generalised anxiety disorder). In these instances, DSM provides a hierarchical rule whereby coding one diagnosis precludes the endorsement of the other.

Concern about labelling that dogged the early days of DSM–III led senior APA delegates to argue vigorously for making sure that conduct disorder, a stigmatising diagnosis that carries with it implications of therapeutic futility, should be a diagnosis given only to very severe cases. A new category, ODD, was retained for mild cases – defying Farr's warnings. The result is that the prevalence of conduct disorder in epidemiological studies was reduced to a vanishingly small number. ICD–10 retained the socialised and unsocialised conduct-disorder subtypes, despite experience that these are difficult criteria to apply. DSM–IV adopted early-onset *v.* late-onset subtypes, for which there are some empirical data indicating that age of onset distinguishes between genders and good and bad prognosis (Loeber *et al,* 1992).

Questions for the future

Although the new generation of classification systems, aided mightily by Michael Rutter, has brought great advances, there are ongoing concerns. The first is that we have almost no understanding of what comorbidity means. The child psychiatry literature is replete with references to it (Angold *et al,* 1999), but what does it mean to have up to 80% of child psychiatric patients with more than one diagnosis? Does it mean that one disorder has led to another and that there is an aetiological relationship between the two? Some have held this to be the case and propose, for example, that the presence of ADHD predisposes to ODD and conduct disorder (Mannuzza, 1989, 1998; Klein & Mannuzza, 1991; Loeber *et al,* 1992, 1995), that the presence of conduct disorder leads to depression (Zoccolillo 1992; Shaffer *et al,* 1996), or that social phobia predisposes to depression (Regier *et al,* 1998; Schatzberg *et al,* 1998). Do disorders co-occur because of common environmental or biological antecedents? Or, more important for nosologists, is comorbidity an artefact of definitional problems? Have DSM and ICD–10 drawn the lines around disorders in the wrong places?

The other major question concerns the differential validity of seemingly related disorders. The three disruptive disorders often co-occur. Anxiety disorders are often comorbid with one another (Shaffer *et al,* 1996; Lewinsohn *et al,* 1997), and the distinction between the PDD disorders has not been tested. These disorders appear to share broadly similar symptoms and risk factors. Are these really different disorders or are they 'varieties' that reflect differences in severity or environmental influence? We need to know whether definitional differences predict different outcomes or whether we have just given them different names for non-scientific reasons. If the latter, how, in an age when phenotype purity is becoming so important for basic research, can we juggle competing scientific and political needs?

Rutter should have the last word:

> "In our present state of knowledge it's likely that any classification will have to be largely based on behavioural manifestations. But it should be noted that the same clinical picture may be due to many different aetiological factors... Disorders can be defined before the aetiology is known … [I]ndeed, advances in our knowledge about aetiology are likely to be slow until we can identify and classify disorders." (Rutter, 1965: p. 73)

References

Aitken, W. (1864) *Science and Practice of Medicine*. London: Charles Griffin.

American Medical Association (1942) *Standard Nomenclature of Disease and Standard Nomenclature of Operations* (ed. E. P. Jordan). Chicago: AMA.

American Psychiatric Association (1952) *Diagnostic and Statistical Manual of Mental Disorders* (1st edn) (DSM–I). Washington, DC: APA Mental Hospital Service.

—— (1968) *Diagnostic and Statistical Manual of Mental Disorders* (2nd edn) (DSM–II). Washington, DC: APA.

—— (1980) *Diagnostic and Statistical Manual of Mental Disorders* (3rd edn) (DSM–III). Washington, DC: APA.

—— (1991) *DSM–IV Options Book: Work in Progress 9/9/91*. Washington, DC: APA.

—— (1994) *Diagnostic and Statistical Manual of Mental Disorders* (4th edn) (DSM–IV). Washington, DC: APA.

—— (1997) *DSM–IV Sourcebook, Vol. 3*. Washington, DC: APA.

—— (1998) *DSM–IV Sourcebook, Vol. 4*. Washington, DC: APA.

Angold, A., Costello, E. J. & Erkanli, A. (1999) Comorbidity. *Journal of Child Psychology and Psychiatry*, **40**, 57–87.

Aristotle (edn 1981) *Aristotle in 23 Volumes. Vol. 20* (transl. H. Rackham). Cambridge, MA, & London: Harvard University Press & William Heinemann. http://www.perseus.tufts.edu/cgi-bin/ptext?doc=Perseus:text:1999.01.0050&layout=&loc=1247a.

Bellevue (1911) *Bellevue Hospital Nomenclature*. New York: Bellevue Board of Trustees.

Bleuler, P. E. (1911) *Dementia Praecox oder Gruppen der Schizophrenia. 4. Abtailung 1. Hälfte der Handbuch der Psychiatrie* (ed. G. Aschaffenburg). Leipzig & Vienna: Franz Deuticke.

Boissier de Sauvages, F. (1760) *Nosologia Methodica*. Montpellier, France.

Cullen, W. (1792) *Cullen's Synopsis: Synopsis and Nosology, Being an Arrangemnt and Definintion of Diseases*. Worcester & Boston, MA: Isaiah Thomas.

Darwin, E. (1809) *Zoonomia or the Laws of Organic Life*. Boston, MA: Thomas and Andrews.

Emerson, H. & Baehr, G. (1933) Preface. In *Standard Nomenclature of Disease* (2nd edn) (National Conference on Nomenclature of Disease, ed. H. B. Logie), pp. xi–xvii. New York: Commonwealth Fund.

Good, J. M. (1824) *The Study of Medicine: With a Physiological System of Nosology. Vol. 5* (2nd edn). Philadelphia, PA: Bennett and Walton.

Gouley, J. W. S. (1888) *Diseases of Man: Data of their Nomenclature, Classification and Genesis*. London: H. K. Lewis.

Group for the Advancement of Psychiatry (1966) *Psychopathological Disorders in Childhood: Theoretical Considerations and a Proposed Classification (GAP Classification)*. New York: GAP.

International Commission (1909) *International List of Causes of Death*. Paris: International Commission.

Jaspers, K. (1913) *Allgemeine Psychopathologie: Ein Leitfaden für Studierende, Ärzte, und Psychologen*. Berlin: Verlag von Julius Springer.

Klein, R. G. & Mannuzza, S. (1991) Long-term outcome of hyperactive children: a review. *Journal of the American Academy of Child and Adolescent Psychiatry*, **30**, 383–387.

Knoff, W. F. (1970) A history of the concept of neurosis, with a memoir of William Cullen. *American Journal of Psychiatry*, **127**, 80–84.

Kraepelin, E. (1883) *Compendium der Psychiatrie*. Leipzig: Verlag von Ambr. Abel.

Lahey, B. B., Applegate, B., Barkley, R. A., *et al* (1994) DSM–IV field trials for oppositional defiant disorder and conduct disorder in children and adolescents. *American Journal of Psychiatry*, **151**, 1163–1171.

Lambert, A. V. S. & Martin, W. (1910) *A Terminology of Disease: To Facilitate the Classification of Histories in Hospitals*. New York: Columbia University Press.

Lewinsohn, P. M., Zinbarg, R., Seeley, J. R., *et al* (1997) Lifetime comorbidity among anxiety disorders and between anxiety disorders and other mental disorders in adolescents. *Journal of Anxiety Disorders*, **11**, 377–394.

Loeber, R., Green, S. M., Lahey, B. B., *et al* (1992) Developmental sequences in the age of onset of disruptive child behaviors. *Journal of Child and Family Studies*, **1**, 21–41.

——, ——, Keenan, K., *et al* (1995) Which boys will fare worse? Early predictors of the onset of conduct disorder in a six-year longitudinal study. *Journal of the American Academy of Child and Adolescent Psychiatry*, **34**, 499–509.

Longrigg, J. (1998) *Greek Medicine from the Heroic to the Hellenistic Age: A Source Book*. New York: Routledge.

Mannuzza, S., Klein, R. G., Konig, P. H., *et al* (1989) Hyperactive boys almost grown up. IV. Criminality and its relationship to psychiatric status [see comments]. *Archives of General Psychiatry*, **46**, 1073–1079.

——, ——, Bessler, A., *et al* (1998) Adult psychiatric status of hyperactive boys grown up. *American Journal of Psychiatry*, **155**, 493–498.

National Conference on Nomenclature of Disease (1933) *A Standard Classified Nomenclature of Disease* (ed. H. B. Logie). New York: Commonwealth Fund.

■ 113

Parr, B. (1819) *The London Medical Dictionary. Vol. 2* (2nd series). Philadelphia, PA: Mitchell, Ames and White.

Raines, G. N. (1951) Foreword. In *Diagnostic and Statistical Manual of Mental Disorders* (1st edn) (DSM–I) (American Psychiatric Association), pp. v–xi. Washington, DC: APA.

Regier, D. A., Rae, D. S., Narrow, W. E., *et al* (1998) Prevalence of anxiety disorders and their comorbidity with mood and addictive disorders. *British Journal of Psychiatry*, **173** (suppl. 34), 24–28.

Royal College of Physicians of London (1869) *The Nomenclature of Diseases (Drawn up by a Joint Committee of the Royal College of Physicians of London)*. London: His Majesty's Stationery Office.

—— (1918) *Nomenclature of Diseases (Drawn up by a Joint Committee Appointed by the Royal College of Physicians of London)*. London: His Majesty's Stationery Office.

Rutter, M. (1965) Classification and categorization in child psychiatry. *Journal of Child Psychology and Psychiatry*, **6**, 71–83.

—— & Shaffer, D. (1980) DSM–III: A step forward or back in terms of the classification of child psychiatric disorders? *Journal of the American Academy of Child and Adolescent Psychiatry*, **19**, 371–394.

——, —— & Shepherd, M. (1975) *A Multi-Axial Classification of Child Psychiatric Disorders*. Geneva: WHO.

Sartorius, N., Jablensky, A., Regier, D. A., *et al* (eds.) (1990) *Sources and Traditions of Classification in Psychiatry*. Toronto: Hogrefe & Huber.

Schatzberg, A. F., Samson, J. A., Rothschild, A. J., *et al* (1998) McLean Hospital Depression Research Facility: early-onset phobic disorders and adult-onset major depression. *British Journal of Psychiatry*, **173** (suppl. 34), 29–34.

Shaffer, D., (1996) A participant's observations: preparing DSM–IV. *Canadian Journal of Psychiatry*, **41**, 325–329.

——, Fisher, P., Dulcan, M. K., *et al* (1996) The NIMH diagnostic interview schedule for children, version 2.3 (DISC–2.3): description, acceptability, prevalence rates, and performance in the MECA study. *Journal of the American Academy of Child and Adolescent Psychiatry*, **35**, 865–877.

Spitzer, R., Endicott, J. E. & Robins, E. (1977) *Research Diagnostic Criteria for a Selected Group of Functional Disorders* (3rd edn). New York: New York State Psychiatric Institute.

Standard Nomenclature of Disease (1933, 1935) *National Conference on Nomenclature of Disease* (ed. H. B. Logie). New York: Commonwealth Fund.

State Board of Health of New York (1883) *Nomenclature of Diseases*. New York: State Board of Health.

US Public Health Service (1916) *Nomenclature of Diseases and Conditions*. Washington, DC: US Public Health Service/Government Printing Office.

Volkmar, F. R., Klin, A., Siegel, B., *et al* (1994) Field trial for autistic disorder in DSM–IV. *American Journal of Psychiatry*, **151**, 1361–1367.

World Health Organization (1968) *International Classification of Diseases* (8th edn) (ICD–8). Geneva: WHO.

—— (1993) *The ICD–10 Classification of Mental and Behavioral Disorders: Diagnostic Criteria for Research* (10th edn) (ICD–10). Geneva: WHO.

Zoccolillo, M. (1992) Co-occurrence of conduct disorder and its adult outcomes with depressive and anxiety disorders: a review. *Journal of the American Academy of Child and Adolescent Psychiatry*, **31**, 547–556.

8 Making sense of the increasing prevalence of conduct disorder

Lee N. Robins

Through follow-up studies in a variety of populations, Michael Rutter has demonstrated that rates of conduct disorder vary by geographical area (Rutter *et al*, 1970, 1975). Yet the predictors of conduct disorder appear to be consistent across areas. Many studies have now shown that conduct disorder is a powerful predictor of adolescent and adult outcomes for both males and females, not only across geographic areas (Robins, 1966; Farrington, 1995), but also in persons born in different eras and members of different subcultures (Robins, 1966, 1978; Robins & Regier, 1991). It is challenging to try to understand why the prevalence rate of conduct disorder varies so markedly over time and place while its predictors and consequences remain stable (Rutter, 1991; Robins, 1999; Silbereisen *et al*, 1995; Kendler *et al*, 1997).

This chapter attempts to shed some light on this mixture of change and consistency by considering possible explanations for changes in conduct disorder rates and what that implies for the outcomes they predict.

Stable predictors and consequences of conduct disorder

The predictors of conduct disorder that Rutter has found consistently in his studies include parental psychiatric disorder and parental discord, parents' poor child-rearing practices, male gender and early behaviour problems (Rutter, 1972). He consistently found that conduct disorder in turn predicts lack of school success, adult antisocial behaviour and depression. He has not followed the pack to study currently fashionable early predictors of adolescent and adult outcomes, such as foetal alcohol syndrome, child abuse, exposure to cocaine *in utero* and exposure to violence on television or in the neighbourhood. His lack of attention to these single causes of conduct problems and adult behaviours is consistent with his view that longitudinal studies should examine a broad range of features of the child's environment and track changes in the whole environment over time (Rutter, 1988), rather than focusing on individual environmental risk factors at a fixed point in time. He would argue that instability of the family or neighbourhood environment is a better predictor of conduct disorder than is any specific family or neighbourhood feature (Rutter, 1989a). He might well argue that mothers who drank heavily or used cocaine during pregnancy, who abuse their children and whose poverty forces them to rear their children in neighbourhoods where violence is an everyday event are the very same parents that he has described as suffering from psychiatric disorder and involved in discordant marriages or liaisons. Further, he does not see the child in such environments as a passive victim, but rather as a person whose response to stressors has an important influence on the level of environmental stressors he or she will experience in the future (Rutter, 1991: p. 195). It is Rutter's attention over the years to a consistent set of predictor variables that has allowed him to note that the same predictors of adolescent behaviour problems and of adult antisocial behaviour work well across communities with high and low rates of poverty, school completion and arrest. Although not a particular focus of his attention, it is also noteworthy that his studies have been carried out over a long and productive research career, and therefore he has also shown that these predictors work as well for recent generations as for those who grew up 20–30 years ago (Rutter *et al*, 1970; Quinton *et al*, 1984).

Study design and the demonstration of cohort effects

Studies of general population samples of adults have asked for retrospective reports of psychiatric symptoms (Robins & Regier, 1991; Kessler *et al*, 1994), conduct disorder and adult antisocial behaviour (Robins *et al*, 1991) and substance abuse (Grant, 1997). These studies have suggested that the prevalence of many disorders, including conduct disorder, has increased over the past 70 years. As conduct disorder has become more common, it appears to have lost none of its power to predict adult antisocial behaviour and substance dependence (Robins & McEvoy, 1990). These observations come from studies that included adults of all ages, representing many birth cohorts. It is a puzzle to understand why conduct disorders have increased and how much of a role this increase has played in increases in the prevalence of adult disorders. The aim of this chapter is to consider how well data from retrospective studies of adults, asked to recall their childhood behaviour, serve to support both the growth of conduct disorder and its undiminished strength as a predictor of adverse adult outcomes, creating a rise in their incidence.

It may seem odd to celebrate Rutter's excellence in follow-up studies of children by citing data obtained from single retrospective interviews with samples from general populations of adults. It would be preferable to have a series of studies of children representative of the total population staggered across 20 or 30 years. Each of these studies would follow its subjects into adulthood. If each study were to select youngsters of the same ages and ask them the same questions, the series would provide prospective follow-up into adulthood of successive birth cohorts, comparably studied. These studies in childhood would show definitively whether conduct disorder has increased over time and whether the prevalence of its predictors has changed. The follow-up into adulthood would discover whether conduct disorder continues to have the same degree of impact on adult disorders as it becomes more common. This evidence would be free of the possible sources of confounding that plague retrospective studies, for example: missing all cases with the most disastrous outcome – death; having reduced access to those alive but with serious disability leading to homelessness or broken contacts with family members; obtaining less complete information from older cohorts, owing either to forgetting long-past events or having reached adulthood before the change in social customs that has probably increased the willingness of younger adults to admit behavioural and psychological problems. Unfortunately, these ideal follow-up studies from childhood into adulthood in successive cohorts have not been done. This was perhaps inevitable. Had similar studies been initiated in different eras, each almost certainly would have asked different questions to assess conduct disorder, because the criteria describing conduct disorder have changed over the years (Robins, 1986). Table 8.1 shows how the North American criteria have varied since their first publication in the second edition of the *Diagnostic and Statistical Manual*, DSM–II, in 1968 (American Psychiatric Association, 1968). The first edition, DSM–I (American Psychiatric Association, 1952), did not even include children's disorders. Only six symptoms have appeared in all four subsequent editions (American Psychiatric Association, 1968, 1980, 1987, 1994): fighting, vandalism, lying, stealing, running away from home and truancy (Robins, 1999).

Rutter has come close to performing the ideal studies described above in a replication of the Isle of Wight study (Rutter *et al*, 1970) 5 years later in children of the same age in inner London, using the same interview (Rutter *et al*, 1975). He found a much higher rate of conduct problems in the second study, but since the settings differed, he believed that this was more likely explained by social disadvantage in the London subjects than by their membership of a slightly later birth cohort.

Offord *et al* (1986) studied children in Ontario some 20 years after the Isle of Wight study. But differences between rates in Rutter's Isle of Wight study of 10-year-olds and in Offord's Ontario study of children aged 4–16 cannot serve to estimate change over

Table 8.1 How criteria for conduct disorder have changed over time

Criterion and symptoms	DSM–IV	DSM–III–R	DSM–III[1]	DSM–II Runaway reaction	DSM–II Unsocialized aggressive	DSM–II Group delinquency
Aggression						
Bullying	✓				✓	
Fighting[2]	✓	✓	(Assault)		✓	
Using weapons	✓	✓				
Using physical cruelty						
People	✓	✓				
Animals	✓	✓				
Robbery	✓	✓	✓			
Rape	✓	✓	✓			
Vandalism						
Setting fires	✓	✓	✓			
Other vandalism[2]	✓	✓	✓		✓	
Deceit or theft						
Breaking in	✓	✓	✓			
Lying[2]	✓	✓	✓		✓	
Stealing[2]	✓	✓	✓	✓	✓	✓
Violation of rules						
Staying out late	✓				✓	✓
Running away[2]	✓	✓	✓	✓		
Truanting[2]	✓	✓	✓			✓
Substance misuse			✓			
Unsocialised						
No lasting friendship			✓	✓		
Lacking altruism			✓			
Blaming others			✓			
No concern for others			✓			
Verbal bad behaviour						
Quarrelsomeness					✓	
Verbal aggression					✓	
Tantrums					✓	

1. Four categories: aggressive non-socialised; non-aggressive non-socialised; aggressive socialised; and non-aggressive socialised.
2. Consistent across all editions of DSM.

time. While the questions are reasonably equivalent, the younger children in Offord's sample will inevitably have lower rates of conduct disorder than do Rutter's 10-year-olds, because young children have not had the time to accumulate the number of symptoms required for the diagnosis of conduct disorder (e.g., they cannot be truant before they attend school), while Offord's 12- to 16-year-olds should have *higher* rates than do Rutter's 10-year-olds, whether or not there are cohort effects, because they have had more years at risk.

Retrospective studies of adults overcome the difficulty of comparing studies of conduct disorder where the children are of different ages, because all adult subjects are past the age of risk for developing the disorder. Retrospective studies also overcome the problem of changing diagnostic criteria. They apply current criteria for conduct disorder to all birth cohorts. They have the additional asset of being able to include cohorts born too long ago to have been studied as children within even so long a research career as Rutter's.

Two major retrospective studies of adults have been done in the USA in the past 20 years, the Epidemiologic Catchment Area (ECA) project (Robins & Regier, 1991), carried out in the early 1980s, and the National Comorbidity Study (NCS; Kessler *et al*, 1994), conducted some 12 years later. Because both had large samples of randomly selected subjects born in different eras and because both covered a broad range of adult psychiatric disorders, they can show which disorders have increased in younger cohorts. Conduct disorder was included in these studies, neither of which was intended to include childhood psychiatric disorders, because three or more behaviour problems before age 15 were required for the diagnosis of antisocial personality in DSM–III (1980) and DSM–III–R (1987).

The ECA showed that later birth cohorts had higher rates of conduct disorder, as well as an increased prevalence of substance misuse (Robins *et al*, 1984; Klerman & Weissman, 1989; Wickramaratne *et al*, 1989; Joyce *et al*, 1990). Many of the publications about cohort effects have centred on depression. Researchers have shown considerable scepticism about interpreting the lower rate of depression in the life time of older than younger cohorts to mean that the rate has risen over the past 70 years (Simon & Von Korff, 1992). There are two arguments that justify these doubts. First, older people may underreport symptoms in interviews, either because they forget them once they remit or because they are less willing to admit to them. Second, affected older people may be less accessible for interviews than affected young people, both because they have been longer at risk of the premature death associated with depression and because older people with psychiatric illness may be particularly resistant to being interviewed.

While both arguments are reasonable, they seem to account only in part for higher rates of disorder among the young. If they were the whole story, we would expect to find lower rates of all disorders in elderly people, except perhaps for disorders associated neither with early death nor remission. We would also expect the same scarcity of affected older people in all parts of the population. Yet the young do not have higher rates than elderly people for all disorders covered by the ECA and NCS. Exceptions include somatisation disorder, obsessive–compulsive disorder, panic disorder, phobia and dysthymia (Robins & Regier, 1991). Nor are lower rates of disorders in elderly people found in all populations. For example, the rate of depressive disorder was not lower among the older sample members in Puerto Rico (Cross-National Collaborative Group, 1992), and in the USA the lower rate in elderly people is more notable among White than among African Americans (Robins & Regier, 1991). Yet affected older Puerto Ricans and African Americans do not experience remission much less often than mainland Whites; they do not have better memories; they are no less likely to have their life span shortened by psychiatric disorder; nor are they known to be less sensitive about reporting symptoms.

Despite arguments that the inverse relationship between age and life-time psychiatric illness may be artefactual, I consider here the cohort effect in three disorders in which it is particularly striking and in which alternative explanations seem least likely: conduct disorder, antisocial personality and substance misuse. A true increase in these disorders is validated by objective records, as well as by interviews. Police records show a dramatic rise over the past 40–50 years in juvenile and adult arrests for assault and homicide, the legal terms for aggression, a symptom of both conduct disorder and adult antisocial personality (Home Office, 1989). While police records show some decline in the past 5 years in both assaults and homicides, rates are still higher than 50 years ago (Office of Juvenile Justice and Delinquency Prevention, 1999). There is a well-documented drug epidemic beginning in the 1960s and leading to an increase in substance-related disorders. Evidence for this comes from police records, coroners' reports, emergency room attendances, the growth in the number of persons in drug treatment and from yearly surveys such as those published by Johnston *et al* (1996) and the Office of Applied Studies (1998). Both surveys show a decline in use rates beginning early in the 1990s, but use has begun to rise again, although it is still not as high as in the late 1970s and early 1980s. There has also been a striking increase in births to unmarried teenagers (although again the rates have declined somewhat in the past few years) and in the proportion of all marriages that end in divorce. The rise in teenage pregnancies may be an indicator of a rise in conduct disorder, and the increase in marital disruption may indicate a rise in both antisocial personality and substance misuse.

Survey results show a large increase in conduct symptoms over recent generations for both men and women (Fig. 8.1). In the ECA, rates of three or more conduct problems before age 15 rose from 2% in men 65 or older to 13% in men under 40, a six-fold difference; female rates rose from less than 0.5% in women over 65 to 5% in women under 40, a ten-fold increase. Although rates were much higher for men than women in every cohort, the male:female ratio has gradually declined, so that in the youngest cohort it is about 2.5:1.

118

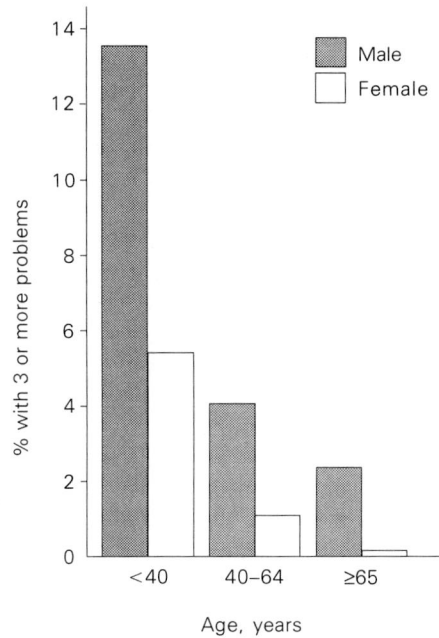

Fig. 8.1 Age and gender as predictors of conduct disorder.

Are these disorders especially likely to be associated with an excess of premature deaths? Follow-up studies carried out with child guidance clinic patients (Robins, 1966) and with young Black men selected from public school records (Robins, 1968) showed that conduct disorder is associated with premature non-natural deaths, as well as with many other adverse adult outcomes. (Note that excess deaths as an outcome is detected only in follow-up studies because cross-sectional studies of adults look only at the survivors.) While deaths are higher when there is a history of conduct disorder, substance misuse and antisocial personality, they are not sufficiently elevated to explain the dramatic increase in rates observed.

To overcome the confounding of cohort effects with effects of forgetting and changing norms regarding what may be told to strangers, we took advantage of the fact that the NCS was carried out 12 years after the ECA. This meant that when members of a birth cohort represented in the ECA were interviewed in the NCS, they had grown up in the same era and shared its culture, but had survived 12 more years and had 12 more years in which to forget early symptoms. For example, someone born in 1960 would have been aged 24 when interviewed for the ECA and 36 when interviewed for the NCS. When the ECA project asked a member of this cohort about conduct problems before age 15, he or she was being asked to recall events at least 9 years earlier, but these same events were at least 21 years earlier when he or she was asked about them in the NCS. As one would expect, there was some effect of the longer survival and recall requirements for NCS subjects. When interviewed in the ECA, they were found to have had conduct disorder before 15 in 26% of cases, but in only 17% when interviewed in the NCS. Not all of this difference was due to the greater time elapsed between conduct disorder symptoms and interview in the NCS than in the ECA. The ECA sample was largely urban, but the NCS sample was representative of the USA with respect to urban:rural proportions; furthermore, the ECA included persons in institutions, while the NCS was entirely a household sample. Both urban residence and institutionalisation were associated with conduct disorder. Despite these sample differences, the cohort effect was so strong that the 1960s NCS cohort had a prevalence of conduct disorder higher than the 1950s ECA cohort for both men and women. Therefore, the increase in prevalence of conduct disorder as age declined appears to be at least in part a cohort effect, with increasing prevalence in each younger cohort.

An increase over time in arrests for violent crime is found in both the UK and the USA, although the UK rates for violent crime are much lower than the US (Langan & Farrington, 1998). The increase is found both for juvenile and adult offenders. The ECA found increased reports of child fighting, adult fighting, adult weapon use and hitting one's

Consequences of conduct disorder

■ 119

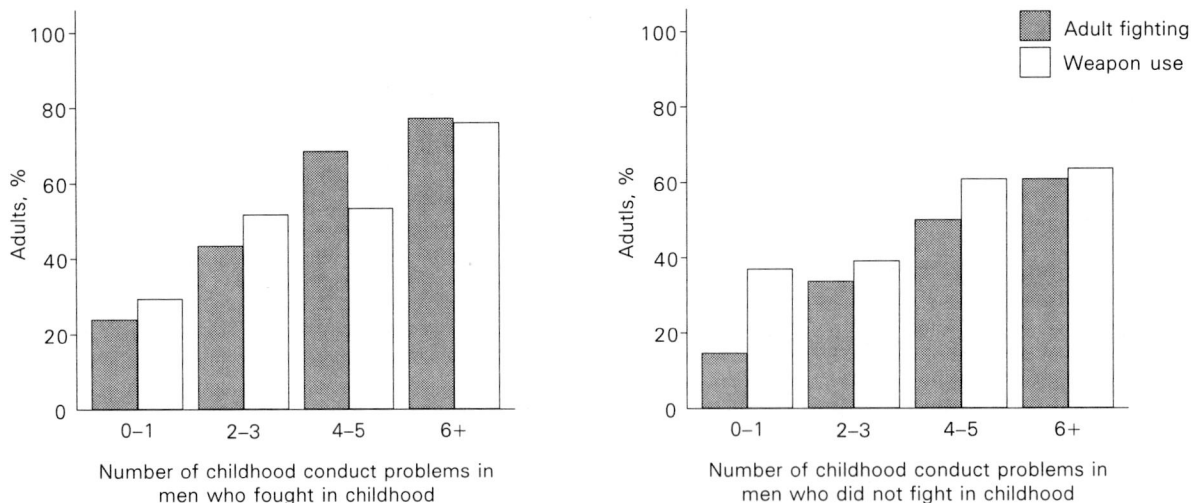

Fig. 8.2 Conduct problems and fighting in childhood as forecast of adult fighting and weapon use in Epidemiologic Catchment Area study: men aged <50 years (n=3051).

120

spouse, indicating an increase in violence, while there has been little increase in multiple traffic tickets or total arrests.

An interesting observation is that conduct disorder predicts adult fighting and weapon use even when the conduct disorder symptoms did not include fighting (Fig. 8.2). Note also that the likelihood of adult fighting is much greater when the child who fights also has conduct disorder problems other than fighting. This is an instance supporting Rutter's view that the total pattern of child behaviour is a better predictor of outcome than is the same activity in childhood as in adulthood. This not to say that there is no specificity of prediction. At every level of conduct disorder in childhood, childhood fighters are more likely to be adult fighters than are childhood non-fighters.

Figure 8.3 shows that the rise in both child and adult fighting across cohorts closely parallels the increase in conduct problems. This suggests that adult violence might not have increased if the frequency of conduct problems had not increased. In fact, about half of all children who met the criteria for conduct disorder were violent as adults, whether they were born in the 1930s or the 1960s (Fig. 8.4). For children who did not meet the criteria for conduct disorder, the frequency of fighting in adulthood was less than 10%, regardless of date of birth. This is a demonstration that the later impact of conduct disorder on adult violence is not influenced by the proportion of children with conduct disorder. These findings also suggest that preventing adult violence may require preventing the development of conduct disorder. This is not to say that the adult environment is unimportant. Adult unemployment and being unmarried are also associated with adult violence, but increased employment opportunities and discouraging

Fig. 8.3 Time trends in childhood and adult fighting in relation to trends in childhood conduct problems in Epidemiologic Catchment Area study subjects from 3 sites (n=11 000).

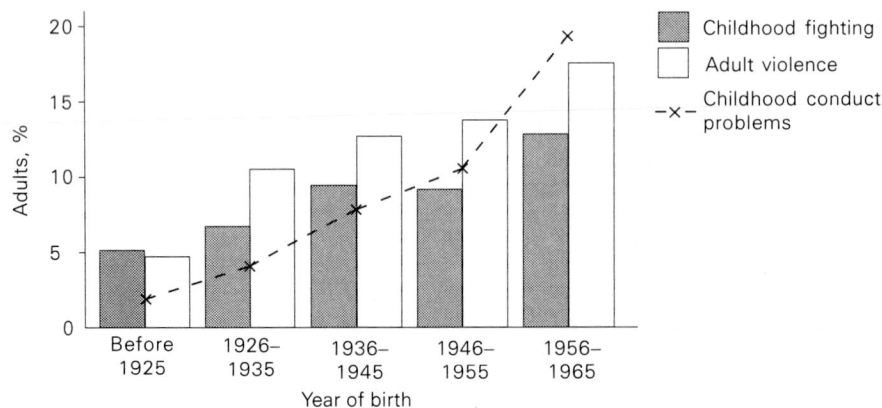

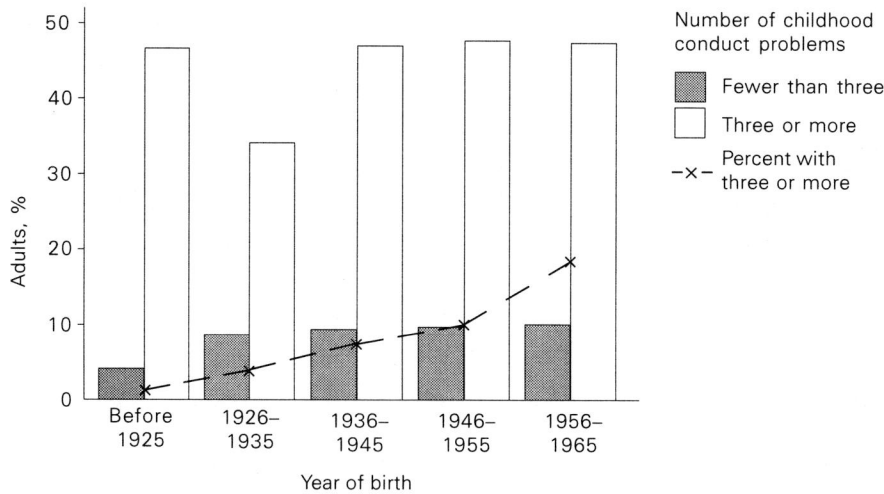

Fig. 8.4 Adult violence
following childhood
conduct problems in birth
cohorts to 1965 for three
sites in Epidemiologic
Catchment Area study
(n=11 000).

postponement and disruption of marriage may be insufficient to reverse the observed increase in violent offences.

Conduct disorder affects many adult outcomes other than violence. Children with conduct disorder grow up to have high rates of the externalising disorders, antisocial personality and substance misuse (Robins & Price, 1991; Robins, 1998), but there are also increased rates of internalising disorders, particularly depression, in women. As Fig. 8.5 shows, women are less likely to develop externalising disorders than men, but the female curve closely parallels the male, indicating that conduct symptoms are as potent predictors for women as for men. The effect of conduct disorder is less striking on internalising than on externalising disorders, but is none the less significant, strikingly so for women. For men, the modest increase in internalising disorders chiefly reflects depression secondary to substance misuse. Note that there is no sharp shift in liability when the official cut-off point of three symptoms needed for a diagnosis of conduct disorder is reached. Even a single conduct problem increases the likelihood of psychiatric disorder. The effect of conduct symptoms is dimensional, with psychiatric liability rising with each addition of another conduct symptom. As Rutter has pointed out, classification-driven research can be misleading. There is no ideal cut-off point for distinguishing between those affected and those not affected by conduct disorder.

The effect of conduct disorder on adult psychiatric status results in an increased frequency of admissions to psychiatric hospitals and more suicide attempts and completions among those who suffer from a history of conduct disorder (Kendler et al, 1997).

■ 121

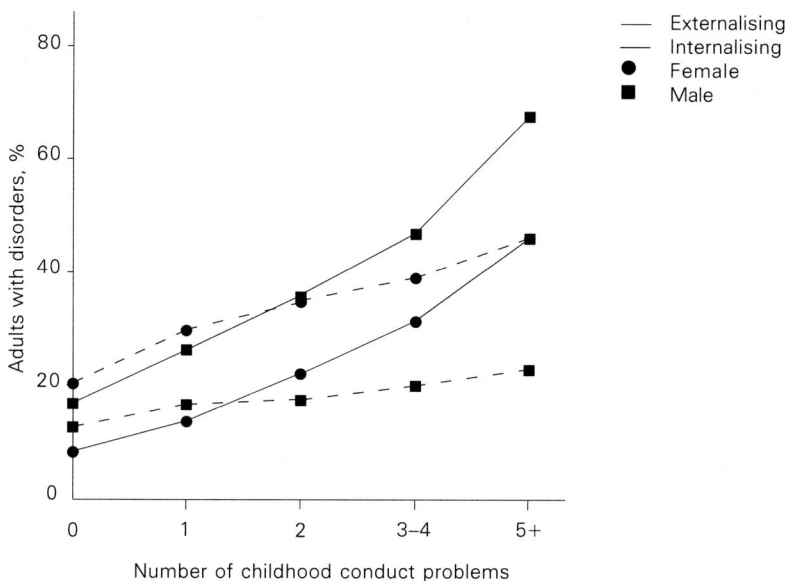

Fig. 8.5 Relationship
between conduct problems
in childhood and
externalising and
internalising disorders in
adults for five sites in
Epidemiologic Catchment
Area study, weighted to US
population.

In addition to this increase in psychiatric problems among adults who had conduct disorder, there are many social problems. These include: family effects – high divorce and separation rates, offspring with a high incidence of conduct problems, more family desertion and failure to support dependants, more extramarital affairs; legal consequences – imprisonment, being cited for spouse or child abuse, unpaid debts and repossession of purchased articles, traffic violations; educational effects – premature school leaving; economic effects – prolonged periods of unemployment, frequent job changes, bad credit ratings, illegal occupations; and finally, excess mortality, particularly non-natural deaths, but also excess natural deaths consequent to substance misuse and AIDS.

Information about this wealth of adverse outcomes comes not only from interviews, but also from record searches for persons known to have had conduct disorder (Robins, 1966). All studies agree that these are the outcomes, regardless of when the studies were conducted, how they assessed conduct disorder and whether the populations studied were former patients or members of the general population.

Explaining the adverse effects of conduct disorder: the case of substance misuse

How can conduct disorder be so powerful a determinant of future outcomes? One hypothesis is that it leads to substance misuse, which has a direct effect on other outcomes. The great advantage of studying substance misuse is that dating the first significant use of substances tells us when the person became at risk. For other psychiatric disorders, there is no information prior to the appearance of the first symptom to indicate risk status. Even knowing that there is a family history of a disorder, suggesting a genetic loading, is insufficient (unless an identical twin has the disorder) because the person may not have inherited the gene. For substance misuse, not only is it possible to establish that exposure has occurred, but the degree of exposure can be determined by measuring the frequency of use, as well as the quantity used for tobacco, alcohol and prescription drugs (Robins, 1998). (The quantity of street drugs used cannot be accurately determined because their purity is unknown.) While the degree of exposure to drugs in humans is strongly influenced by the subject's prior characteristics, which in turn may be associated with the likelihood of becoming dependent on substances, the importance of exposure *per se* to the development of dependence has been demonstrated in animal studies in which the investigator, rather than the user, determines the dose and its frequency (Ahmed & Koob, 1997). In animals, dependence can be demonstrated by the occurrence of well-established withdrawal symptoms when the drug is stopped.

Age at first exposure predicts problem use

In an early study of African American men born and reared in St Louis, the occurrence of heavy drinking was strongly predicted by the age at which the first drink was taken (Robins *et al*, 1968). Of the men who said they had had a first drink before age 12, 80% became heavy drinkers, as compared with only 12% of those who had waited until age 17 or later to begin drinking. The effect of age at exposure was regular, with increasing percentages becoming heavy drinkers with every decline in age of first exposure. Twenty years later, in the ECA study, age at first substance use, whether that was the first time the respondent ever drank enough to become intoxicated or the first exposure to an illicit drug, strongly predicted whether symptoms of misuse would occur in at least three of four categories of psychoactive substances: alcohol; cannabis; heroin or cocaine; and other types of illicit drug (Fig. 8.6; Robins & Przybeck, 1985; Robins & McEvoy, 1990). Age at first use of substances predicted the amount and variety that would be used, and also whether that use would become symptomatic. Substance misuse occurred at three times the rate for the total sample in persons who first got drunk or used illicit drugs before age 15 (44% v. 15%), while drug misuse or dependence occurred at seven times the rate for the total sample. This association between early use and problem use has been noted frequently (D'Avanzo *et al*, 1994).

Conduct disorder predicts early use

In the ECA, early use of substances occurred primarily among those with an already established history of conduct problems: the more conduct problems, the earlier use

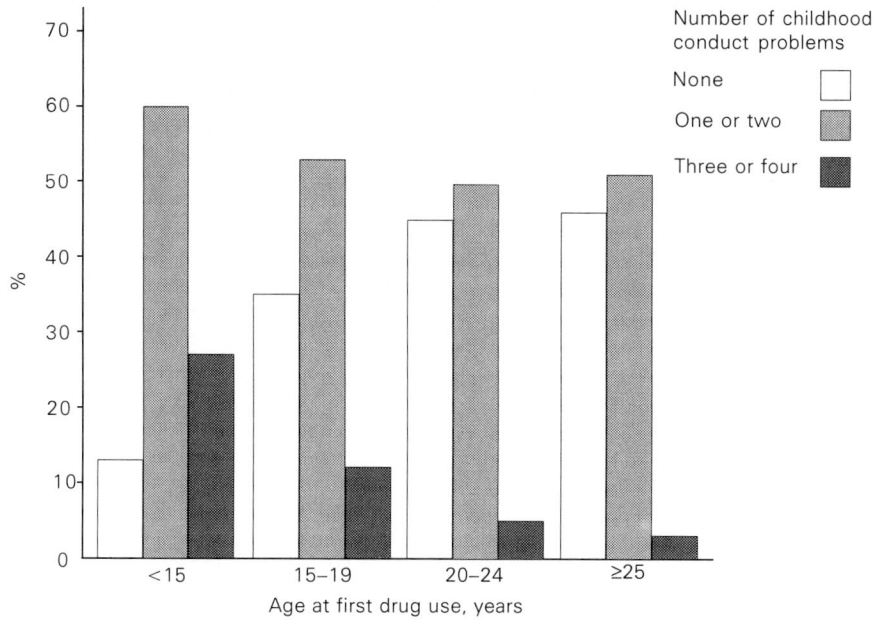

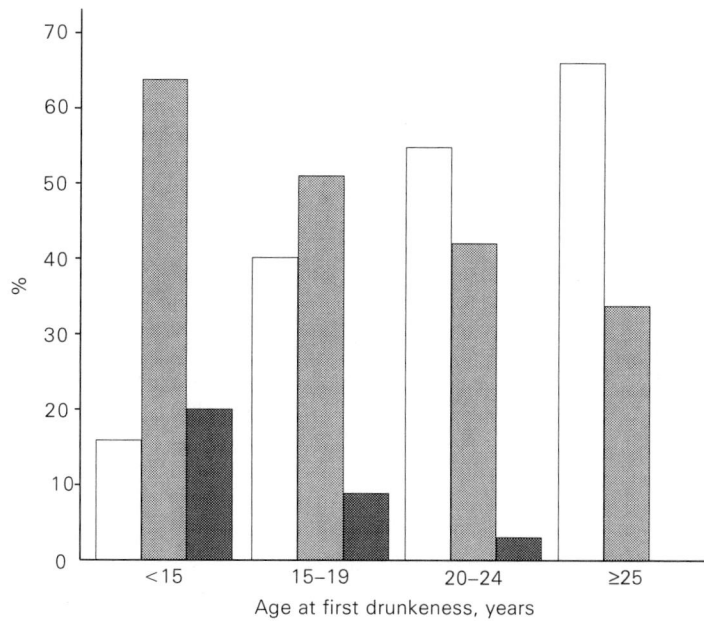

Fig. 8.6 Relationship
between number of
childhood conduct
problems and age of first
misuse of drugs and
alcohol.

began (Fig. 8.7). Among those with no conduct problems in childhood, the average age
at first alcohol intoxication was 17 years and at first drug use it was 21. At the other end
of the continuum, among youngsters with nine conduct problems, the average age at
first intoxication was 12 and at first illicit drug use, 14. Again, the dimensional nature of
conduct problems is seen: with each increase in the number of conduct problems, there
is a corresponding decline in the age of first exposure to substances.

To test the proposition that it was the type of children who use early rather than
early use *per se* that accounted for the bad consequences of substance misuse, we divided
the ECA sample according to both age at first use of illicit drugs and whether that first
use occurred before 1974, an era when use typically began in the late teens or early 20s,
or later than 1974, when illicit drug use was no longer rare among children in grades
8 and 9 (typically aged 13–14 years) (Johnston *et al*, 1993). If the apparent effect of
early first use on later problems with drugs was simply due to its role as an indicator
of unusual daring and the flouting of existing norms, very early first use should be a
better predictor of outcomes during the era prior to 1974 than later. But as Fig. 8.8
shows, early age of first use continued to be a potent predictor of developing dependence
or misuse after 1974, although as one would expect, as youngsters with less prior

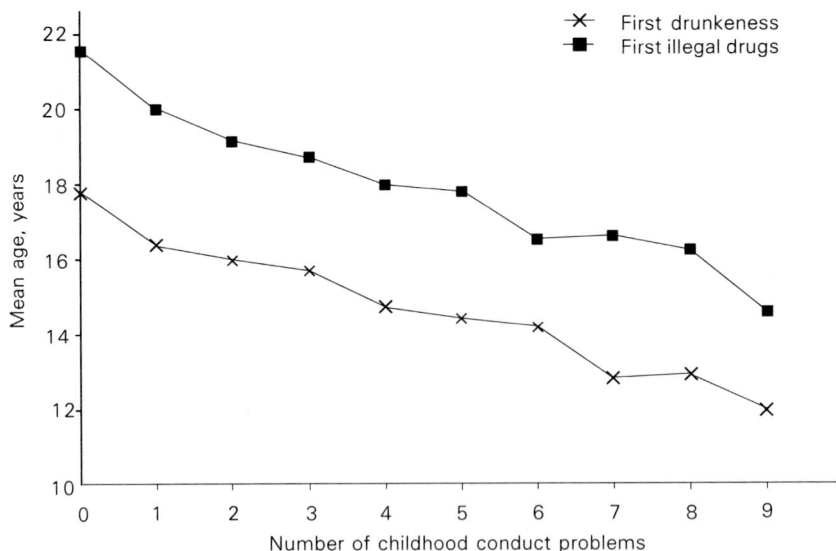

Fig. 8.7 Relationship between childhood conduct problems and age of first alcohol and drug misuse.

deviance were recruited into drug use, the proportion of users developing substance misuse problems declined.

It is interesting to note that before 1974, when use by girls was even more unusual than use by boys, girls who did use were as prone as boys to develop a substance misuse disorder. After 1974, when girls used drugs about as frequently as boys, the protective effect of female gender on susceptibility to substance misuse problems can be seen.

Additional impact of conduct disorder

The influence of conduct disorder on age of exposure to substances does not exhaust its effect on the liability to problems with substances. Even controlling for age at first use, those with more symptoms of conduct disorder have increased risks of developing problems with a variety of substances. As Fig. 8.9 shows, if there are only one or two conduct symptoms, age of first use is unimportant: the incidence of developing problems with multiple substances is negligible. The converse is that if use is delayed to age 20 or later, there is little risk of problems with multiple substances no matter the number of conduct problems. A very large number of conduct problems might predict problems even in those who began substance use that late, but such children are hard to find; children with a substantial number of conduct problems virtually never put off substance use until age 20. Among children with three or more conduct problems who initiate first drunkenness or first illicit drug use early, the number of conduct problems remains predictive of substance misuse problems. Whether or not initiation is delayed past age 15, those with a large number of conduct symptoms

Fig. 8.8 Consequences of first drug use by men and women pre-1974 and later.

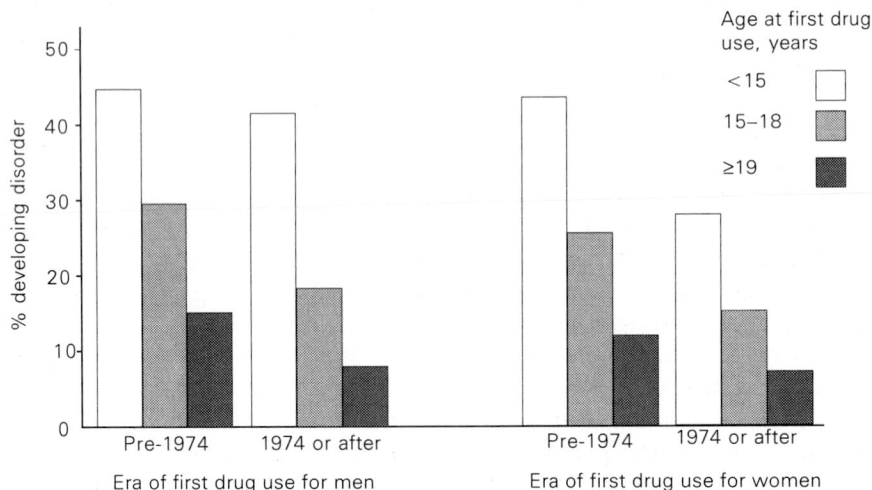

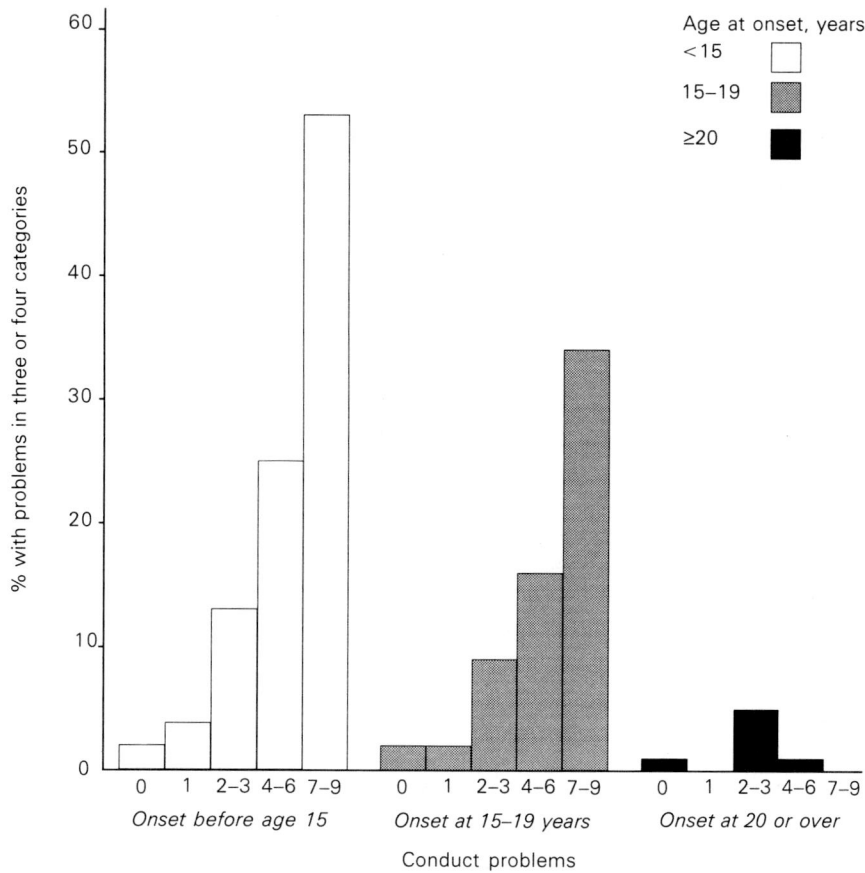

Fig. 8.9 Relationship between conduct disorder and age of first substance misuse

are far more at risk of misuse of multiple substances than are those with fewer conduct problems.

Discussion

How does this exploration of the relationship between conduct disorders and substance misuse help in understanding the progressive increase in conduct disorder and adult antisocial behaviour over the past two generations? Here is one possible explanation. When the rates of adult antisocial behaviour and substance misuse first increased in parents, for whatever reason, the rates of conduct problems and early substance use rose in their children. This rising rate of conduct disorder led to a further increase in antisocial personality and substance misuse when these children became adults. They then functioned less well as parents than their own parents had, leading to a further increase in their children's conduct problems and early substance use.

How did this cycle get started? Several major social changes could be implicated. First, an increase in divorce and separation, fuelled in part by the trend towards a convergence of male and female roles, which led to acceptance of mothers' working outside the home and using alcohol. Second, the drug epidemic that began among North American inner-city Black youth in the 1950s spread to the White middle class in the late 1960s, involving more and more youngsters up to 1980. As drug use grew, the age of introduction to drugs fell from the 20s to the early teens, without diminishing the use of alcohol. The combination of less supervision and more and earlier exposure to substances meant that more youngsters became at risk of delinquent behaviour and substance use problems. While an increase in antisocial personality and substance misuse would themselves be associated with rising rates of violence, this trend was enhanced by the increasing availability of firearms.

Even if this explanation is correct, the effects of single parenting, lack of supervision, parents' substance misuse, access to firearms and early exposure to drugs are probably inadequate to explain fully the increasing rates of conduct disorder and its adult consequences. Other changes that may help to explain the upward trend are an increased tolerance of conceiving or adopting a child as a single parent, increasing urbanisation, the decline in entry-level jobs for unskilled persons and ghettoisation of the minority poor as middle-class minorities became free to live elsewhere.

This sketch of the possible causes of rising rates of conduct disorder in the past two generations does not offer an optimistic view of the future. However, in the USA there has been a small drop in drug use, delinquency and crimes of violence in the 1990s. The National Commission on Civic Renewal finds that while measurements of political participation, trust, strength of the family, group membership and personal security fell between 1984 and 1994, since then gains have occurred in all five categories (Communitarian Network, 1994). In addition, substance misuse by teenagers in 1998 was only half that in 1979, the peak year.

While encouraging, these improvements may not continue. Use of marijuana has been increasing since 1993 (Substance Abuse and Mental Health Services Administration, 1999). The involvement of youth in crimes involving firearms showed no decline until 1995 and remains twice as high as in 1987 (MacKenzie, 1999). Further, the proportion of delinquents who are female and below age 16 continues to rise, suggesting a growing rate of female conduct disorder and an earlier onset or more rapid escalation of symptoms of conduct disorder. However, if this recent drop in substance use and delinquency rates should persist, it will be important to try to explain it and to build programmes based on that explanation to achieve further reductions. At present, solutions that interrupt this rise in conduct disorder and its consequences are at best uncertain. For example, they have led to the confinement of increasing numbers of young antisocial or drug-misusing men in jail.

The finding of an increase in conduct and antisocial personality disorders could be questioned if the apparent increase in later-born cohorts can be attributed to forgetting by older people or their greater relcutance to report disapproved behaviour. Yet there is hard evidence, based on objective records as well as interviews, for an increase in antisocial behaviour and its consequences. Perhaps its level is no higher now than it has been at times in the more distant past, but it is clearly higher than it was just 50 years ago. Compared with 50 years ago, there are more murders, more aggravated assaults, more children reared out of wedlock and more ruptured families.

If it is correct that a single rise in the prevalence of poor parenting is sufficient to initiate a higher rate of conduct disorder in offspring, which in turn generates a still higher rate in the next generation, this implies that the impact of conduct disorder on parenting problems, antisocial behaviour and substance misuse is unchanging over time. If so, we might expect to find an even higher rate of conduct disorder than we actually find. Missing from our ability to forecast rates is an understanding of why most children have survived this era of increased disruption of the traditional family and of a decline in parental supervision without developing conduct disorder. In the ECA's youngest age group (18–29 years), only 26% of men and 10% of women had at least three symptoms of conduct disorder before age 15 (Robins & Regier, 1991: p. 269, Fig. 11.2). One explanation for why these rates, although higher than in older persons, are not still higher may be the fact that most heavy users of alcohol and drugs in their teens reduce or quit their use in their early 20s, and so do not serve as deviant models for their children during the children's vulnerable pre-teen years. Nor does childhood conduct disorder invariably result in equally high rates of antisocial personality. Most children with conduct disorder do not grow up to be antisocial adults and ineffective parents (Robins, 1966).

That so many children of antisocial parents do not develop conduct disorder, and that so many children with conduct disorder do not grow up to be antisocial or poor parents, means that there must be protective factors at work to mitigate transmission from parent to child and continuity between behaviours in childhood and adulthood (Rutter, 1985). As yet there have not been adequate studies of changes in the prevalence of protective factors and their impact on intergenerational transmission. Parental divorce may be less traumatic for children when it is common among their peers, who provide a support group of youngsters with the same experience. Whether a higher frequency of poor parenting in the community makes surviving it in one's own family similarly easier, or has the opposite effect, is still unknown. It is time to evaluate and measure these possibly countervailing factors so that they can be entered into our calculations for risks of continuity between generations and from childhood to adulthood.

No one has been a more ardent advocate of studying discontinuities across generations than Michael Rutter (1989a). He suggests studying total sets of offspring, instead of the common practice of studying one child per family, to highlight differences between those who do and do not survive intact when experiencing equally poor parenting. He also urges utilising the power of prospective studies to specify when discontinuities occur and their apparent causes. He warns us that interpretations of continuity between generations as a simple consequence of socialisation failures and poor role models may be incorrect: there might be shared psychiatric illness of genetic origin that creates similar impairments in parent and adult offspring. Absence of an underlying illness in the parents may account for the many children who show early conduct problems because of poor socialisation in the home, but recover when they are exposed to better adult models at school or in a step- or foster-parent.

As Rutter has noted, prediction from childhood to adult life must be multi-factorial. Such factors include not only genetic liabilities and the experience of parental inadequacy, but also environmental and social circumstances such as practices with regard to removal of children from abusive parents, minimum age for legal access to alcohol, availability and price of illicit drugs and the community's tolerance of their use. It remains for the epidemiologist to determine how much these factors vary in prevalence over time and place.

References

Ahmed, S. H. & Koob, G. F. (1997) Cocaine- but not food-seeking behavior is reinstated by stress after extinction. *Psychopharmacology*, **132**, 289–295.

American Psychiatric Association (1952) *Diagnostic and Statistical Manual of Mental Disorders* (1st edn) (DSM–I). Washington, DC: APA.

—— (1968) *Diagnostic and Statistical Manual of Mental Disorders* (2nd edn) (DSM–II). Washington, DC: APA.

—— (1980) *Diagnostic and Statistical Manual of Mental Disorders* (3rd edn) (DSM–III). Washington, DC: APA.

—— (1987) *Diagnostic and Statistical Manual of Mental Disorders* (3rd edn, revised) (DSM–III–R). Washington, DC: APA.

—— (1994) *Diagnostic and Statistical Manual of Mental Disorders* (4th edn) (DSM–IV). Washington, DC: APA.

Communitarian Network (1994) *Communitarian Update*. Washington, DC: Communitarian Network.

Cross-National Collaborative Group (1992) The changing rate of major depression: cross-national comparisons. *Journal of the American Medical Association*, **268**, 3098–3105.

D'Avanzo, B., La Vecchia, C. & Negri, E. (1994) Age at starting smoking and number of cigarettes smoked. *Annals of Epidemiology*, **4**, 455–459.

Farrington, D. P. (1995) The Twelfth Jack Tizard Memorial Lecture. The developing of offending and antisocial behaviour from childhood. *Journal of Child Psychology and Psychiatry and Allied Disciplines*, **36**, 929–967.

Grant, B. F. (1997) Prevalence and correlates of alcohol use and DSM–IV alcohol dependence in the United States: results of the National Longitudinal Alcohol Epidemiologic Survey. *Studies on Alcohol*, **58**, 464–473.

Home Office (1989) *Criminal and Custodial Careers of those Born in 1953, 1958 and 1963*. London: Home Office.

Johnston, L., O'Malley, P. M. & Bachman, J. G. (1993) *National Survey Results on Drug Use from Monitoring the Future Study, 1975–1992*, Rockville, MD: National Institute on Drug Abuse.

——, —— & —— (1996) *National Survey Results on Drug Use from the Monitoring the Future Study, 1975–1995*. Rockville, MD: National Institute on Drug Abuse.

Joyce, P. R., Oakley-Browne, M. A., Wells, J. E., *et al* (1990) Birth cohort trends in major depression. *Journal of Affective Disorder*, **18**, 83–89.

Kendler, S. K., Davis, C. G. & Kessler, R. C. (1997) The familial aggregation of common psychiatric and substance abuse disorders in the National Comorbidity Survey: A Family History Study. *British Journal of Psychiatry*, **170**, 541–548.

Kessler, R. C., McGonagle, K. A., Zhao, S., *et al* (1994) Lifetime and 12-month prevalences of DSM–III–R psychiatric disorders in the United States. *Archives of General Psychiatry*, **51**, 8–19.

Klerman, G. L. & Weissman, M. M. (1989) Increasing rates of depression. *Journal of the American Medical Association*, **261**, 2229–2395.

Langan, P. A & Farrington, D. P. (1998) *Crime and Justice in the United States and in England and Wales, 1981–96. Bureau of Justice Statistics Executive Summary*. Washington, DC: US Department of Justice.

MacKenzie, L. R. (1999) *Detention in Delinquency Cases, 1987–1996*. Fact Sheet. Washington, DC: US Department of Justice, Office of Justice Programs, Office of Juvenile Justice and Delinquency Prevention.

■127

Offord, D. R., Alder, R. J. & Boyle, M. H. (1986) Prevalence and sociodemographic correlates of conduct disorder. *American Journal of Social Psychiatry*, **4**, 272–278.

Office of Juvenile Justice and Delinquency Prevention (1999) *Research: Making a Difference for Juveniles*, p. 14. Washington, DC: Office of Justice Programs.

Quinton, D. & Rutter, M. (1984) Parents with children in care. II. Intergenerational continuity, *Journal of Child Psychology and Psychiatry and Allied Disciplines*, **25**, 231–250.

——, —— & Liddle, C. (1984) Institutional rearing, parenting difficulties, and marital support. *Psychological Medicine*, **14**, 107–124.

Robins, L. (1966) *Deviant Children Grown Up: A Sociological and Psychiatric Study of Sociopathic Personality*. Baltimore: Williams & Wilkins. Reprinted (1974) Huntington, NY: Robert E. Krieger.

—— (1968) Negro homicide victims – Who will they be? *Transaction*, **5**, 15–19.

—— (1978) Sturdy childhood predictors of adult outcomes: replications from longitudinal studies. *Psychological Medicine* **8**, 611–622.

—— (1986) Changes in conduct disorder over time. In *Intellectual and Psychosocial Development* (eds D. C. Farran & J. D. McKinney), pp. 227–257. New York: Academic Press.

—— (1998) The intimate connection between antisocial personality and substance abuse. *Social Psychiatry and Psychiatric Epidemiology*, **33**, 393–399.

—— (1999) A 70-year history of conduct disorder: variations in definition, prevalence and correlates. In *Time, Place and Psychopathology* (eds P. Cohen, C. Slomkowski & L. N. Robins), pp. 37–56, Table 3.5. Mahwah, NJ: Lawrence Erlbaum.

—— & McEvoy, L. T. (1990) Conduct problems as predictors of substance abuse. In Robins LN and Rutter, M. (eds) *Straight and Devious Pathways from Childhood to Adulthood*, pp. 182–204. New York & Cambridge: Cambridge University Press.

—— & Price, R. (1991) Adult disorders predicted by childhood conduct problems: results from the NIMH Epidemiologic Catchment Area Project. *Psychiatry*, **54**, 116–132.

—— & Przybeck, T. R. (1985) Age of onset of drug use as a factor in drug and other disorders. In *Etiology of Drug Abuse: Implications for Prevention* (eds C. L. Jones & R. J. Battjes) (NIDA Research Monograph 56, DHHS Pub. No. (ADM)85-1335), pp. 178–192. Washington, DC: DHHS.

—— & Regier, D. (eds) (1991) *Psychiatric Disorders in America*. New York: Free Press.

——, Murphy, G. E. & Breckenridge, M. B. (1968) Drinking behavior of young urban Negro men. *Quarterly Journal of Studies on Alcohol*, **29**, 657–684.

——, Helzer, J. E., Weissman, M., *et al* (1984) Lifetime prevalence of specific psychiatric disorders in three sites. *Archives of General Psychiatry*, **41**, 949–958.

——, Tipp, J. & Przybeck, T. (1991) Antisocial personality. In *Psychiatric Disorders in America* (eds L. N. Robins & D. Regier), pp. 258–290. New York: Free Press.

Rutter, M. (1972) Relationships between child and adult psychiatric disorders. *Acta Psychiatrica Scandinavica*, **48**, 3–21.

—— (1985) Resilience in the face of adversity. Protective factors and resistance to psychiatric disorder. *British Journal of Psychiatry*, **147**, 598–611.

—— (1988) Longitudinal data in the study of causal processes. In *Studies of Psychosocial Risk* (ed. M. Rutter), pp. 1–28. Cambridge: Cambridge University Press.

—— (1989a) Intergenerational continuities and discontinuities in serious parenting difficulties. In *Child Maltreatment: Theory and Research on the Causes and Consequences of Child Abuse* (eds D. Cicchetti & V. Carlson), pp. 317–348. Cambridge: Cambridge University Press.

—— (1989b) Isle of Wight revisited: 25 years of child psychiatric epidemiology. *American Academy of Child and Adolescent Psychiatry*, **28**, 633–653.

—— (1991) Childhood experiences and adult psychosocial functioning. In *The Childhood Environment and Adult Disease* (eds G. Bock & J. Whelan), p. 195. Chichester: John Wiley & Sons.

——, Tizard, J. & Whitmore, K. (1970) *Education, Health and Behaviour; Psychological and Medical Study of Childhood Development*. London: Longman.

——, Cox, A., Tupling, C., *et al* (1975) Attainment and adjustment in two geographical areas. I. The prevalence of psychiatric disorder. *British Journal of Psychiatry*, **126**, 413–509.

Silbereisen, R. K., Robins, L. N. & Rutter, M. (1995) Secular trends in substance abuse: concepts and data on the impact of social change on alcohol and drug abuse. In *Psychosocial Disorders in Young People: Time Trends and their Causes* (ed. M. Rutter), pp. 490–543. Cambridge, John Wiley & Sons.

Simon, G. E. & Von Korff, M. (1992) Reevaluation of secular trends in depression rates. *American Journal of Epidemiology*, **135**, 1411–1422.

Substance Abuse and Mental Health Services Administration (SAMHSA) Office of Applied Studies (1998) *Preliminary Results from the 1997 National Household Survey on Drug Abuse*. Rockville, MD: US Department of Health and Human Services.

—— (1999) *Summary Findings from the 1998 National Household Survey on Drug Abuse*, Tables 2.6, 2.8. Rockville, MD: US Department of Health and Human Services.

Wickramaratne, P. J., Weissman, M. M., Leaf, P. I., *et al* (1989) Age, period and cohort effects on the risk of major depression. *Journal of Clinical Epidemiology*, **92**, 333–343.

9 Psychosocial adversity and child psychopathology

Michael Rutter

Behaviour geneticists have expressed scepticism about the importance of psychosocial influences except at the extremes (Scarr, 1992; Rowe, 1994). Attention has been drawn to the role of genetic influences in individual differences in psychosocial risk exposure (Plomin & Bergeman, 1991), and it has been argued that shared environmental effects are quite minor with respect to most psychological traits (Plomin & Daniels, 1987). Strong claims have been made that 'genetic theory' should replace 'socialisation theory' (Bouchard, 1997; Scarr, 1997). It might seem that psychosocial research has been put on the defensive, with questions raised on its methodologies and basic tenets, as well as on its findings. However, the evidence suggests a more positive appraisal. In this chapter I seek to re-evaluate our understanding of psychosocial influences on childhood psychopathology, by considering developments over the past half century or so, taking as the starting point 1948.

Three main movements in the first half of the 20th century provided the basis for **1948** thinking about the influence of psychosocial factors on mental disorders in childhood.

The mental hygiene movement

First, the mental hygiene movement had played a major role in the development of child guidance services in both North America and the UK (Kanner, 1959), with its emphasis on the ways in which interpersonal relationships at home and at school played a part in shaping children's behaviour, both normal and abnormal. This movement had led to a series of systematic studies seeking to relate patterns of family relationships and child rearing to patterns of children's behaviour (see, e.g., Hewitt & Jenkins' (1946) classic study of child guidance clinic records).

Psychoanalysis

Second, there was the influence of psychoanalysis. Seemingly paradoxically, this was associated with two contrasting trends. On the one hand, a focus on intra-psychic mental mechanisms led to a downplaying of the role of real-life experiences. Therapeutic interventions focused much more on children's inner thought processes than on what

---

Reprinted, with amendments and with permission, from Rutter (1999a).

was happening to them at home or at school. On the other hand, psychoanalytic theories concerned with the child's transition through the early psychosexual stages led to a focus on the importance of whether or not the child had been breast-fed or bottle-fed, on the timing of weaning and on the ways in which toilet training was managed. In both these features, however, the emphasis was very much on the role of past experiences in shaping current behaviour and, hence, on the need in treatment to concentrate on the past rather than the present (Baldwin, 1968; Dare, 1976). Alongside the concern with the specifics of child-rearing practices, there was also a focus on the role of maladaptive parent–child relationships in the genesis of mental disorder. The concepts of the schizophrenogenic mother (Reichard & Tillman, 1950) and of 'refrigerator' parenting of children with autism (Kanner, 1949) were beginning to make their mark.

Developmental studies

The third set of influences derived from developmental studies. Although some of the methodologies may appear crude by present-day standards, the quality of much of the work was high. The extent to which the research ideas of the first half of the 20th century adumbrated much of what was to be rediscovered later is striking. Two examples serve to illustrate the point. Levy (1943), in his pioneering study of maternal overprotection, emphasised the importance of assessing parents' behaviour as it impinged on one particular child and not just on children in general; he noted the ways in which characteristics of the child served to influence parental behaviour; and he commented on the observation that one relationship (as between parents) could affect others (as between parent and child). Jones (1946) brought together the findings in the Burks (1928) and Leahy (1935) studies of foster-children to note that the correlations between biological parents and their children were substantially stronger than those between foster-parents and their children. He concluded that a part of what seemed to be an environmental influence on mental development was actually genetically mediated.

Developmental researchers also appreciated the value of experimental methods for the testing of hypotheses about environmental mediation. Thus, Lewin and his colleagues (Lewin *et al*, 1939; Lippitt & White, 1943) took the notion of social ethos or climate and studied the effects of adult behaviour in groups of 11-year-old boys, comparing 'democratic', 'authoritarian' and 'laissez-faire' leadership styles. Similarly, Skeels and colleagues (Skeels *et al*, 1938; Skeels & Dye, 1939) used an experimental design to examine the effects of improving the circumstances of children being reared in an institutional orphanage. Experimental animal research, too, was making its mark. Hebb's (1949) studies of the effects of environmental restriction and enrichment on the development of rats were particularly important and served as a major theoretical and empirical base for later work on infant stimulation in humans (Hunt, 1979).

Longitudinal studies

The 1930s and 1940s were also the time when many long-term longitudinal studies were first established (see Bronfenbrenner & Crouter, 1983; Cairns, 1983), as well as various major centres for the study of child development in the USA. Both were accompanied by an increasing attention to methodological issues with respect to sampling and measurement (Anderson, 1946). Most of this focused on the assessment of children, rather than of the environment, but it is noteworthy that Baldwin *et al* (1945) had been innovative in combining observations in the home with interviews and questionnaires given to parents.

Measurement

This was also a period during which developmental researchers became increasingly aware of measurement issues in relation to the source of information. Becker and colleagues (Becker, 1960; Becker *et al*, 1962) showed important differences depending on who made ratings. It became evident that parental attitude measures were strongly influenced by social class (Zuckerman *et al*, 1960) and might have little to do with how parents actually treated their children. Bronfenbrenner (1961) began to explore the use of children's reports on parental behaviour, and Hoffman (1957, 1960) made use of detailed descriptions of actual family interactions, rather than relying on ratings by either parents or children.

Behaviourism

Although psychoanalysis had undoubtedly constituted the major influence on research into psychosocial influences on psychopathology, the 1930s were also marked by the growth of behaviourism, led especially by Hull (1943) and Skinner (1938, 1953). On the eve of the Second World War, Dollard and Miller (Dollard *et al*, 1939; Miller & Dollard, 1941) brought these traditions together under the broad concept of social learning. The scene was set for a major strengthening and expansion of developmental research and, indeed, it ushered in what Cairns (1983) has described as the golden age, extending until the late 1970s.

The second half of the 20th century began with Bowlby's (1951) World Health Organization monograph on the effects of 'maternal deprivation'.

The 1950s and early 1960s

Maternal deprivation

Bowlby asserted that,

> "mother love in infancy and childhood is as important for mental health as are vitamins and proteins for physical health". (1951)

■ 131

Strong claims were made for the supposedly severely damaging effects of even short separations of mother and child, and it was argued that the damage was both pervasive and irreversible. These claims ran into a storm of criticism on the quality of the evidence and on the inferences drawn (O'Connor, 1956; Wootton, 1959; O'Connor & Franks, 1960; Casler, 1961; Yarrow, 1961).

In laudable fashion, Bowlby went on to test the hypothesis of the profoundly damaging effects of separation by assessing children admitted to a tuberculosis sanatorium and comparing their outcome with a matched control group (Bowlby *et al*, 1956). The results showed that the claims that prolonged separation *usually* resulted in affectionless psychopathy were mistaken. Although Bowlby maintained his view that a continuous loving relationship with the mother was crucial for mental health, empirical research findings indicated that the damage was not as inevitable or as irreversible as first thought (Ainsworth, 1962). Despite the obvious need for epidemiological studies to quantify the psychopathological risks associated with different forms of parent–child separation, Ainsworth & Bowlby (1954) dismissed the value and the need. Wootton (1959: p. 151) scathingly castigated this as "a counsel of despair as well as a grave breakdown in logic". As she argued, it is not possible to conclude that separation is a pathogenic factor until it can be shown that pathological problems are more frequent among children who have experienced separation than among those who have not.

It was by no means only Bowlby's maternal deprivation hypothesis that came under attack at this time. Much the most thoughtful and well-informed critique was that by Wootton (1959). She reviewed the evidence on psychosocial influences on crime and personality disorder, concluding that the quality of the evidence allowed very few generalisations. There was a need for rigorous scientific study, with much better attention to epidemiological sampling, to measurement, to concepts and to testing causal inferences. Nevertheless, Wootton emphasised the importance of the issues and was optimistic about what social science could deliver.

Child rearing

Empirical studies of child-rearing practices during this era (e.g., Sears *et al*, 1957) cast doubt on the influence of the specifics of feeding, weaning and toileting practices. The value of counselling to counter the adverse psychosocial influences predisposing to delinquency was also called in question by the Cambridge–Somerville study (Powers & Witmer, 1951). Although the treatment lasted some half a dozen years, systematic evaluations failed to show any benefits.

Animal studies

Despite an accumulation of discouraging findings and increasing methodological criticisms, the 1950s also included some rather more encouraging research features. Most strikingly, animal studies were consistent in showing that early experiences could have important lasting effects. For example, both Scott's (Scott, 1963; Scott & Fuller, 1965) studies of social isolation in dogs and Harlow's (Harlow, 1958, 1963) studies of monkeys showed the profound effects on social functioning of a lack of contact with parents or peers in the early period of rearing. Hubel & Wiesel (1965; Wiesel & Hubel, 1965a,b) demonstrated the neural effects of visual deprivation in kittens. All these animal studies dealt with much more marked environmental changes than ordinarily applied to the human situation, but the findings were nevertheless important in showing that early experiences could have important effects on later development. Moreover, other studies, such as those by Levine (1962) in rats, showed far-reaching psychological and physical effects of relatively minor stress experiences in early infancy. Somewhat later, Hinde's careful experimental studies in monkeys similarly showed persistent effects from separation experiences (Hinde & McGinnis, 1977).

Peer relationships

Human research in this period was mainly characterised by a focus on parenting as the most important psychosocial influence. However, there was an influential small clinical study by Freud & Dann (1951) of six concentration-camp children who came to the UK. Despite their horrendous experiences and loss of parents, they showed remarkable resilience and it seemed that the peer relationships among them had constituted the main protective factor.

Social groups

Bandura's experimental studies of imitation showed its importance in human social learning, at least under laboratory conditions (Bandura & Walters, 1963). Experimental approaches to social groups were taken further through innovative studies by Sherif (Sherif & Sherif, 1953; Sherif et al, 1961) using a mixture of qualitative and quantitative methods in what came to be known as the Robbers' Cave experiments. Findings were informative with respect to how social groups developed and operated but, in some respects, the research was even more important in showing how experiments could be undertaken in the natural environment. The work of Barker & Wright (1955) was also important in its focus on the school as a social context and as an influence on children's functioning.

Reappraisal of psychosocial influences

The 15 years or so after the establishment of the National Health Service (NHS) in the UK in 1948 saw a major reappraisal of psychosocial influences on mental disorder in childhood. It involved a fading of interest in the role of variations in child-rearing practices with respect to feeding, toileting and the minutiae of discipline. Bowlby's 1951 monograph, although overstating the case in some respects, led to a major change in the approach to experiences during the pre-school years. His argument that the quality of parent–child relationships was the key influence altered the focus of research. At a practical level, it also led, in time, to a revolution in how both hospitals and residential nurseries dealt with children in their care. In addition, developmentalists were beginning to consider social influences outside parent–child relationships and interaction. Animal studies were decisive in showing that early experiences could have marked effects, and the challenge was to determine how such experiences actually operated in the ordinary living conditions of children. It was accepted, however, that if this challenge was to be met successfully, there would have to be a very considerable improvement in the strategies and tactics employed.

Methodological issues continued to be a concern during the next decades, and the 1960s and 1970s were characterised by a range of developments designed to meet the challenges of establishing sensitive measures and rigorous research designs.

The 1960s and 1970s

Retrospective recall

Radke-Yarrow *et al* (1968, 1970), in a highly influential study, noted the many problems with respect to both the reliability of retrospective recall and the biases in the measures that it provided. Robbins (1963), using data from the New York longitudinal study, also highlighted the problems of bias in recall. Most crucially, the findings showed that the biases were of a kind that were likely to lead to an artefactual confirmation of prevailing views regarding child development and influences on it.

Children's effects on parents

A rather different sort of challenge was provided by the evidence on the importance of children's effects on their parents. The New York longitudinal study of children undertaken by Thomas *et al* (1968) pointed to the importance of children's temperamental characteristics, and Bell (1968), in a seminal paper, argued that many of the effects attributed to parents might actually reflect the reverse direction of causation. Clearly, there was a need to develop research designs that could both assess the direction of influences and also test, in rigorous fashion, hypotheses about environmental risk mediation.

■ 133

Interview measures

George Brown and I developed the Camberwell interview to assess family life and relationships (Brown & Rutter, 1966; Rutter & Brown, 1966) . It was innovative in making a careful distinction between events and happenings on the one hand, and people's feelings about those events on the other, while recognising that both were important. In so far as the former were concerned, a style of interviewing was developed that relied on obtaining detailed descriptions of actual behaviour, rather than informants' perceptions and ratings. Criteria for codings were investigator-based and operationalised. In so far as feelings were concerned, there was reliance on the affect *shown* by the informant during the interview when talking about specific family members. The notion of negative expressed emotion came into being. The method also focused on parental behaviour as shown to individual children, rather than relying only on measures of the general family situation. Despite being concerned with features such as warmth and hostility that might be thought to be quite subtle and open to cultural variations and interpretation, a high degree of reliability and validity was established. Later studies also showed the predictive validity of these measures (Quinton *et al*, 1976).

Observational measures

During the same era there were major advances in the development of improved observational measures for studying family interaction in the home (Hinde & Herrmann, 1977). Many of these were concerned with either the frequency or the duration of particular behaviours. In addition, however, technological advances made possible the study of sequences of behaviour as they applied to dyadic interactions. The technique made possible a more direct study of the ways in which the behaviour of one individual affected the subsequent behaviour of another individual in the home. Patterson *et al* (1973; Patterson, 1979) were pioneers in the development of this approach to understanding how vicious cycles of coercive interchange develop in families. It proved necessary, however, to consider individuals' prior behaviour as a self-regulatory component in order to separate out interactive influences (Thomas & Martin, 1976; Thomas & Malone, 1979; Martin, 1981). Most especially, during this period, the use of multi-method, multi-informant assessments became firmly established. These became the norm for most major programmes of research concerned with the study of psychosocial influences on children's development.

Risk indicators and risk mechanisms

One of the key issues in consideration of the effects of maternal deprivation concerned the suggestion that the main risk lay in the child's separation from its parents (Rutter, 1972). It was clear, however, that much of the evidence derived from separation experiences that were associated with a wide range of other psychosocial risks. Accordingly, it was necessary to ask whether the risk derived from the separation *per se* or from other adverse experiences with which separation happened to be associated. I tackled this issue by comparing the effects of parental divorce and parental death, as well as by comparing separations that appeared to represent neutral or pleasurable experiences and those that reflected stress or discord (Rutter, 1971). The findings were clear, as they were from other studies, that separation itself constituted only a minor risk factor, but that the accompanying family discord and disruption were probably the key risk factors. This study, and others like it, emphasised the importance of differentiating between risk indicators and risk mechanisms.

Cohort studies

Epidemiological studies, and especially those that constituted the initiation of a prospective longitudinal study, were established in many countries (Mednick & Baert, 1981; Mednick *et al*, 1984). Major national longitudinal studies of birth cohorts born in 1946 (Douglas, 1964), 1958 (Pringle *et al*, 1966) and 1970 (Osborn *et al*, 1984) were set up in the UK. Because the samples were geographically scattered, there was a need to rely primarily on questionnaires and structured interviews. In addition, however, good use was made of health and social service records, capitalising on the research potential provided by the NHS. In addition, local or regional epidemiological studies, using more detailed standardised interviews with parents, children and teachers, were established in Newcastle (Kolvin *et al*, 1988; Kolvin *et al*, 1990), the Isle of Wight (Rutter *et al*, 1970) and London (West & Farrington, 1973; Rutter *et al*, 1975; Rutter & Quinton, 1977). It was shown that quite detailed measures of the psychosocial environment could be applied on a population-wide basis and that the findings could be used to study psychosocial risk factors. Findings also underlined the crucial importance of representative samples for the testing of causal hypotheses (Cox *et al*, 1977; Berk, 1983), which is critical in the study of nature–nurture interplay (see Rutter *et al*, 1999*b*, 2000).

Broadening of risk features

One of the most striking features of psychosocial research during the 1960s and 1970s was the broadening of the range of psychosocial risk factors that were studied as possible influences on the development of psychopathology. I focused on the role of parental mental disorder as a factor associated with family disruption and dysfunction, as well as serious impairments in parenting (Rutter, 1966). This study drew attention to the finding that the main risks to the child seem to derive from personality disorders in the parents, rather than from parental psychosis. It was necessary to differentiate between genetic and environmental mediation, and I contrasted the effects of mental disorder in step-parents with those of similar disorders in biological parents. Child-specific effects in particular had to be considered, and I found an immense heterogeneity in children's responses. Reviewing a broader research literature, I argued that determination of the factors leading to individual differences in children's response to stress and adversity constituted one of the key priorities (Rutter, 1972).

Research into the development of social relationships and the effects of such relationships on risk of psychopathology advanced in several key respects during the late 1970s. Five advances warrant special emphasis. First, there was Ainsworth's discovery of the importance of attachment security in parent–child relationships, and her development of the 'strange situation' in order to measure security (Ainsworth *et al*, 1978). The rather diffuse concept of mother-love was transformed into a two-way relationship with qualities that were susceptible to measurement. Second, a seminal book by Hinde (1979) did much to bring conceptual clarity to the study of human relationships. Third, Dunn opened up the field of study of sibling relationships and showed their importance for children's psychological development (Dunn & Kendrick, 1982). Research into peer relationships also underwent a renaissance during the 1970s, having declined markedly during the 1950s and 1960s, when the emphasis was almost entirely on parent–child relationships (Asher & Gottman, 1981; Hartup, 1983). From a psychopathological perspective, two foci were of particular importance. On the one hand, studies began to address the question of the extent to which the personal experience of social isolation and rejection could create an increased risk of mental disorder (Parker & Asher, 1987). On the other, there was a growing awareness that the peer group, as a social influence, might be important. From the outset, the need to differentiate between selection effects (i.e, people choose the peer group that they enter) and socialisation effects (i.e., the influence exerted by the particular ethos of that peer group) was appreciated. Kandel's study (1978a,b) was seminal in its demonstration of the value of studying changes over time in peer similarity as a means of differentiating these two effects. Finally, longitudinal studies of children in divorcing families were important in their demonstration that the event of divorce needed to be re-conceptualised in terms of a process that usually began a long time before the family break-up and often continued quite some time afterwards (Hetherington et al, 1982; Wallerstein, 1983). The findings showed, among other things, the importance of conflict, rivalries and insecurity in relationships. The findings also re-emphasised the very important variations among children in how they responded to both conflict and divorce.

Schooling

Up to the mid-1970s, the conventional wisdom held it that schooling had minimal effects on children's psychological development and functioning (see, e.g., Coleman et al, 1966; Jensen, 1969; Jencks et al, 1972). Of course, people had been aware that some schools had high levels of problem behaviour and poor achievement, whereas in others pupil success was the order of the day. It was just that an assumption was made that these variations between schools reflected little more than differences in the intake of pupils to them. Questioning this assumption, colleagues and I studied children's progress through secondary schools in inner London, and we found that school qualities did indeed make a difference (Rutter et al, 1979). We recognised that school effects could be studied satisfactorily only if three conditions were met. First, adequate account needed to be taken of the qualities of the children before they entered secondary school; second, the children's functioning had to be studied as it changed over time during their period at the school; and third, variations in pupil progress had to be related to systematically measured qualities of the school environment. Using a design with these features, the findings showed substantial school effects on both pupil behaviour and scholastic attainments. Subsequent research has confirmed this conclusion (Maughan, 1994; Mortimore, 1995).

Residential care

During the 1970s, there was also a growth in the broader field of research into the ways in which children's behaviour is influenced by the characteristics of residential institutions such as group homes providing substitute parental care, institutions for children with disabilities, special schools and hostels for delinquent youths. Tizard et al (1975) brought together these diverse studies and, in so doing, emphasised both that it was possible to assess the qualities of institutions in a reliable, meaningful and quantified fashion, and also that children's experiences in such institutions influenced their behaviour. In the adult field, Wing & Brown's (1970) studies of mental hospitals carried the same message.

Area influences

Throughout the course of the 20th century, there had been numerous observations that some geographical areas were characterised by unusually high rates of crime or of mental disorder. Surprisingly little was known, however, about the mechanisms underlying this finding, and there had been very little study of geographical variations in child mental disorder. The systematic comparison of the Isle of Wight and of a borough in inner London (Rutter *et al*, 1975; Rutter & Quinton, 1977) opened up the topic in several ways. Because the investigation covered the total general population, and because the same detailed standardised methods of measurement were used in both areas, confidence could be placed on the reality of the finding that the rate of psychopathology was twice as high in inner London. It was also possible to show that the difference was not a function of selective in- or out-migration. It seemed that there was some sort of area risk factor operating but it was also apparent that, in so far as child psychopathology was concerned, it largely operated through the family, rather than directly on the child. Thus, the difference between the two areas in rates of psychopathology was largely explicable in terms of family risk factors. Moreover, the area differences applied most strongly to mental disorders that had begun in early or middle childhood, rather than those with an onset in adolescence (Rutter, 1979). The study left open, however, just what it was about life in an inner city that created risks for families (Quinton, 1994).

Life events

The study of acute life events as precipitants of psychiatric disorder was also revolutionised during the 1970s, primarily as a result of the work by Brown and his colleagues with adults (Brown *et al*, 1973; Brown & Harris, 1978). The notion that stressful experiences create a psychopathological risk goes right back to the beginnings of psychiatry, and was put on a firm footing by Meyer (1957), although until the 1970s the research had been rather inconclusive in testing the causal hypothesis. Brown brought new clarity to the field, as well as introducing a range of crucial methodological features in the study of life events. Four features were particularly important.

(i) It was recognised that because many life events are brought on by the ways in which people behave, it was crucial to differentiate between life events that were independent of people's actions and those that they might have brought about themselves.

(ii) Because people's recognition of stress experiences is likely to be influenced by their mental state, it was necessary to assess life events independently of people's perception of their impact on them.

(iii) The psychopathological risk was likely to be affected by the long-term implications of the acute event, which was rather more important than what happened at the immediate time of its occurrence. Thus, the impact of events was likely to be influenced by their social-contextual meaning for that individual.

(iv) The causal inference could be made more strongly if a temporal connection could be shown between the timing of the life event and the timing of onset of psychiatric disorder. The early studies provided evidence that life events that carried long-term threat did indeed play a role in precipitating the onset of disorder. As with all other psychosocial factors that have been studied, however, there was enormous individual variation in response. Most life events did not result in the onset of disorder.

It is clear that the 1970s was a most exciting decade for psychosocial research. There were crucial advances in measurement, the range of psychosocial factors extended well beyond the parent–child relationship and there was a marked improvement in the quality of the research designs used to test causal inferences. Before proceeding to consider research during the next decade, it should be noted that there was something of a divergence in the psychosocial features being studied in relation to adult mental disorder and those being investigated in relation to child psychopathology. In the adult field, the main emphasis was on acute life events and on their importance with respect to the timing of the onset of disorder. By contrast, studies with children focused much more on chronic psychosocial adversities and their effects on the overall liability to disorder, rather than the timing of onset.

The 1980s and early 1990s

The period of the 1980s and early 1990s saw a consolidation of some aspects of psychosocial research and an opening up of new topics, but also a set of challenges from behaviour geneticists who queried the reality of environmental influences other than at the extremes of psychosocial adversity.

Vulnerability factors

Research with adults during this period provided many confirmations of the temporal association between negative life events carrying long-term threat and the onset of psychiatric disorder (Brown & Harris, 1990). The same research also showed, however, the importance of vulnerability factors, such as the experience of poor parenting in their own upbringing, that predisposed individuals to react adversely to life events. Studies by Goodyer et al (1985; Goodyer, 1990, 1995) showed somewhat similar associations in childhood and adolescence, although questions were raised about the extent to which the risk effects mainly applied to the time period immediately preceding the onset of disorder. The 1980s also saw a re-evaluation of the possible long-term effects of adverse life experiences. Reviews at the beginning of the 1980s (Clarke & Clarke, 1976; Rutter, 1981a) concluded that, on the whole, there were few serious long-term sequelae of adverse experiences in early life that were independent of adverse experiences when older.

Indirect long-term effects

The inference seemed empirically secure, but it came to be realised that the question had been posed the wrong way (Rutter, 1989). That was because one of the ways in which early experiences exerted long-term effects stemmed from their influences both in making negative experiences more likely to occur later and in rendering individuals more vulnerable to such experiences (Rutter et al, 1995). There were long-term sequelae of early experiences, but they mainly arose through indirect chain effects rather than direct effects that permanently damaged the child at the time. It was necessary to pose the question of what adverse experiences did to the organism and how the effects of such experiences were carried forward into later phases of development. Did the mechanisms lie in alterations in ways in which the individuals processed their experiences, or in effects on the neuroendocrine system, or in the creation of vicious cycles through which individuals shaped and selected their environments in maladaptive ways that created risks for them? Increasingly, research began to focus on testing hypotheses about these and other possible mechanisms underlying indirect chain effects.

■ 137

Distal and proximal processes

Traditionally, social scientists had been concerned with the seemingly increased risks of psychiatric disorder associated with broad concepts such as poverty, social disadvantage or parental loss. It had become clear, however, that it was unlikely that such broad variables were directly implicated in the causal processes for psychopathology. A distinction came to be drawn between distal and proximal risk processes, meaning those that operate indirectly through effects that occur earlier in the causal chain, and those that are more directly implicated in the immediate risk process that brings about the psychopathology. Evidence started to accumulate that it was necessary to view the causal processes in more dynamic terms. Thus, it seems that the risks of antisocial behaviour associated with poverty derive from the fact that poverty makes good parenting more difficult and the proximal risk processes derive from problems in parenting rather than from the economic factors as such (Conger et al, 1992, 1994).

Person–environment interplay

Scarr & McCartney (1983), in a seminal paper focusing on the role of genetics, pointed to the importance of a person's own actions in determining the risk experiences that they encountered. Such effects had been shown most dramatically nearly two decades earlier by Robins (1966) in her pioneering, and crucially important, long-term follow-up of children who had attended a child guidance clinic. Her findings had shown that people exhibiting antisocial behaviour in childhood had a greatly increased likelihood in adult life of such psychosocial risk experiences as unemployment, quarrels with friends, lack of social support and break-up of love relationships. Several long-term follow-up studies of high-risk samples have both confirmed and extended these findings. In a study of institution-reared girls (Quinton & Rutter, 1988), Quinton & I showed the importance of teenage pregnancies and a tendency to marry spouses exhibiting behavioural deviance from a similarly disadvantaged background. The girls' maladaptive responses to family stress served to put them in new family situations in adult life that recreated serious stresses for them. Champion *et al*'s (1995) long-term follow-up of a general population sample in inner London similarly showed that antisocial behaviour at age 10 was associated with more than a doubling of the likelihood of both acute and chronic psychosocial adversities in adult life. Farrington *et al*'s (1996) longitudinal study of boys in inner London also emphasised the very strong tendency for antisocial individuals to marry people showing similar antisocial behaviour.

These longitudinal studies focused on effects as they were seen over long periods of time. In addition, a range of different designs were used to examine the various ways in which children's behaviour affected other people's responses to them (Bell & Chapman, 1986). Thus, in addition to naturalistic studies (Maccoby & Jacklin, 1983; Lee & Bates, 1985), experimental studies were undertaken in which children were trained to behave in oppositional ways in order to see how this affected their interactions with other people (Brunk & Henggeler, 1984), children's interactions with their own parents were compared with their interactions with other children's parents in ingenious ways that served to separate child and parent effects (Anderson *et al*, 1986), and the effects of stimulant medication on children's hyperactive behaviour were used to examine effects on parental behaviour that were mediated by changes in child behaviour (Barkley & Cunningham, 1979; Schachar *et al*, 1987). The findings were consistent in showing important effects of children's behaviour on other people's responses, but the research left open the question of the significance of these effects for children's later psychological development or risks of psychopathology (Rutter *et al*, 1997).

Active processing of experiences

At one time, life experiences were thought about in terms of stimuli impinging on a passive organism. Both human and animal research during the 1960s and 1970s brought about a realisation that that was a very misleading way of conceptualising psychosocial effects (Rutter, 1981*b*; Rutter & Rutter, 1993). Even quite young children actively process their experiences, think about what happens to them and develop concepts about the meaning of such experiences. Kagan (1984), in developing this point, argued that experiences in the period after infancy were likely to have greater effects simply because of children's enhanced capacity to undertake cognitive processing of them.

Several rather separate bodies of research serve to demonstrate the extent to which cognitive biases in processing were associated with psychopathology. For example, these have been well demonstrated with respect to depressive disorders in adult life (Teasdale & Barnard, 1993), and research by Dodge *et al* (1990, 1995) has shown a somewhat different set of biases associated with antisocial behaviour in childhood. In both cases the research has only begun to address the question of how such variations in cognitive and affective processing influence people's responses to defined psychosocial experiences, but their strong potential relevance is obvious. One of the most ambitious attempts to take this matter further is represented by the study undertaken by Dodge *et al* (1990, 1995) looking at the possible mechanisms by which the experience of being abused made it more likely that children would themselves come to exhibit antisocial behaviour. Results suggest that effects on cognitive biases in processing may constitute part of the mediating mechanism.

'Planning' tendency

Longitudinal studies that Clausen (1991) and that Quinton & I undertook (Quinton & Rutter, 1988; Quinton *et al*, 1993) both showed the importance of what was called a 'planning' tendency. Institution-reared youngsters showed a markedly diminished tendency to think that they could influence what happened to them by planning, for example, in relation to marital choice or work careers. As a consequence, they tended to act impulsively without thinking ahead and, by so doing, landed themselves in further risk situations.

Internal working models

Over this same time period, attachment theorists came to place an increasing emphasis on what they called 'internal working models' (Main *et al*, 1985; Bretherton, 1987). The proposition started with the recognition that, as a result of experiences, people build up models to represent both their own self-concept and their expectations of relationships with others. The hypothesis has been that how people think about negative experiences and relationships may make a big difference to whether or not these predispose to later psychopathology. The adult attachment interview was developed by Main *et al* (1985; Main, 1991) to focus on the nature of such models; studies have shown both marked individual variations in such models and that they can be assessed with a reasonable degree of reliability (van IJzendoorn, 1995). It is certainly very plausible that variations in how experiences are processed may account for individual differences in the sequelae of adverse relationships in early life, but the hypothesis has yet to be put to a decisive test, although research is beginning to accumulate evidence (Patrick *et al*, 1994; Phelps *et al*, 1998).

Testing causal hypotheses

■ 139

Methodological teaching from the undergraduate years onwards has always driven home the message that correlations cannot prove causation. Taken at face value, however, this negative message is in danger of being misleading. After all, within experimental designs, correlations are regularly used to infer causation, and if the experiment has been well designed, the inferences are well based. Although it is certainly the case that most psychological risk experiences are not of a kind that can be studied in the laboratory, at least not in humans, nevertheless, naturally occurring circumstances do provide real-life experiments that can do much to pull apart risk and protective factors that ordinarily go together (Rutter, 1981*b*, 1994).

Farrington (1988) has emphasised the value of studying changes within the individual over time in this connection, and I have drawn attention to the power of 'natural experiments', provided that the research is planned appropriately to put the causal hypotheses to the test (Rutter, 1981*b*, 1994). In so doing, use can be made of non-replications in order to test causal hypotheses (Rutter, 1974). That is, it is useful to identify circumstances in which effects should *not* be found if the causal mechanism has been identified appropriately. Among the elements needed in order to use epidemiological findings to test causal hypotheses are reversal effects (i.e., do the risks go down when the adverse experiences are alleviated?), consistent dose–response relationships (i.e., is there a consistent tendency across the range for the risks to go up progressively according to the severity or duration of risk experiences?), identification of a plausible biological mediating mechanism (both in terms of the element in the experience that creates the risk and its effects on the organism) and treatment effects. In so far as the last of these is concerned, the issue is not whether treatment of psychopathology is effective but, rather, whether within a treated group changes in the postulated mediating mechanism are consistently associated with benefits in terms of symptomatology. Surprisingly few treatment studies have tackled this issue, but the work of Patterson and his colleagues (Dishion *et al*, 1992; Patterson *et al*, 1993) in the field of antisocial behaviour and of Murray & Cooper (1997) in relation to maternal depression constitute notable exceptions.

One important element in the use of epidemiological methods to test causal hypotheses is the pitting of one postulated mechanism against another. Twin and adoptee studies provide just such an opportunity for differentiating between genetic and environmental mediation, and there is a similar need to use natural experiments to differentiate between different forms of environmental mediation. Thus, for example, longitudinal data have been used to determine whether the psychopathology associated with parental divorce was present before the divorce took place (Block *et al*, 1986; Cherlin *et al*, 1991). The finding that it was suggests that the mechanism is likely to lie in the conflict and discord that preceded and led to the divorce rather than in the parent–child separation that followed the marital break-up. Comparisons of the effects of family change and family conflict have led to the same conclusion (Fergusson *et al*, 1992).

Similarly, in our study of children from Romanian orphanages adopted into UK families, colleagues and I contrasted the effects of malnutrition with the effects of psychological privation. Both played a role, but the importance of psychological privation was indicated by findings that both its duration and its severity had significant effects even after the degree of malnutrition had been taken into account (O'Connor *et al*, 1998*b*; Rutter & ERA Study Team, 1998; Castle *et al*, 1999). Longitudinal data were also able to differentiate between the effects of duration of institutional care and the length of time in the adoptive home (Castle *et al*, 1999). Roy *et al* (2000) used the natural experiment of the contrast between institutional care and family fostering as a way of dealing with a breakdown of parenting in order to examine the effects of variations in pattern of rearing. The findings showed that these two groups were closely similar in parental characteristics (both being high risk) and in leaving their biological families in the early months of life. The effects of rearing were evident in the finding that hyperactivity/inattention and unsociability were much more common in the institution-reared group than in the family-fostered group.

Turning-point and accentuation effects

The study of intra-individual change over time has been informative in showing the importance of both 'turning-point' and 'accentuation' effects (Caspi & Moffitt, 1993; Sampson & Laub, 1993; Rutter, 1996). Turning-point effects refer to the phenomenon of a change from a maladaptive to an adaptive life trajectory as a result of some set of life experiences. They have been shown to occur following experiences as diverse as a harmonious marriage (Zoccolillo *et al*, 1992; Sampson & Laub, 1993; Rutter *et al*, 1997; Laub *et al*, 1998), a period of army service providing educational and career advantages (Elder, 1986; Sampson & Laub, 1996) and a geographical move from a high-risk inner-city area (Osborn, 1980). In each case, the power of the research has lain in the demonstration of within-individual change that was not a function of prior behavioural or psychosocial risk features, nor of measurement error. The findings have been particularly important in their demonstration that experiences in adult life may make a decisive difference to people who have been placed at risk as a result of adverse experiences in childhood, and also in their indication that experiences that people bring about themselves through their own behaviour may nevertheless have important effects on them (Rutter, 1986).

Turning-point effects concern discontinuities in development, but Caspi & Moffitt (1993) have emphasised that life experiences may be just as important in their role in promoting continuity. Again, experiences brought about by the individuals themselves may be important here, as shown by delinquency findings in relation to the adverse effects of imprisonment, heavy drinking and unemployment (Sampson & Laub, 1993). There has sometimes been a tendency to consider life stresses as something that change the individual, and it has now become clear that, although this may happen, it is at least as frequent for them to enhance or accentuate pre-existing psychological characteristics, rather than change them.

Challenges from genetics

Over this time period, evidence on the importance of genetic influences on psychopathology had been accumulating steadily. In addition, behaviour geneticists increasingly challenged what they saw as some of the key assumptions of psychosocial research. Three challenges seemed to be particularly important. First, Plomin & Daniels (1987) argued, on the basis of genetic evidence, that shared environmental effects were much less important than non-shared effects. In other words, findings suggested that, on the whole, environmental influences tended to make children within the same family different, rather than similar. The implication was that there needed to be more of a focus on the ways in which psychosocial risk factors impinged differentially on individual children. That message had already been apparent in developmental research many decades earlier, but the point certainly needed re-emphasis because the lessons had been overlooked in much research. This corrective was clearly helpful, but the findings were misleadingly overgeneralised by some reviewers to argue that environmentally mediated family influences were rather unimportant (Scarr, 1992; Rowe, 1994). The main reason for the misunderstanding was that the findings were thought to mean that family-wide variables such as discord, disruption or disorganisation were of little importance. However, that did not follow logically from the findings. Rather, they suggested that in so far as these family-wide risk factors had effects, they varied from child to child even within the same family. Thus, it may well be that it is more important that a particular child is scapegoated in the family or treated disparagingly in relation to siblings, than that the home as a whole is a quarrelsome one (Dunn & Plomin, 1990; Reiss *et al*, 1995). It should be added that the dismissal of psychosocial influences as of little importance failed to pay adequate attention to the fact that the twin and adoptee studies on which the argument rested tended to underrepresent families likely to present the greatest environmental risks (Rutter *et al*, 1999*a*,*b*).

The second challenge was that some of the associations that seemed to reflect environmental risks were partially genetically mediated (Plomin & Bergeman, 1991). Studies had shown a familial aggregation of stressful life events (McGuffin *et al*, 1988), and twin studies had shown the importance of genetic influences on individual variations in environmental risk exposure (Kendler *et al*, 1996; Kendler & Karkowski-Shuman, 1997). In addition, there were indications that genetically influenced aspects of children's behaviour were responsible for provoking negative responses in other people (Ge *et al*, 1996; O'Connor *et al*, 1998*a*). Plomin & Bergeman (1991) rightly argued that the fact that a variable seemed to represent an environmental risk did not necessarily mean that that risk was environmentally mediated. Clearly, there was a need for designs that could provide an effective test of environmental risk mediation hypotheses.

There was little recognition at that time, however, of the extent to which psychosocial researchers were already developing strategies for just that purpose. Also, it was unfortunate that the focus was placed on the genetic component in environmental *measures*, with the implication that 'purer' environmental measures were needed. Although unbiased environmental assessment was obviously needed, that was not the most important issue. Rather, the crucial point was that the individual differences in environmental risk exposure reflected, in part, genetically influenced aspects of people's own behaviour in influencing their environments.

The third challenge derived from the evidence that genetic influences on the liability over time to psychopathology tended to be rather greater than those for any single episode of disorder (Kendler *et al*, 1993*a*). Epidemiological and longitudinal data have emphasised the extent to which many psychiatric disorders are recurrent or chronic. This is evident, for example, with respect to both antisocial behaviour (Rutter *et al*, 1998) and depressive disorders (Harrington *et al*, 1996). The implication was that more attention needed to be paid to the role of psychosocial risk factors in relation to people's experience of mental disorders over time, rather than to the timing of the onset of an individual episode of disorder.

■141

The mid- to late-1990s

The mid- to late-1990s saw a reappraisal of several factors thought to influence child psychopathology in the light of new approaches, revised beliefs and the coming to fruition of longitudinal studies from earlier decades.

Time trends in disorder

It might be thought that by this time psychosocial researchers had been put on the defensive. However, this was also the time when the evidence on the huge rise in psychosocial disorders among young people over the previous 50 years was gathered together (Rutter & Smith, 1995), and the claims of psychosocial research began to be substantiated. In the half-century since the Second World War, there had been a great increase in the rates of antisocial disorder, suicidal behaviour, depressive disorders and abuse of drugs and alcohol among young people. Clearly, environmental factors must have been responsible for this major secular change. Whatever the importance of genetics in relation to individual differences, it is quite implausible that a change in the genetic pool could have arisen so rapidly as to bring about this increase in rates of psychopathology in young people. It should be noted, however, that the evidence suggests that the rise in psychopathology largely applied to disorders in young people (and not older age groups). The study of possible causes of changes over time in rates of disorder has received very little attention so far from psychosocial researchers and it constitutes a clear priority for the future.

Multi-factorial causation

Much psychosocial research has seemed to assume that single risk factors may be largely responsible for the causation of disorder. The empirical evidence is consistently against that assumption. The usual finding has been that the increase in psychopathological risk associated with any single psychosocial risk factor occurring truly in isolation is quite low (Rutter, 1979; Kolvin *et al*, 1988, 1990). Fergusson & Lynskey's (1996) findings from the Christchurch longitudinal study illustrate the point well. There was a 100-fold difference in the rate of antisocial disorder between those who were at the extremes of a composite risk index built up of 39 individual factors (some of which will have reflected genetic as well as environmental influences), but the separate effect of each individual risk factor was quite low. Other research delivers much the same message (Rutter *et al*, 1998). Exactly the same applies to genetic risk factors (Plomin *et al*, 1997). That is to say, the overall genetic or environmental effect on any form of psychopathology is quite high, but most individual risk factors are likely to account for a tiny proportion of the variance.

Resilience

The implication of this is that research needs to take seriously the probability that risk factors operate in combination. As research findings on resilience illustrate well (Rutter, 1999*b*, 2000), there is huge individual variability in responses to stress and adversity which derives from complex mixes of risk and protective influences. The easy part of psychosocial risk research has been the identification of psychosocial risk factors. Already, we know a great deal about these. What remains to be understood satisfactorily, however, is why and how these lead to psychopathology in some children but not in others. I identified this as a key issue in 1972 (Rutter, 1972) but, although some progress has been made, there is still a long way to go before there can be an adequate understanding of risk and protective processes.

Reappraisal of life events

In that connection, it seems important to go beyond a focus on factors involved with precipitation of an episode of disorder. When the role of negative life events as precipitants of disorder was first shown through the conceptual and methodological advances of Brown and his colleagues, it constituted an important discovery. However, it is necessary now to pay attention to four key concerns (Rutter & Sandberg, 1992; Sandberg *et al*, 2001). First, typically the timing of life events is done on the basis of timing of onset, which might result in biases that bring the two closer together than they were in reality. It is also necessary to recognise that too little attention has been paid to what is meant by onset: most disorders do not have a single moment when it can be said that the condition began. Second, inadequate attention has been paid to the extent to which acute events are part of more long-standing psychosocial adversities: the relative importance of the acute event and the long-standing difficulties must be differentiated. Third, in so far as children are concerned, parent and child accounts of both symptomatology and life events show only modest agreement. Finally, and most important of all, the key issue is not so much when disorders begin, but why people vary so greatly in the extent to which they show a persistent or recurrent liability to psychopathology. The factors involved in the timing of onset are not necessarily synonymous with those that are most important with respect to tendencies to persist or recur (Brown *et al*, 1994). Life-events research is only just beginning to come to terms with these crucial conceptual and methodological issues (Rutter & Sandberg, 1992; Sandberg *et al*, 1998, 2001), and there is a need to shift attention from a focus on timing to a focus on psychosocial factors that may be influential with respect to liability over time.

New studies on regional areas

Although it had been known for a long time that there are major differences between areas in rates of crime and of mental disorder (see, e.g., Freeman, 1985; Rutter *et al*, 1998), few studies had included adequate controls for individual and family characteristics and little was known on how area influences operated. Systematic investigations during the 1990s began to remedy both lacks (Brooks-Gunn *et al*, 1997; Sampson *et al*, 1997; Macintyre & Ellaway, 2000). It may be concluded that there are true area effects and that these warrant systematic study (Rutter *et al*, 1998).

Non-shared environmental effects

Empirical findings over the past few years have forced behaviour geneticists to modify their claims regarding the much greater importance of non-shared than shared environmental effects (Rutter *et al*, 1999b, 2000). Two main findings have forced the reappraisal. First, the usual univariate estimate of non-shared environmental effects includes measurement error. Once this error had been taken into account, it was apparent that the strength of non-shared effects tended to fall dramatically. Second, the original findings were based on one-off assessments. It now seems that non-shared effects are less important with respect to psychological traits measured over time. That is likely to be because psychosocial influences that impinge on individuals tend to be specific to a particular time. Cumulative effects are more likely to derive from genetic variables and, to a lesser extent, from shared environmental influences. Good measures of child-specific psychosocial influences are still needed, and it is useful that there have been improvements in interview measures for this purpose (Carbonneau *et al*, 2001). However, parents, especially parents of younger children, are not particularly good at reporting the ways in which they treat their children differently, and therefore child reports, together with measures of parental expressed emotion (Leff & Vaughn, 1985; Magaña *et al*, 1986) and observational measures, should be used. The study of child-specific psychosocial influences should also pay particular attention to the possibility that the children's own behaviour has caused the parents to treat them differently.

Gene–environment correlations and interactions

In recent years, geneticists have sought to consider the issue of differential parental treatment of children almost entirely in terms of gene–environment correlations of an active or evocative kind (Scarr, 1992; Plomin, 1994a,b). From a genetic perspective, it is important to know how far genetic effects are indirect, rather than direct. That is, the implications are rather different if the genetic effects are dependent, at least in part, on the fact that they either bring about environmental risks (gene–environment correlations) or cause an increased vulnerability to such risks (gene–environment interactions). From the point of view of understanding psychosocial risk factors, however, this constitutes much too narrow a focus. The testing of environmental risk hypotheses requires the differentiation between effects of the environment on people's behaviour and the effects of people's behaviour on the environment. This is the case irrespective of whether that behaviour is largely genetically influenced or due to some other environmental risk factor. The most crucial need is to understand the role of person–environment correlations. The question of the extent to which personal characteristics are genetically influenced arises only after person effects have been determined. Findings from the Colorado adoption study suggest that, as regards antisocial behaviour, most of the person effects remain after genetic influences have been taken into account in so far as measures allow

■ 143

(O'Connor *et al*, 2000). Psychosocial researchers need to consider bidirectional effects between psychosocial influences and people's behaviour, but as yet few studies have done this adequately.

Tests of environmental mediation

It is important to appreciate the range of research strategies that are available to test hypotheses about environmental risk mediation. Geneticists have been inclined to emphasise the need to use twin and adoptee designs in order to exclude the possibility of the genetic mediation of effects that seem on the surface to be environmental. Genetically sensitive designs have a vitally important place in psychosocial risk research, but on their own they provide an inadequate solution. Adoption strategies are severely limited by the fact that adoptive parents have been chosen deliberately to exclude environmental risks so far as possible. As a result, they provide a very limited opportunity to study the psychosocial risks that are likely to be of greatest relevance for psychopathology. Twin studies can be used to study both shared (Kendler *et al*, 1996) and non-shared (Pike *et al*, 1996) environmental effects but both have their constraints. The former has to rely on assumptions that cannot be tested directly (Meyer *et al*, 2000) and the latter is constrained by the fact that the environments of twins are likely to be more similar than those of singleton siblings because the former are of the same age. Also, the importance of gene–environment correlations will mean that it will be unusual for the environments of pairs of identical twins to differ substantially. In addition, some twin samples are seriously biased with respect to environmental high-risk groups (Rutter *et al*, 1999*b*, 2000). As already noted, solutions should include the use of longitudinal data with 'natural experiments' that pull apart variables that ordinarily go together and of treatment studies designed to test mediating mechanisms (Rutter, 1994; Rutter *et al*, 1997). Migration designs (McKenzie & Murray, 1999) and the analysis of geographically varying time trends in disorder (Rutter & Smith, 1995) provide other possibilities. The challenge from behavioural genetics has been healthy in forcing psychosocial researchers to take much more seriously the need to put environmental mediation hypotheses under rigorous tests, but it is essential that we do not make the mistake of thinking that genetic designs provide the only way forward.

Reappraisal of genetic influences

The 1990s also saw something of a reappraisal of the role of genetic factors in liability to psychiatric disorder. Several seemingly contradictory trends are identifiable.

First, the evidence supporting the power of genetic influences on most types of psychopathology in both childhood and adult life has strengthened (Rutter *et al*, 1999*a*, 2000). The same evidence has, however, shown that the importance of genetic influences varies considerably according to the type of psychiatric disorder. Also, it has become increasingly evident that the great majority of psychiatric disorders are multi-factorial in origin, with environmental factors playing a substantial role in aetiology. We therefore need not so much to identify the tiny proportion of psychiatric disorders that are purely genetic as to understand the mechanisms involved in nature–nurture interplay.

Second, it is becoming increasingly evident that gene–environment correlations and interactions are likely to be influential with many types of psychopathology. Again, the need is to understand the processes underlying this interplay. A variety of rather disparate causal mechanisms are likely to be involved and research must focus on what these are. Knowing that there is a genetic or an environmental contribution is of very little use in its own right. Virtually all forms of psychopathology involve both, and therefore it is necessary to move on to the question of which genes have which effects, which psychosocial risk factors are most important and, in both cases, how they operate and how they combine or interact with each other.

Third, and most crucially, it has become very clear that the future lies in delineating the range of specific mechanisms involved in nature–nurture interplay with respect to different forms of psychopathology. Geneticists have become unduly excited about the rediscovery of the role of genetic factors in individual differences in environmental risk exposure, and psychosocial researchers have become unnecessarily defensive on the same topic. It is crucial to appreciate that the origins of a risk factor and its mode of risk mediation are not necessarily synonymous (Rutter *et al*, 1993). Smoking provides an obvious example of such divergence. Because genetic analyses tend to assume that the two are the same, quantifications of genetic effects will be misleading, since they do not take on board the crucial importance of the involvement of environmental factors. The challenge for geneticists lies in understanding these indirect genetic effects as much as the direct ones. The challenge for psychosocial researchers, however, lies in recognising that the operation of psychosocial risk factors cannot be understood without appreciating the importance of gene–environment correlations and interactions.

The 21st century

At the start of a new century, it is appropriate that we consider what we have learned from psychosocial risk research and what are the challenges ahead. There is every reason to accept the importance of psychosocial risk and protective factors in relation to most forms of child and adolescent psychopathology. The dismissal of environmental influences by genetic evangelists is not justified. The rise during the past 50 years in rates of many disorders in young people makes it clear that environmental factors of some kind must be influential. Twin and adoptee studies also emphasise that non-genetic factors play a substantial role. Moreover, an increasing number of studies using a range of different research strategies show the effect of psychosocial influences on psychopathology. The topic is therefore of undoubted importance.

■ 145

On the other hand, it is equally necessary to accept that all is not well in the study of psychosocial influences. Substantial progress has been made in the development of research strategies that can put environmental mediation hypotheses to rigorous test, but not enough use has been made of them. We know a good deal about psychosocial risk indicators, but much less about the actual environmental mechanisms or processes underlying risk mediation. Also, remarkably little is known about possible diagnostic specificities in psychosocial risk processes. Most research has been concerned with antisocial behaviour (Rutter *et al*, 1998), and much less is known about the role of environmental factors in the genesis of, say, depressive (Harrington, 1994) or anxiety disorders (March, 1995) in childhood. Too little attention has been paid to the factors involved in individual differences in environmental risk exposure, and there is a need for much better research designed to differentiate environmental effects on the person and person effects on the environment. Too much research has neglected the importance of gene–environment correlations and interactions in shaping individual differences in responses to psychosocial stress and adversity. It has long been obvious that these individual differences are of crucial importance and that the study of resilience should be rewarding, but more research designed to identify the mechanisms involved in resilience is certainly required. In that connection, the focus needs to shift from the precipitants of the onset of disorder to an understanding of the processes that operate over time in the initiation and course of disorders as they remit and relapse. The importance of indirect chain reactions is obvious, but much has still to be learned about how they operate. Perhaps the least well understood of all issues is what psychosocial risks do to the organism. How do they bring about their effects and what determines whether these effects persist or fade? More than anything else, this last question requires that psychosocial research be part of biological psychiatry. In looking into the future, it is to be hoped that the absurd dualisms of the past can be put behind us.

References

Ainsworth, M. D. (1962) The effects of maternal deprivation: a review of findings and controversy in the context of research strategy. In *Deprivation of Maternal Care: A Reassessment of Its Effects*, pp. 97–165. Geneva: World Health Organization.

—— & Bowlby, J. (1954) Research strategy in the study of mother–child separation. *Courier*, **4**, 105–131.

——, Belhar, M. C., Waters, E., *et al* (1978) *Patterns of Attachment*. Hillsdale, NJ: Erlbaum.

Anderson, J. E. (1946) Methods of child psychology. In *Manual of Child Psychology* (ed. L. Carmichael), pp. 1–42. New York: John Wiley & Sons.

Anderson, K. E., Lytton, H. & Romney, D. M. (1986) Mother's interactions with normal and conduct-disordered boys: Who affects whom? *Developmental Psychology*, **22**, 604–609.

Asher, S. R. & Gottman, J. M. (eds) (1981) *The Development of Children's Friendships*. Cambridge: Cambridge University Press.

Baldwin, A. L. (1968) *Theories of Child Development*. New York: John Wiley & Sons.

——, Kalhorn, J. & Breese, F. H. (1945) Patterns of parent behavior. *Psychological Monographs*, **58**, 1–75.

Bandura, A. & Walters, R. H. (1963) *Social Learning and Personality Development*. New York: Holt, Rinehart & Winston.

Barker, R. G. & Wright, H. F. (1955) *Midwest and Its Children*. New York: Harper & Row.

Barkley, R. A. & Cunningham, C. E. (1979) The effects of methylphenidate on the mother–child interactions of hyperactive children. *Archives of General Psychiatry*, **36**, 201–208.

Becker, W. C. (1960) The relationship of factors in parental ratings of self and each other to the behaviour of kindergarten children as rated by mothers, fathers, and teachers. *Journal of Consulting Psychology*, **6**, 507–527.

——, Peterson, D. B., Luria, Z., *et al* (1962) Relations of factors derived from parent interview ratings to behaviour problems of five-years-olds. *Child Development*, **33**, 509–536.

Bell, R. Q. (1968) A reinterpretation of the direction of effects in studies of socialization. *Psychological Review*, **75**, 81–95.

—— & Chapman, M. (1986) Child effects in studies using experimental or brief longitudinal approaches to socialization. *Developmental Psychology*, **22**, 595–603.

Berk, R. A. (1983) An introduction to sample selection bias in sociological data. *American Sociological Review*, **48**, 386–398.

Block, J. H., Block, J. & Gjerde, P. F. (1986) The personality of children prior to divorce: a prospective study. *Child Development*, **57**, 827–840.

Bouchard, T. J. (1997) IQ similarity in twins reared apart: findings and responses to critics. In *Intelligence, Heredity and Environment* (eds R. J. Sternberg & E. Grigorenko), pp. 126–160. New York: Cambridge University Press.

Bowlby, J. (1951) *Maternal Care and Mental Health*. Geneva: World Health Organization.

——, Ainsworth, M. D., Boston, M., *et al* (1956) The effects of mother–child separation: a follow-up study. *British Journal of Medical Psychology*, **29**, 211–247.

Bretherton, I. (1987) New perspectives on attachment relations: security, communication, and internal working models. In *Handbook of Infant Development* (3rd edn) (ed. J. Osofsky), pp. 1061–1100. New York: John Wiley & Sons.

Bronfenbrenner, U. (1961) Toward a theoretical model for the analysis of parent–child relationships in a social context. In *Parental Attitudes and Child Behaviour* (ed. J. Glidewell), pp. 90–109. Springfield, IL: Charles C. Thomas.

—— & Crouter, A. C. (1983) The evolution of environmental models in developmental research. In *Handbook of Child Psychology. Vol. I. History, Theory, and Methods* (4th edn) (ed. W. Kessen), pp. 357–414. New York: John Wiley & Sons.

Brooks-Gunn, J., Duncan, G. J. & Aber, J. L. (1997) *Neighborhood Poverty. Vol. 1. Context and Consequences for Children*. New York: Russell Sage Foundation.

Brown, G. W. & Harris, T. O. (1978) *Social Origins of Depression: A Study of Psychiatric Disorder in Women*. London: Tavistock.

—— & —— (1990) *Life Events and Illness*. New York: Guilford.

—— & Rutter, M. (1966) The measurement of family activities and relationships: a methodological study. *Human Relations*, **19**, 241–263.

——, Harris, T. & Peto, J. (1973) Life events and psychiatric disorders. Part 2. The nature of the causal link. *Psychological Medicine*, **3**, 159–179.

——, —— & Hepworth, C. (1994) Life events and endogenous depression: a puzzle reexamined. *Archives of General Psychiatry*, **51**, 525–534.

Brunk, M. A. & Henggeler, S. W. (1984) Child influences on adult controls: an experimental investigation. *Developmental Psychology*, **20**, 1074–1081.

Burks, B. S. (1928) The relative influence of nature and nurture upon mental development: a comparative study of foster parent–foster child resemblance and true parent–true child resemblance. *Yearbook of the National Society for the Study of Education*, **27**, 219–316.

Cairns, R. B. (1983) The emergence of developmental psychology. In *Handbook of Child Psychology. Vol. I. History, Theory, and Methods* (4th edn) (ed. W. Kessen), pp. 41–102. New York: John Wiley & Sons.

Carbonneau, R., Rutter, M., Simonoff, E., *et al* (2001) The Twin Inventory of Relationships and Experience (TIRE): psychometric properties of a measure of the nonshared environmental experiences of twins and singletons. *International Journal of Methods in Psychiatric Research*, in press.

Casler, L. (1961) Maternal deprivation: a critical review of literature. *Monographs of the Society for Research in Child Development*, **26**(2), serial no. 80.

Caspi, A. & Moffitt, T. E. (1993) When do individual differences matter? A paradoxical theory of personality coherence. *Psychological Inquiry*, **4**, 247–271.

Castle, J., Groothues, C., Bredenkamp, D., *et al* (1999) Effects of qualities of early institutional care on cognitive attainment. E.R.A. Study team. English and Romanian Adoptees. *American Journal of Orthopsychiatry*, **69**, 424–437.

Champion, L. A., Goodall, G. M. & Rutter, M. (1995) Behavioural problems in childhood and stressors in early adult life: a 20-year follow-up of London school children. *Psychological Medicine*, **25**, 231–246.

Cherlin, A. J., Furstenberg Jr., F. F., Chase-Lansdale, P. L., *et al* (1991) Longitudinal studies of effects of divorce on children in Great Britain and the United States. *Science*, **252**, 1386–1389.

Clarke, A. M. & Clarke, A. D. B. (eds) (1976) *Early Experience: Myth and Evidence*. London: Open Books.

Clausen, J. (1991) Adolescent competence and the shaping of the life course. *American Journal of Sociology*, **96**, 805–842.

Coleman, J. S., Campbell, E. Q., Hobson, C. J., *et al* (1966) *Equality of Educational Opportunity*. Washington: US Government Printing Office.

Conger, R. D., Conger, K. J., Elder, G. H. Jr, *et al* (1992) A family process model of economic hardship and adjustment of early adolescent boys. *Child Development*, **63**, 526–541.

——, Ge, X., Elder, G. H. Jr, *et al* (1994) Economic stress, coercive family process, and developmental problems of adolescents. *Child Development*, **65**, 541–561.

Cox, A., Rutter, M., Yule, B., *et al* (1977) Bias resulting from missing information: some epidemiological findings. *Journal of Epidemiology and Community Health*, **31**, 131–136.

Dare, C. (1976) Psychoanalytic theories. In *Child Psychiatry: Modern Approaches* (eds M. Rutter & L. Hersov), pp. 255–268. Oxford: Blackwell Scientific.

Dishion, T. J., Patterson, G. R. & Kavanagh, K. A. (1992) An experimental test of the coercion model: linking theory, measurement and intervention. In *Preventing Antisocial Behaviour: Intervention from Birth through Adolescence* (eds J. McCord & R. E. Tremblay), pp. 253–282. New York: Guilford.

Dodge, K. A., Bates, J. E. & Pettit, G. S. (1990) Mechanisms in the cycle of violence. *Science*, **250**, 1678–1683.

——, Pettit, G. S., Bates, J. E., *et al* (1995) Social information-processing patterns partially mediate the effect of early physical abuse on later conduct problems. *Journal of Abnormal Psychology*, **104**, 632–643.

Dollard, J., Miller, N. E., Doob, L. W., *et al* (1939) *Frustration and Aggression*. New Haven, CT: Yale University Press.

Douglas, J. W. B. (1964) *The Home and the School*. London: MacGibbon & Kee.

Dunn, J. & Kendrick, C. (1982) *Siblings: Love, Envy and Understanding*. Cambridge, MA: Harvard University Press.

—— & Plomin, R. (1990) *Separate Lives: Why Siblings Are So Different*. New York: Basic Books.

Elder, G. H. Jr (1986) Military times and turning points in men's lives. *Developmental Psychology*, **22**, 233–245.

Farrington, D. P. (1988) Studying changes within individuals: the causes of offending. In *Studies of Psychosocial Risk: The Power of Longitudinal Data* (ed. M. Rutter), pp. 158–183. Cambridge: Cambridge University Press.

——, Barnes, G. C. & Lambert, S. (1996) The concentration of offending in families. *Legal and Criminological Psychology*, **1**, 47–63.

Fergusson, D. M. & Lynskey, M. T. (1996) Adolescent resiliency to family adversity. *Journal of Child Psychology and Psychiatry*, **37**, 281–292.

——, Horwood, L. J. & Lynskey, M. T. (1992) Family change, parental discord and early offending. *Journal of Child Psychology and Psychiatry*, **33**, 1059–1075.

Freeman, H. L. (1985) *Mental Health and the Environment*. London: Churchill Livingstone.

Freud, A. & Dann, S. (1951) An experiment in group upbringing. *Psychoanalytical Study of the Child*, **6**, 127–168.

Ge, X., Conger, R. D., Cadoret, R. J., *et al* (1996) The development interface between nature and nurture: a mutual influence model of child antisocial behavior and parenting. *Developmental Psychology*, **32**, 574–589.

Goodyer, I. M. (1990) *Life Experiences, Development and Child Psychopathology*. Chichester: John Wiley & Sons.

—— (1995) Life events and difficulties: their nature and effects. In *The Depressed Child and Adolescent: Developmental and Clinical Perspectives* (ed. I. M. Goodyer), pp. 171–193. Cambridge: Cambridge University Press.

——, Kolvin, I. & Gatzanis, S. (1985) Recent undesirable life events and psychiatric disorder in childhood and adolescence. *British Journal of Psychiatry*, **147**, 517–523.

Harlow, H. F. (1958) The nature of love. *American Psychologist*, **13**, 673–685.

—— (1963) The maternal affectional system. In *Determinants of Infant Behaviour. Vol. 2* (ed. B. M. Foss), pp. 3–33. London: Methuen.

Harrington, R. (1994) *Depressive Disorders in Childhood and Adolescence*. Chichester: John Wiley & Sons.

——, Rutter, M. & Fombonne, E. (1996) Developmental pathways in depression: multiple meanings, antecedents, and endpoints. *Development and Psychopathology*, **8**, 601–616.

Hartup, W. W. (1983) Peer relations. In *Handbook of Child Psychology. IV. Socialization, Personality, and Social Development* (ed. M. Hetherington), pp. 103–196. New York: John Wiley & Sons.

Hebb, D. O. (1949) *The Organization of Behavior*. Chichester: John Wiley & Sons.

Hetherington, E. M., Cox, M. & Cox, R. (1982) Effects of divorce on parents and children. In *Nontraditional Families* (ed. M. Lamb), pp. 233–288. Hillsdale, NJ: Erlbaum.

Hewitt, L. E. & Jenkins, R. L. (1946) *Fundamental Patterns of Maladjustment*. Michigan, IL: Michigan Child Guidance Institute.

Hinde, R. A. (1979) *Towards Understanding Relationships*. London: Academic Press.

—— & Herrmann, J. (1977) Frequencies, durations, derived measures and their correlations in studying dyadic and triadic relationships. In *Studies in Mother–Infant Interaction* (ed. H. R. Schaffer), pp. 19–46. London: Academic Press.

—— & McGinnis, L. (1977) Some factors influencing the effect of temporary mother–infant separation: some experiments with rhesus monkeys. *Psychological Medicine*, **7**, 197–212.

Hoffman, M. L. (1957) An interview method for obtaining descriptions of parent–child interaction. *Merrill-Palmer Quarterly*, **3**, 76–83.

—— (1960) Power assertion by the parent and its impact on the child. *Child Development*, **31**, 129–143.

Hubel, D. H. & Wiesel, T. N. (1965) Binocular interaction in striate cortex of kittens reared with artificial squint. *Journal of Neurophysiology*, **28**, 1041–1049.

Hull, C. L. (1943) *Principles of Behavior*. New York: Appleton-Century-Crofts.

Hunt, J. McV. (1979) Psychological development: early experience. *Annual Review of Psychology*, **30**, 103–143.

Jencks, C., Smith, M., Acland, H., *et al* (1972) *Inequality: A Reassessment of the Effect of Family and Schooling in America*. New York: Basic Books.

Jensen, A. R. (1969) How much can we boost IQ and scholastic achievement? *Harvard Educational Review*, **39**, 1–123.

Jones, H. E. (1946) Environmental influences on mental development. In *Manual of Child Psychology* (ed. L. Carmichael), pp. 582–632. New York: John Wiley & Sons.

Kagan, J. (1984) *The Nature of the Child*. New York: Basic Books.

Kandel, D. (1978a) Homophily, selection, and socialization in adolescent friendships. *American Journal of Sociology*, **84**, 427–436.

—— (1978b) Similarity in real-life adolescent friendship pairs. *Journal of Personality and Social Psychology*, **36**, 306–312.

Kanner, L. (1949) Problems of nosology and psychodynamics in early infantile autism. *American Journal of Orthopsychiatry*, **19**, 416–426.

—— (1959) The thirty-third Maudsley Lecture: trends in child-psychiatry. *Journal of Mental Science*, **105**, 581–593.

Kendler, K. S. & Karkowski-Shuman, L. (1997) Stressful life events and genetic liability to major depression: genetic control of exposure to the environment? *Psychological Medicine*, **27**, 549–564.

——, Neale, M., Kessler, R., *et al* (1993a) A longitudinal twin study of personality and major depression in women. *Archives of General Psychiatry*, **50**, 853–862.

——, ——, ——, *et al* (1993b) A twin study of recent life events and difficulties. *Archives of General Psychiatry*, **50**, 789–796.

——, ——, Prescott, C. A., *et al* (1996) Childhood parental loss and alcoholism in women: a causal analysis using a twin-family design. *Psychological Medicine*, **26**, 79–95.

Kolvin, I., Miller, F. J., Fleeting, M., *et al* (1988) Social and parenting factors affecting criminal-offence rates. Findings from the Newcastle Thousand Family Study (1947–1980). *British Journal of Psychiatry*, **152**, 80–90.

——, ——, Scott, D. M., *et al* (1990) *Continuities of deprivation? The Newcastle Thousand-Family Survey*. Aldershot: Avebury.

Laub, J. H., Nagin, D. S. & Sampson, R. J. (1998) Trajectories of change in criminal offending: good marriages and the desistance process. *American Sociological Review*, **63**, 225–238.

Leahy, A. M. (1935) Nature–nurture and intelligence. *Genetic Psychology Monographs*, **17**, 236–308.

Lee, C. L. & Bates, J. E. (1985) Mother–child interaction at age two years and perceived difficult temperament. *Child Development*, **56**, 1314–1325.

Leff, J. & Vaughn, C. (1985) *Expressed Emotion in Families: Its Significance for Mental Illness*. New York: Guilford Press.

Levine, S. (1962) The effects of infantile experience on adult behavior. In *Experimental Foundations of Clinical Psychology* (ed. A. J. Bachrach), pp. 139–169. New York: Basic Books.

Levy, D. M. (1943) *Maternal Overprotection*. New York: Columbia University Press.

Lewin, K., Lippitt, R. & White, R. K. (1939) Patterns of aggressive behavior in experimentally created 'social climates'. *Journal of Social Psychology*, **10**, 271–299.

Lippitt, R. & White, R. K. (1943) The 'social climate' of children's groups. In *Child Behavior and Development* (eds R. G. Barker, J. S. Kounin & H. F. Wright), pp. 485–508. New York: McGraw-Hill.

Maccoby, E. E. & Jacklin, C. N. (1983) The 'person' characteristics of children and the family as environment. In *Human Development: An International Perspective* (eds D. Magnusson & V. L. Allen), pp. 76–91. New York: Academic Press.

McGuffin, P., Katz, R., Aldrich, J., *et al* (1988) The Camberwell Collaborative Depression Study. II. Investigation of family members. *British Journal of Psychiatry*, **152**, 766–774.

Macintyre, S. & Ellaway, A. (2000) Ecological approaches: rediscovering the role of the physical and social environment. In *Social Epidemiology* (eds L. Berkman & I. Kawachi), pp. 332–348. Oxford: Oxford University Press.

McKenzie, K. & Murray, R. M. (1999) Risk factors for psychosis in the UK African–Caribbean population. In *Ethnicity: An Agenda for Mental Health* (eds D. Bhugra & V. Bahl), pp. 48–59. London: Gaskell.

Magaña, A. B., Goldstein, M. J., Karno, M., *et al* (1986) A brief method for assessing expressed emotion in relatives of psychiatric patients. *Psychiatric Research*, **17**, 203–212.

Main, M. (1991) Metacognitive knowledge, metacognitive monitoring and singular (coherent) vs multiple (incoherent) model of attachment: findings and directions for future research. In *Attachment Across the Life Cycle* (eds C. M. Parkes, J. Stevenson-Hinde & P. Marris), pp. 127–159. London: Routledge.

——, Kaplan, N. & Cassidy, J. (1985) Security in infancy, childhood and adulthood: a move to the level of respresentation. In *Growing Points in Attachment Theory* (eds I. Bretherton & E. Waters). *Monographs of the Society for Research in Child Development*, **50**, 66–106.

March, J. S. (ed.) (1995) *Anxiety Disorders in Children and Adolescents*. New York: Guilford Press.

Martin, J. A. (1981) A longitudinal study of the consequences of early mother–infant interaction: A microanalytic approach. *Monographs of the Society for Research in Child Development*, **46**(3), serial no. 190.

Maughan, B. (1994) School influences. In *Development Through Life: A Handbook for Clinicians* (eds M. Rutter & D. F. Hay), pp. 134–158. Oxford: Blackwell Scientific.

Mednick, S. A. & Baert, A. E. (1981) *Prospective Longitudinal Research: an Empirical Basis for the Primary Prevention of Psychosocial Disorders*. Oxford: Oxford University Press.

——, Harway, M. & Finello, K. M. (eds) (1984) *Handbook of Longitudinal Studies*. Westport, CT: Praeger Publications.

Meyer, A. (1957) *Psychobiology: A Science of Man*. Springfield, IL: Charles C. Thomas.

Meyer, J. M., Rutter, M., Simonoff, E., *et al* (2000) Familial aggregation for conduct disorder symptomatology: The role of genes, marital discord, and family adaptability. *Psychological Medicine*, **30**, 759–774.

Miller, N. E. & Dollard, J. (1941) *Social Learning and Imitation*. New York: McGraw-Hill.

Mortimore, P. (1995) The positive effects of schooling. In *Psychosocial Disturbance in Young People: Challenges for Prevention* (ed. M. Rutter), pp. 333–363. New York: Cambridge University Press.

Murray, L. & Cooper, P. J. (1997) *Postpartum Depression and Child Development*. New York: Guilford Press.

O'Connor, N. (1956) The evidence for the permanently disturbing effects of mother–child separation. *Acta Psychologica*, **12**, 174–191.

—— & Franks, C. M. (1960) Childhood upbringing and other environmental factors. In *Handbook of Abnormal Psychology: An Experimental Approach* (ed. H. J. Eysenck), pp. 393–416. London: Pitman Medical Publishing.

O'Connor, T. G., Deater-Deckard, K., Fulker, D., *et al* (1998a) Genotype–environment correlations in late childhood and early adolescence: Antisocial behavioral problems and coercive parenting. *Developmental Psychology*, **34**, 970–981.

O'Connor, T., Rutter, M., Beckett, C., *et al* (2000) The effects of global severe privation on cognitive competence: Extension and longitudinal follow-up. *Child Development*, **72**, 376–390.

Osborn, A. F., Butler, N. R. & Morris, A. C. (1984) *The Social Life of Britain's Five-Year-Olds. A Report of the Child Health and Education Study*. London: Routledge & Kegan Paul.

Osborn, S. G. (1980) Moving home, leaving London and delinquent trends. *British Journal of Criminology*, **20**, 54–61.

Parker, J. G. & Asher, S. R. (1987) Peer relations and later personal adjustment: are low-accepted children at risk? *Psychological Bulletin*, **102**, 357–389.

Patrick, M., Hobson, P., Castle, D., *et al* (1994) Personality disorder and the mental representation of early social experience. *Development and Psychopathology*, **6**, 375–388.

Patterson, G. R. (1979) A performance theory for coercive family interaction. In *The Analysis of Social Interactions: Methods, Issues and Illustrations* (ed. R. B. Cairns), pp. 119–162. Hillsdale, NJ: Erlbaum.

——, Cobb, J. A. & Ray, R. S. (1973) A social engineering technology for retraining the families of aggressive boys. In *Issues and Trends in Behavior Therapy* (eds H. E. Adams & I. P. Unikel), pp. 139–224. Springfield, IL: Charles C Thomas.

■ 149

——, Dishion, T. J. & Chamberlain, P. (1993) Outcomes and methodological issues relating to treatment of antisocial children. In *Handbook of Effective Psychotherapy* (ed. T. R. Giles), pp. 43–87. New York: Plenum.

Phelps, J. L., Belsky, J. & Crnic, K. (1998) Earned security, daily stress and parenting: a comparison of five alternative models. *Development and Psychopathology*, **10**, 21–38.

Pike, A., Reiss, D., Hetherington, E. M., *et al* (1996) Using MZ differences in the search for nonshared environmental effects. *Journal of Child Psychology and Psychiatry*, **37**, 695–704.

Plomin, R. (1994*a*) Genetic research and identification of environmental influences: Emanuel Miller Memorial Lecture (1993). *Journal of Child Psychology and Psychiatry*, **35**, 817–834.

—— (1994*b*) *Genetics and Experience: The Interplay Between Nature and Nurture*. Thousand Oaks, CA: Sage Publications.

—— & Bergeman, C. S. (1991) The nature of nurture: Genetic influence on 'environmental' measures. *Behavioral and Brain Sciences*, **14**, 373–427.

—— & Daniels, D. (1987) Why are children in the same family so different from one another? *Behavioral and Brain Sciences*, **10**, 1–15.

——, DeFries, J. C., McClearn, G. E., *et al* (1997) *Behavioral Genetics* (3rd edn). New York: W. H. Freeman.

Powers, E. & Witmer, H. (1951) *An Experiment in the Prevention of Delinquency: The Cambridge-Somerville Youth Study*. New York: Columbia University Press.

Pringle, M. K., Butler, N. & Davie, R. (1966) *11,000 Seven Year Olds*. London: Longman/National Children's Bureau.

Quinton, D. (1994) Cultural and community influences. In *Development Through Life: A Handbook for Clinicians* (eds M. Rutter & D. F. Hay), pp. 159–184. Oxford: Blackwell Scientific.

—— & Rutter, M. (1988) *Parenting Breakdown: The Making and Breaking of Inter-Generational Links*. Aldershot: Avebury.

——, —— & Rowlands, O. (1976) An evaluation of an interview of marriage. *Psychological Medicine*, **6**, 577–586.

——, Pickles, A., Maughan, B., *et al* (1993) Partners, peers, and pathways: assortative pairing and continuities in conduct disorder. *Development and Psychopathology*, **5**, 763–783.

Radke-Yarrow, M., Campbell, J. D. & Burton, R. V. (1968) *Child Rearing: An Inquiry in Research and Methods*. San Francisco, CA: Jossey-Bass.

——, —— & —— (1970) Recollections of childhood: a study of the retrospective method. *Monographs of the Society for Research in Child Development*, **35**(5), serial no. 138.

Reichard, S. & Tillman, C. (1950) Patterns of parent–child relationships in schizophrenia. *Psychiatry*, **13**, 247–257.

Reiss, D., Hetherington, R., Plomin, R., *et al* (1995) Genetic questions for environmental studies: differential parenting and psychopathology in adolescence. *Archives of General Psychiatry*, **52**, 925–936.

Robbins, L. C. (1963) The accuracy of parental recall of aspects of child development and of child rearing practices. *Journal of Abnormal and Social Psychology*, **66**, 261–270.

Robins, L. (1966) *Deviant Children Grown Up*. Baltimore, MD: Williams and Wilkins.

Rowe, D. C. (1994) *The Limits of Family Influence: Genes, Experience, and Behavior*. New York: Guilford Press.

Roy, P., Rutter, M. & Pickles, A. (2000) Institutional care: Risk from family background or pattern of rearing? *Journal of Child Psychology and Psychiatry and Allied Disciplines*, **41**, 139–149.

Rutter, M. (1966) *Children of Sick Parents*. Oxford: Oxford University Press.

—— (1971) Parent–child separation: psychological effects on the children. *Journal of Child Psychology and Psychiatry*, **12**, 233–260.

—— (1972) *Maternal Deprivation Reassessed*. Harmondsworth: Penguin.

—— (1974) Epidemiological strategies and psychiatric concepts in research on the vulnerable child. In *The Child in His Family: Children at Psychiatric Risk. Vol. 3* (eds E. Anthony & C. Koupernik), pp. 167–179. New York: John Wiley & Sons.

—— (1979) *Changing Youth in a Changing Society: Patterns of Adolescent Development and Disorder*. London: Nuffield Provincial Hospitals Trust.

—— (1981*a*) *Maternal Deprivation Reassessed* (2nd edn). Harmondsworth: Penguin.

—— (1981*b*) Epidemiological/longitudinal strategies and causal research in child psychiatry. *Journal of the American Academy of Child Psychiatrists*, **20**, 513–544.

—— (1986) Meyerian psychobiology, personality development and the role of life experiences. *American Journal of Psychiatry*, **143**, 1077–1087.

—— (1989) Pathways from childhood to adult life. *Journal of Child Psychology and Psychiatry*, **30**, 23–51.

—— (1994) Beyond longitudinal data: causes, consequences, changes and continuity. *Journal of Consulting and Clinical Psychology*, **62**, 928–940.

—— (1996) Transitions and turning points in developmental psychopathology: as applied to the age span between childhood and mid-adulthood. *International Journal of Behavioral Development*, **19**, 603–626.

—— (1999a) Psychosocial adversity and child psychopathology. *British Journal of Psychiatry*, **174**, 480–493.

—— (1999b) Resilience, concepts and findings: implications for family therapy. *Journal of Family Therapy*, **21**, 119–144.

—— (2000) Resilience reconsidered: conceptual considerations and empirical findings. In *Handbook of Early Childhood Intervention* (2nd edn) (eds J. P. Shonkoff & S. J. Meisels), pp. 651–682. New York: Cambridge University Press.

—— & Brown, G. W. (1966) The reliability and validity of measures of family life and relationships in families containing a psychiatric patient. *Social Psychiatry*, **1**, 38–53.

—— & ERA (English and Romanian Adoptees) Study Team (1998) Developmental catch-up, and deficit, following adoption after severe global early privation. *Journal of Child Psychology and Psychiatry*, **39**, 465–476.

—— & Quinton, D. (1977) Psychiatric disorder – ecological factors and concepts of causation. In *Ecological Factors in Human Development* (ed. H. McGurk), pp. 173–187. Amsterdam: North-Holland.

—— & Rutter, M. (1993) *Developing Minds: Challenge and Continuity across the Lifespan*. Harmondsworth: Penguin.

—— & Sandberg, S. (1992) Psychosocial stressors: concepts, causes and effects. *European Child and Adolescent Psychiatry*, **1**, 3–13.

—— & Smith, D. J. (1995) *Psychosocial Disorders in Young People: Time Trends and Their Causes*. Chichester: John Wiley & Sons.

——, Tizard, J. & Whitmore, K. (eds) (1970) *Education, Health and Behaviour*. London: Longmans.

——, Yule, B., Quinton, D., *et al* (1975) Attainment and adjustment in two geographical areas. III. Some factors accounting for area differences. *British Journal of Psychiatry*, **126**, 520–533.

——, Maughan, B., Mortimore, P., *et al* (1979) *Fifteen Thousand Hours: Secondary Schools and Their Effects on Children*. Cambridge, MA: Harvard University Press.

——, Silberg, J. & Simonoff, E. (1993) Whither behavioral genetics? A developmental psychopathology perspective. In *Nature, Nurture, and Psychology* (eds R. Plomin & G. E. McClearn), pp. 433–456. Washington, DC: APA Books.

——, Champion, L., Quinton, D., *et al* (1995) Understanding individual differences in environmental risk exposure. In *Examining Lives in Context: Perspectives on the Ecology of Human Development* (eds P. Moen, G. H. Elder, Jr. & K. Lüscher), pp. 61–93. Washington, DC: American Psychological Association.

——, Dunn, J., Plomin, R., *et al* (1997) Integrating nature and nurture: implications of person–environment correlations and interactions for developmental psychology. *Development and Psychopathology*, **9**, 335–364.

——, Giller, H. & Hagell, A. (1998) *Antisocial Behavior by Young People*. New York: Cambridge University Press.

——, Silberg, J., O'Connor, T., *et al* (1999a) Genetics and child psychiatry. I. Advances in quantitative and molecular genetics. *Journal of Child Psychology and Psychiatry*, **40**, 3–18.

——, ——, ——, *et al* (1999b) Genetics and child psychiatry. II. Empirical research findings. *Journal of Child Psychology and Psychiatry*, **40**, 19–55.

Sampson, R. J. & Laub, J. H. (1993) *Crime in the Making: Pathways and Turning Points Through Life*. Cambridge, MA: Harvard University Press.

—— & —— (1996) Socioeconomic achievement in the life course of disadvantaged men: military service as a turning point, circa 1940–1965. *American Sociological Review*, **61**, 347–367.

——, Raudenbush, S. W. & Earls, F. (1997) Neighborhoods and violent crime: a multilevel study of collective efficacy. *Science*, **277**, 918–924.

Sandberg, S., McGuinness, D., Hillary, C., *et al* (1998) Independence of childhood life events and chronic adversities: a comparison of two patient groups and controls. *Journal of the American Academy of Child and Adolescent Psychiatry*, **37**, 728–735.

——, Rutter, M., Pickles, A., *et al* (2001) Do stressful life events really provoke onset of child psychiatric disorder? *Journal of Child Psychology and Psychiatry and Allied Disciplines*, in press.

Scarr, S. (1992) Developmental theories for the 1990s: development and individual differences. *Child Development*, **63**, 1–19.

—— (1997) Behavior-genetic and socialization theories of intelligence: truth and reconciliation. In *Intelligence, Heredity and Environment* (eds R. J. Sternberg & E. L. Grigorenko), pp. 3–41. Cambridge: Cambridge University Press.

—— & McCartney, K. (1983) How people make their own environment: a theory of genotype→environmental effects. *Child Development*, **54**, 424–435.

Schachar, R., Taylor, E., Wieselberg, M., *et al* (1987) Changes in family function and relationships in children who respond to methylphenidate. *Journal of the American Academy of Child and Adolescent Psychiatry*, **26**, 728–732.

Scott, J. P. (1963) The process of primary socialization in canine and human infants. *Monographs of the Society for Research in Child Development*, **28**, serial no. 85.

■ 151

—— & Fuller, J. L. (1965) *Genetics of the Social Behavior of the Dog*. Chicago, IL: University of Chicago Press.

Sears, R. R., Maccoby, E. E. & Levin, H. (1957) *Patterns of Child Rearing*. Evanston, IL: Row, Peterson.

Sherif, M., Harvey, O. J., White, B. J., *et al* (1961) *Intergroup Conflict and Cooperation: The Robbers' Cave Experiment*. Norman, OK: University of Oklahoma Press.

—— & Sherif, C. W. (1953) *Groups in Harmony and Tension*. New York: Harper.

Skeels, H. M. & Dye, H. (1939) A study of the effects of differential stimulation on mentally retarded children. *Proceedings of the American Association of Mental Deficiency*, **44**, 114–136.

——, Updegraff, R., Wellman, B. L., *et al* (1938) A study of environmental stimulation: an orphanage preschool project. *Universtiy of Iowa Studies in Child Welfare*, **15**(4), serial no. 362.

Skinner, B. F. (1938) *The Behavior of Organisms: An Experimental Analysis*. New York: Appleton-Century-Crofts.

—— (1953) *Science and Human Behavior*. New York: Macmillan.

Teasdale, J. D. & Barnard, P. J. (1993) *Affect, Cognition and Change: Re-Modelling Depressive Thought*. Hove: Erlbaum.

Thomas, A., Chess, S. & Birch, H. G. (1968) *Temperament and Behavior Disorders in Childhood*. New York: New York University Press.

Thomas, E. A. C. & Malone, T. W. (1979) On the dynamics of two-person interactions. *Psychological Review*, **86**, 331–360.

—— & Martin, J. A. (1976) Analyses of parent–infant interaction. *Psychological Review*, **83**, 141–156.

Tizard, J., Sinclair, I. & Clarke, R. V. G. (1975) *Varieties of Residential Experience*. London: Routledge & Kegan Paul.

van IJzendoorn, M. H. (1995) Adult attachment representations, parental responsiveness, and infant attachment: a meta-analysis on the predictive validity of the Adult Attachment Interview. *Psychological Bulletin*, **116**, 387–403.

Wallerstein, J. S. (1983) Children of divorce: stress and developmental tasks. In *Stress, Coping, and Development in Children* (eds N. Garmezy & M. Rutter), pp. 265–302. New York: McGraw-Hill.

West, D. J. & Farrington, D. P. (1973) *Who Becomes Delinquent?* London: Heinemann Educational Books.

Wiesel, T. N. & Hubel, D. H. (1965*a*) Comparison of the effects of unilateral and bilateral eye closure on cortical unit responses in kittens. *Journal of Neurophysiology*, **28**, 1029–1040.

—— & —— (1965*b*) Extent of recovery from the effects of visual deprivation in kittens. *Journal of Neurophysiology*, **28**, 1060–1072.

Wing, J. & Brown, G. (1970) *Institutionalism and Schizophrenia: A Comparative Study of Three Mental Hospitals, 1960–1968*. Cambridge: Cambridge University Press.

Wootton, B. (1959) *Social Science and Social Pathology*. London: Allen & Unwin.

Wright, H. F., Barker, R. G., Null, J., *et al* (1955) Toward a psychological ecology of the classroom. In *Readings in Educational Psychology* (ed. A. Coladarci). New York: Holt, Rinehart & Winston.

Yarrow, L. J. (1961) Maternal deprivation: toward an empirical and conceptual re-evaluation. *Psychological Bulletin*, **58**, 459–490.

Zoccolillo, M., Pickles, A., Quinton, D., *et al* (1992) The outcome of childhood conduct disorder: implications for defining adult personality disorder and conduct disorder. *Psychological Medicine*, **22**, 971–986.

Zuckerman, M., Barrett, B. H. & Bragiel, R. M. (1960) The parental attitudes of parents of child guidance cases. 1. Comparisons with normals, investigations of socio-economic and family constellation factors, and relations to the parents' reaction to the clinic. *Child Development*, **31**, 401–417.

10 Appreciation of Professor Sir Michael Rutter

Ann Le Couteur

Michael Rutter has played a unique part in the development of child and adolescent psychiatry. He has a most distinguished worldwide reputation and an extraordinary number and diversity of achievements. His breadth of knowledge and ability to formulate research questions that advance and clarify the complexities of our understanding; his emphasis on child development and life-span opportunities for individual and family growth; his abiding focus on the clinical relevance of research findings for the child, the family and the community (however defined): all have advanced child and adolescent psychiatry and mental health immeasurably over the past 40 years.

In Chapter 1, Barbara Maughan acknowledged that she was a partial heir to Mike's rigour and clinical understanding. I would suggest that, directly or indirectly, we are all his heirs, and I have been given the task and pleasure on behalf of us all to express an appreciation of Mike. In this brief chapter I would like to highlight some of his many achievements and consider some of his special skills.

I have been both taught and supervised by Mike at different times: from registrar and research worker through to lecturer and honorary consultant. Professor John Corbett (while I was on my medical student elective) had said that if I wanted to do child and adolescent psychiatry I should come to the Maudsley Hospital and work with Michael Rutter – good advice indeed.

Brief biography

Michael Rutter qualified from the University of Birmingham in 1955. He became a Member of the Royal College of Physicians in 1958, and in the same year had his first paper published and came to the Maudsley Hospital. Professor Aubrey Lewis is credited with choosing child and adolescent psychiatry as a career for Mike and encouraged him to visit the USA after Mike had heard Herb Birch talk at the Maudsley and had expressed a wish to study with him.

This year in the USA (1961–1962) was spent on a research fellowship at the Department of Pediatrics, Albert Einstein College of Medicine, New York. Mike worked directly with Herb Birch, Alex Thomas and Stella Chess. He was very impressed by all three and, with their encouragement, he was able to meet academics and clinicians from all over the country (including Lee Robins, Leon Eisenberg and many others). This period was enormously informative, and Mike learnt both through the direct experience of participating in a research team and through energetic debates with colleagues on a

■153

Based on a paper presented at the inaugural meeting of the Royal College of Psychiatrists' Faculty of Child and Adolescent Psychiatry, 24–26 September 1998, Bristol.

broad range of topics. The use of research data to challenge accepted knowledge and the intellectual excitement of being able to develop new research designs to answer specific questions have become hallmarks of Mike's approach to research in child psychiatry.

After a brief period in England following this 1-year fellowship, Mike returned to the USA on a Belding Scholarship and again met colleagues from a broad range of backgrounds: Ernest Gruenberg, Julius Richmond, Ed Zigler, Jerry Kagan, Judy Wallerstein, Lee Cronbach and Robert Plomin to name but a few.

Mike returned to the Medical Research Council's (MRC's) Social Psychiatry Research Unit at the Institute of Psychiatry in London, where he worked until 1965. It was here that he met and worked with Jack Tizard, George Brown, Beata Hermelin, Neil O'Connor, Kenneth Rawnsley and others. As in the USA, Mike learnt most from those colleagues who challenged accepted practice or contemporary theory and from the opportunities for multi-disciplinary creative debate and argument. He was struck by the practice implications of epidemiological research to influence policy development and the innovative experimental designs developed by colleagues, including Hermelin and O'Connor. This was also the time that Mike's collaboration with George Brown on the Camberwell Interview (Brown & Rutter, 1966) and measures of expressed emotion first began.

In 1963 Mike took a statistics course at the London School of Hygiene and in the same year his MD thesis was published (see Rutter, 1966). His first academic appointment at the Institute of Psychiatry was in 1965. He was appointed Honorary Consultant the following year. This was also the time of the Isle of Wight Study (1964–1969) – the project on which Mike worked most closely with Jack Tizard. It was a very ambitious study (Mike was able to incorporate his recent US research experience in epidemiology) and involved many key collaborators, including Philip Graham, Bill Yule, Kingsley Whitmore and Tony Cox.

The research team would travel from London to the Isle of Wight each week, coordinate the assessments, record the findings and hold a research meeting each evening. For everyone it was an intensive training experience that cemented lifelong academic and personal friendships. The Isle of Wight Study (Rutter *et al*, 1970*a*) and the subsequent South London Urban Comparison Study (Rutter *et al*, 1975*b,c*) are seminal studies in the epidemiology of child and adolescent psychiatric disorders. The findings have stood the test of time and continue (30 years later) to be referenced in in the literature: an extraordinary achievement for all who contributed to the project.

In 1973 Mike was appointed the first Professor in Child and Adolescent Psychiatry in the UK and Commonwealth. The Academic Department of Child and Adolescent Psychiatry, Institute of Psychiatry, was founded in 1975. Thus, Mike's career coincided with the establishment of child and adolescent psychiatry as an academic discipline in the UK: there are now over 20 professorial chairs around the country.

In 1984 the MRC Child Psychiatry Unit was established, with Mike as its first Honorary Director. When in 1994, the Social, Genetic and Developmental Psychiatry Research Centre opened at the Institute of Psychiatry, Mike again took the challenge of being a first Honorary Director, a position he held for 4 years.

From 1979 to 1980 Mike was again in the USA. It would be impossible to do justice to all the significant relationships he forged at that time. He was based in Stanford, where he had honorary appointments in five different academic departments, reflecting his diverse areas of interest. Colleagues included Gerry Patterson, Jerry Kagan, Julie Segal, Judy Wallerstein, Herb Leiderman and Norman Garmezy. (Mike had first met Norman Garmezy in the early 1970s, when the latter had spent a year at the Maudsley Hospital. Indeed, their early joint thinking contributed to the later establishment of the Stress, Coping and Development Group (1979–1980; Garmezy & Rutter, 1983).) Mike also made links with educational researchers such as Lee Sholman, the linguist Eve Clark, Seymour Levine (at that time working on stress) and Al Hastorff (a social psychologist). During this year he first met Eleanor Maccoby, Mavis Hetherington, Marian Jadke-Yarrow, Ernie Werner and Bill Hartup. Each represented different areas of psychology and child development research. These contacts resulted in successful collaborations that have continued for more than 20 years.

It was soon after Mike's return from Stanford that I first met him (I was a junior registrar in child psychiatry on a 6-month clinical attachment from another training scheme). I expressed an interest in research in autism and was encouraged to develop this, and so began a rewarding ongoing collaboration that I trust will continue for many years to come.

Michael Rutter's publications span more than 40 years: the first, a report on two cases of juvenile amaurotic familial idiocy, appeared in 1958 (Jefferson & Rutter, 1958) and his first genetics paper was published in 1963 (Rutter et al, 1963). In preparing this appreciation I received a 51 page summary of Mike's publications (Taylor & Green, 2001). This included more than 36 books, 142 chapters and in excess of 300 scientific papers. Mike continues to be extraordinarily productive, with a stream of written work awaiting publication and in preparation. I will highlight a few of these publications – books from various stages of his career that may be of particular interest (see the reference list for full publishing details).

1966 *Children of Sick Parents: An Environmental and Psychiatric Study*
M. Rutter

I have chosen this early publication because, although the key finding has been replicated repeatedly over the intervening years, the *inferences* drawn from the results have undergone revisions and led to more specific research hypotheses. The original study finding was the strength of the association between parental mental disorder and risk for the child. This finding has stood the test of time, even though it is likely that the risk involves mechanisms that go beyond the diagnostic specific features of the parents. Later studies (e.g., the Family Illness Study; Rutter & Quinton, 1984, 1987) have shown that the risk factors apply to the general population in much the same way as in the parental mental disorder sample.

■ 155

1970 *A Neuropsychiatric Study in Childhood*
M. Rutter, P. Graham & W. Yule

This book also reports findings that have influenced clinical practice. The study showed that brain dysfunction is a significant risk factor for child and adolescent mental disorder and that active brain dysfunction is probably more important than loss of brain function. There was no evidence, however, of stereotypic syndrome. (See Chapter 5 in this Festschrift for a consideration of this study.)

1970 *Education, Health and Behaviour*
M. Rutter, J. Tizard & K. Whitmore (eds)

This landmark text emphasises the crucial importance of education and schools for children and their families. It was reprinted in 1981 and continues to be referenced in academic and grant applications focusing on the role of education in child and adolescent mental health.

1971 *Infantile Autism: Concepts, Characteristics and Treatment*
M. Rutter (ed.)

This collaboration, of which Mike was editor, was his first book on autism.

1972 *Maternal Deprivation Re-Assessed*
M. Rutter

This book has always attracted readership from a very wide professional and non-professional audience – it was written as Mike's response to the debate about the impact on children of separation from, or loss of, their biological mother. Mike was certain that separation/loss had important effects on children but that there were problems with the then current theoretical explanations. He sent a draft of the book to Robert Hinde (whom he had never met), who generously returned to Mike a 17 page commentary. Mike concluded that it is not the separation as such, but the associated factors – discord, disruption of child care, poverty and so forth – that provide the risk for the child. These findings are now well accepted and have been widely replicated. At the time, however, the book generated a great deal of discussion, controversy and overt hostility.

In the revised second edition (1981) Mike took the topic further and concluded that there were few long-term effects that were independent of later experiences. Although this is true, it soon became obvious to Mike and others that this inference had things the wrong way round. Later experience is rarely, if ever, independent of earlier experiences. For any individual, there are significant indirect links over time, and an individual's behaviour will in turn shape later experiences. Subsequent writings with colleagues such as David Quinton and Lorna Champion (see, e.g., Quinton & Rutter, 1988; Champion *et al*, 1995) discuss these phenomena in more detail.

1975 *A Guide to a Multi-Axial Classification Scheme for Psychiatric Disorders in Childhood and Adolescence*
M. Rutter, D. Schaffer & C. Sturge

I have included this booklet as it represents the impact that a framework for a multi-dimensional approach to child and adolescent psychiatric diagnosis and formulation has had on facilitating both clinical and research work. The systematic recording of information about all children attending the child and adolescent psychiatry department at the Maudsley Hospital was established in the 1970s. This, together with the computerisation of the item sheets, has produced a unique live database – an invaluable resource for successful research and audit initiatives.

1975 *Helping Troubled Children*
M. Rutter

Helping Troubled Children is (arguably) one of Mike's most successful publications in terms of reaching the widest professional and lay audience. At the time, it proved enormously popular with a variety of health and other professionals and adults involved in childcare work.

1977 *Child Mental Health and Psychosocial Development: Report of a WHO Expert Committee*
World Health Organization

Throughout Mike's career he has been involved in a number of innovative committees and working parties. He played a key role in the work of the WHO Expert Committee, which reviewed all available knowledge on child and adolescent psychiatry research and clinical practice. (David Schaffer, in Chapter 7 of this Festschrift, considers the development of classification systems.)

1977 *Child and Adolescent Psychiatry: Modern Approaches*
M. Rutter & L. Hersov (eds)

This significant reference book was a joint venture with Lionel Hersov. Rereading the preface to the first edition, I noted the emphasis that the editors gave to the Maudsley and Bethlem Royal Hospitals (the Joint Hospitals) in the development of child and adolescent psychiatry as a speciality. All the chapter authors in the first edition had worked at the Joint Hospitals or the Institute of Psychiatry. This preface also highlighted the development of standards for clinical practice and research. The concluding sentence reads:

> "We will be satisfied if (in the words of Sir Aubrey Lewis) [the book] also helps the psychiatrist in training to acquire 'reasoning and understanding' and fits him 'to combine the scientific and humane temper in his studies as the psychiatrist needs to'."

In the third edition (1994), Eric Taylor joined as editor, and the book is now an international venture containing 64 chapters. Many of the contributors trained and have worked or are currently working at the Bethlem Royal and Maudsley Hospitals. Mike is referenced in at least three-quarters of all chapters in the current edition, a tribute to his breadth of knowledge and wide-ranging achievements. This textbook has an international reputation as the reference book of our speciality.

1979 *15,000 hours: Secondary Schools and their Effects on Children*
M. Rutter, B. Maughan, P. Mortimer, J. Ouston & A. Smith

This book, the last I have chosen from the 1970s, presents the findings of a research project that was successfully completed against a background of criticism about the viability of the study (and the added difficulty of a teachers' strike). It is still in print: a reminder of the continuing relevance of the findings. It was intended to be accessible to scientists and non-scientists alike, unambiguously conveying the message that schools can make a significant contribution to child and adolescent mental health. Unfortunately, over the intervening 20 years, insufficient emphasis has been given to this important 'therapeutic' role of schools. In retrospect, the authors probably underestimated the full extent of the school effect. At the time of the study, the work questioned existing accepted theory – another hallmark of Mike's chosen areas of study. He has always seemed keen to question accepted wisdom or theory-driven practices. This has often meant that, in collaboration with colleagues usually from other disciplines, he has developed new methodologies and statistical techniques to enable the investigation of specific research hypotheses, often of a developmental nature, or to test proposed causal mechanisms.

1983 *Stress, Coping and Development*
N. Garmezy & M. Rutter (eds)

This work was the culmination of Mike's year at Stanford, during which he was considering how stress and adversity affect development. The book discussed the effects of individual differences, possible age-related vulnerabilities and the impact of experience. The findings led to subsequent work that has furthered our understanding of both risk and protective factors and the important concepts of resilience and competence.

■ 157

1983 *Juvenile Delinquency: Trends and Perspectives*
M. Rutter & H. Giller

This is one of a number of publications by Mike and colleagues considering areas that have enormous social and health consequences for groups of vulnerable young people (not necessarily seen by mainstream child and adolescent psychiatry services as 'core business').

1987 *Treatment of Autistic Children*
P. Howlin & M. Rutter, with M. Berger, R. Helmsley,
L. Hersov & W. Yule

This book describes in detail the findings of a study of home-based treatment of autism. Outcomes showed that home-based therapeutic interventions could produce a broad range of benefits for the individual child. However, the findings also emphasised substantial individual variations (for children and families). The study found that the group of children with the poorest outcome comprised those who had had an early and prolonged admission to residential services. The challenge seemed to be that dedicated residential services were not always providing therapeutic opportunities and protection for the children. The mainstay of therapeutic intervention for children and young people with autism has continued to be educational and behavioural approaches but with a community focus, working with children and parents in their own home. The project emphasised the essential role that parents play as 'co-therapists' for their children and the need for professionals to work in close collaboration with parents.

1988 *Parenting Breakdown: The Making and Breaking*
of Intergenerational Links
D. Quinton & M. Rutter

Mike has always said that he never places a lot of weight on a single finding: a characteristic of many of his research collaborations has been his enthusiasm for having several ways of tackling the same question. This might include the need to develop new and different strategies, measures or analyses. Perhaps it is this attention to detail in coordinated programmes of interrelated study that has contributed to Mike's research success. As far as I am aware very few of his research findings have not stood the test of time.

In this more recent publication, David Quinton and Mike Rutter clarify how indirect chain effects may be a powerful mechanism for the perpetuation of risk. They also analyse potential protective and facilitating experiences that may provide turning points for a young person, for example, school experiences, an ability to plan or a harmonious marriage.

1990 *Straight and Devious Pathways from Childhood to Adulthood*
L. Robins & M. Rutter (eds)

Lee Robins, in Chapter 8 of this Festschrift, has considered the significance of this rewarding collaboration with Mike, so I shall not elaborate here.

1993 *Developing Minds: Challenge and Continuity*
Across the Life Span
M. Rutter & M. Rutter

I have chosen this as it is the only collaboration between Mike and his wife Marjorie. Both were pleased with the success of the book, which focuses on the clinical implications of developmental concepts across the life span and so challenges professionals to think in a different way about the nature–nurture interplay and the provision of clinical services.

1994 *Stress, Risk and Resilience in Children and Adolescents:*
Processes, Mechanisms and Interventions
R. J. Haggerty, H. J. Sherrod, N. Garmezy & M. Rutter

The concepts of risk and resilience are further developed in this book. These concepts are now central to our understanding of child and adolescent mental health, which has important implications for social policy developments and commissioned guidelines for service provision.

Research themes

The authors of the chapters in this Festschrift publication have considered many of Mike's research themes. Consistently he seems prepared to take on a challenge that he considers to be important and that will increase our understanding of causal mechanisms. He particularly enjoys undertaking studies that others say cannot be done or that require the development of new methodological techniques or statistical analyses to answer the question or test the hypothesis. His work is not theory driven. Many studies, such as the Isle of Wight and inner-city studies, have been based on epidemiological and longitudinal strategies. Other themes include longitudinal studies of high-risk groups, for example: those in institutional care; families with a parent with mental health problems; children at risk from school effects; those with clinical conditions such as severe mental health disorders; and controversial topics including maternal deprivation and parenting by lesbian mothers. In addition to this focus on psychopathology, he has increasingly engaged in genetic studies, including the establishment of the International Collaborative Molecular Genetic Study of Autism.

Another important aspect (exemplified by Mike's involvement with the MRC Child Psychiatry Unit) has been collaborations he has developed with a broad range of scientists, from behaviour geneticists and psychologists to statisticians and social anthropologists. The Social, Genetic and Developmental Psychiatry Research Centre, directed by Professor Peter McGuffin, will (with Mike taking a collaborating role) continue the "scientific enterprise of understanding the nature/nurture interplay" (Kolvin, 1990*b*).

Many of Mike's most successful collaborations have been ones that have continued over many years and often with colleagues outside the UK.

Despite the undoubted success of Mike's research work, funding has at times been difficult. As a young researcher I remember thinking what a waste of time and opportunity that Mike had to spend so long either applying for research support or rethinking strategy when a bid was turned down. Indeed, some projects proceeded without funding and some, as I have already mentioned, were undertaken amid controversy and even hostility.

Underpinning much of Mike's research and academic progress has been his role in the development of new diagnostic instruments. Early on in my joint work with Mike it became clear that to proceed with research in the field of autism there was a need for a reliable investigator-based semi-structured interview. This recognition led to a very rewarding collaboration for me with Mike Rutter, Catherine Lord and numerous other international colleagues, which culminated in the Autism Diagnostic Interview – Revised (ADI–R; Le Couteur *et al*, 1989; Lord *et al*, 1994), the Autism Diagnostic Observation Schedule (ADOS; Lord *et al*, 1989, 2000) and other related measures.

The ADI–R and ADOS use a creative combination of qualitative and quantitative methodologies that enable the researcher to derive reliable quantitative data and, at the same time, record unique individual behavioural characteristics. The detailed attention to individual behaviours recorded in a standardised systematic format with known reliability and validity has enabled new research developments in the field of autism. In a number of other areas of child and adolescent mental health research Mike with colleagues (including George Brown, Tony Cox, Jonathon Hill, Adrian Angold and Emily Simonoff) has pioneered new diagnostic assessment instruments with many of the same strengths. These have included the Camberwell Interview (Brown & Rutter, 1966), the Adult Personality Functioning Assessment (APFA; Hill *et al*, 1989, 1995) and the Child and Adolescent Psychiatric Assessment (CAPA; Angold *et al*, 1995).

For each of these (and there are many more research assessment measures, including some developed for epidemiological screening (Rutter & Graham, 1968)), Mike's clarity of thinking and ability to link conceptual issues with actual behaviour have undoubtedly contributed to their scientific rigour and success (Cox *et al*, 1981*a,b,c*). There is no doubt that the availability of comprehensive and appropriate assessment tools has led to new research initiatives and advanced knowledge and understanding in our field.

Finally in this section I would like to consider Mike's research training and supervision style. All of his research teams are interdisciplinary. His leadership approach is that of the questioning scientist. He values independent thinking and expects autonomy and the ability to take responsibility. He is supportive and encourages reasoned argument, but he is less than tolerant of colleagues who do not show a willingness to work hard and accept criticism. He is impatient for research findings but will delay publication to rework and reconsider the accuracy or meaning of data. Despite these pressures for completion of work he has supported many of his younger colleagues (myself included) in combining career development and caring for their families – at times another reason for delay.

Under Mike's leadership the Academic Department of Child and Adolescent Psychiatry provided many opportunities to link with colleagues working in different areas of research – a reflection of Mike's breadth of experience. When first appointed as research assistant I worked alongside Barbara Maughan, David Quinton, Adrian Angold, Janet Ouston, Dale Hay, Ann Hagell and later Andrew Pickles in addition to child and adolescent psychiatry colleagues. For everyone the opportunities for innovative collaborations, exposure to tough critiques of research work, memorable presentations by visiting academics and multi-disciplinary academic journal clubs were tremendously stimulating.

Mike, incredibly busy, always seemed to have his finger on the pulse. He managed the department, steering a course through NHS and academic demands, led the research and found time to support researchers worldwide. For some (including senior academic scientists in our field) his mentorship at a distance has been invaluable, even though there may never have been a direct working relationship.

In addition to all of this, Mike has always had other national and international responsibilities. I will mention just a few.

Between 1970 and 1974 he was on the Education Research Board and later the Social Services Research Board and in the 1970s he was a member of a group studying transmitted deprivation. At that time, as a young researcher, he remembers the intellectual challenge posed by experienced committee members from various professional backgrounds, who asked probing questions about the practical implications of findings and how ideas could realistically be tested.

In 1972 he became the first chair of the Child Psychiatry Research Society. When founded this group was a society of few members devoted to peer support and advice in a small academic speciality. More recently (since 1992) Mike has been a trustee of the Nuffield Foundation and in 1996 he became a governor of the Wellcome Trust. He has been a vice-president of Young Minds since 1991. He is also on the editorial and advisory boards of many journals and book series. In this brief overview I cannot do justice to the

■ 159

number of memorial lectures, invited lectures, endowed professorships and inaugural lectures (including the Inaugural Faculty Lecture of the Royal College of Psychiatrists' Child and Adolescent Psychiatry Section; see Chapter 9) that Mike has given.

Mike has honorary degrees from universities worldwide. Among the many prestigious awards he has received are The Society for Research in Child Development Distinguished Scientist Award (1989), The American Psychological Association Distinguished Scientist Award (1995) and The Helmut Horten Foundation Research Award (1997). The award that perhaps has given Mike particular satisfaction came in 1987, when he was made a Fellow of the Royal Society. He received his knighthood in 1992.

Contribution to training and standards

Mike was the first chair of the Child and Adolescent Psychiatry Specialist Accreditation Committee (CAPSAC), which he and colleagues, in particular Lionel Hersov, were invited to set up. Throughout his career Mike has been keen to influence training standards, but he has made no secret of his concern about the limitations of rigidity in training and the need for flexibility. He emphasises the importance of freedom to learn, believing that trainees should have some responsibility for their own learning. He also taught me the need for 'protected time' to reflect on learning, clinical work and research ideas and for supervision.

Clinical work

The enduring nature of Mike's academic contributions is also a tribute to his clinical skills and the emphasis he places on clinical work. Throughout his career he has worked in both a specialist and a general clinical capacity. When he first returned from the USA in 1962 with no prior training in child and adolescent psychiatry he led his own team. He has always maintained that his skills are in assessment and diagnosis, and although he would not describe himself primarily as a therapist, he enjoys therapeutic work. His clinical style is rather similar to his approach to research – questioning and hypothesis driven. In turn his research has always been influenced by his clinical experience. With children and families Mike has an honest open approach – I always found him straightforward and confident to share both what he knew and what he was less sure about with parents and professionals alike.

The secret of his success in working in all clinical areas linked to his research topics is that he has never worked in isolation; he has always found collaborators, all with fields of specialist interest. Furthermore, he has not had to keep up any particular area of work over the long term: over the years he has assessed young lesbian couples for court reports, he has consulted to schools, and he has seen neurology and neurological referrals, children with conduct disorder, hyperactivity and so on. More recently, he has assessed a considerable number of the Romanian orphans adopted by UK families. Throughout he has maintained his long-term clinical link with autism, even though he has had less dedicated clinical time since the MRC unit opened.

Mike's clinical career has always been based at the Maudsley Hospital, although (perhaps surprisingly as the Professor of Child and Adolescent Psychiatry) he has never led the in-patient service. His out-patient work informed his research hypotheses and led to the development of some innovative community initiatives – most particularly the Home-Based Autism Service. Mike taught me the importance of continuity and long-term commitment to patients. He does not accept theory-driven practice, as he stressed in the Robina Addis Memorial Lecture Given for Young Minds (London, 1997; further details available from A.L.C. upon request). He expects a clinical multi-disciplinary team to value individual variation, regularly review diagnostic formulations in the light of clinical outcome and search for positive change.

Personal perspectives

Issy Kolvin has recently written about Mike's contribution to child mental health and interviewed him about, among other things, his creativity (Kolvin, 1999a,b). Characteristically, Mike talks about his own mentors, including Robert Cawley and Aubrey Lewis, and the skills he learnt from them. Reading the interview, I was struck by Mike's enthusiasm about what he has gained throughout his career from professionals outside of psychiatry. Mike has an insatiable appetite for new research hypotheses, further analyses and pushing beyond the existing limit to think how concepts can be tested with novel approaches. He has a restless confidence that he will be able to get there with the right expertise to assist him (his collaborations with Andrew Pickles are testament to this). Mike has a talent for knowing what should be done and ensuring that others get involved. He is fair, at times demanding, intolerant of scientific dishonesty, ruthless with his critical appraisal but, irritatingly, usually right. He thrives on debate and argument about academic matters. He describes himself as "an inveterate reader" and gets great pleasure from his hobbies. These include music, the theatre and wine-tasting. He enjoys achievement on the tennis court, and hill and mountain walking in the Lake District and abroad.

Mike has always maintained that we learn most when we are proved wrong (Rutter, 1990): the challenge is to recognise when you are wrong. In Mike's case his research findings have stood the test of time, although occasionally (for example, in his early work on autism and on the impact of behaviour on later experiences) he has needed to change research approach when it became clear that his original inferences were incorrect.

Mike has always been a loyal colleague, valuing continuity of relationships, especially as they change over time. He has also always valued his family life and the devoted support of his wife Marjorie. But for his parents, children and now grandchildren it could perhaps be seen as a mixed blessing to be related to such an eminent child psychiatrist. He maintains he does not work on holiday – but I know that he explained to Philip Graham many years ago that he sees himself as working all the time when he is not doing anything else. And when work and home do meet, he and his wife are generous hosts – at the end of collaborator meetings or training courses, many of us have benefited from extremely enjoyable and productive social functions at their home.

Mike Rutter is an example to us all of the importance of having a breadth of interest, an informed strategic vision and the ability to maximise knowledge gained through the study of natural experiments.

■ 161

For the future Mike is pleased to have given up all administrative responsibilities. In his current post as Research Professor at the Insitute of Psychiatry, he remains involved in several major pieces of research. Much of his work is at the interface of science and policy. He divides his time between his significant Wellcome Trust responsibilities (he is currently the Deputy Chairman and Chair of the Scientific Committee) and all these other activities. He is also involved in a large number of other agencies, including the Nuffield Foundation (UK), the Jacob Foundation (Switzerland) and the Novartis Foundation (London). He is a member of the National Academy of Sciences (USA).

Michael Rutter's work has made lasting contributions to our understanding of child and adolescent development and child and adolescent mental health. His work and his commitment to new research endeavours will continue to benefit a wide range of people – the international scientific and clinical communities across many different disciplines and, perhaps most important, disadvantaged and distressed children and their families worldwide.

References

Angold, A., Prendergast, M., Cox, A., *et al* (1995) The Child and Adolescent Psychiatric Assessment (CAPA). *Psychological Medicine*, **25**, 739–753.

Brown, G. W. & Rutter, M. (1966) Camberwell Interview for the measurement of family activities and relationships: a methodological study. *Human Relations*, **19**, 241–263.

Champion, L., Goodall, G. M. & Rutter, M. (1995) Behavioural problems in childhood and stressors in early adult life: a 20 year follow up of London school children. *Psychological Medicine*, **25**, 231–246.

Cox, A., Hopkinson, K. F. & Rutter, M. (1981*a*) Psychiatric interview techniques. II. Naturalistic study: eliciting factual information. *British Journal of Psychiatry*, **138**, 283–291.

——, Rutter, M. & Holbrook, D. (1981*b*) Psychiatric interview techniques. V. Experimental study: eliciting factual information. *British Journal of Psychiatry*, **139**, 29–37.

——, Holbrook, D. & Rutter, M. (1981*c*) Psychiatric interviewing techniques. VI. Experimental study: eliciting feelings. *British Journal of Psychiatry*, **139**, 144–152.

Garmezy, N. & Rutter, M. (eds) (1983) *Stress, Coping and Development*. New York: McGraw-Hill. Reprinted 1988, New York: John Hopkins University Press.

Haggerty, R. J., Sherrod, H. J., Garmezy, N., *et al* (eds) (1994) *Stress, Risk and Resilience in Children and Adolescents: Processes, Mechanisms and Interventions*. New York: Cambridge University Press.

Hill, J., Harrington, R., Fudge, H., *et al* (1989) Adult Personality Functioning Assessment (APFA). An investigator-based standardised interview. *British Journal of Psychiatry*, **155**, 24–35.

——, Fudge, H., Harrington, R., *et al* (1995) The Adult Personality Functioning Assessment (APFA): factors influencing agreement between subject and informant. *Psychological Medicine*, **25**, 263–275.

Howlin, P., Rutter, M., Berger, M., *et al* (1987) *Treatment of Autistic Children*. Chichester: John Wiley & Sons.

Jefferson, M. & Rutter, M. (1958) A report of two cases of the juvenile form of amaurotic familial idiocy (cerebromacular degeneration). *Journal of Neurology, Neurosurgery and Psychiatry*, **21**, 31–37.

Kolvin, I. (1999*a*) The contribution of Michael Rutter. *British Journal of Psychiatry*, **174**, 471–475.

—— (1999*b*) Talking with Michael Rutter. *British Journal of Psychiatry*, **174**, 494–499.

Le Couteur, A., Rutter, M., Lord, C., *et al* (1989) The Autism Diagnostic Interview – Revised (ADI–R): a standardised investigator-based instrument. *Journal of Autism and Developmental Disorders*, **19**, 363–387.

Lord, C., Rutter, M., Good, S., *et al* (1989) Autism Diagnostic Observation Schedule (ADOS): a standardised observation of communicative and social behaviour. *Journal of Autism and Developmental Disorders*, **19**, 185–212.

——, —— & Le Couteur, A. (1994) Autism Diagnostic Interview – Revised (ADI–R): a revised version of a diagnostic interview for care givers of individuals with possible pervasive developmental disorders. *Journal of Autism and Developmental Disorders*, **24**, 659–685.

——, Risi, S., Lambrecht, L., *et al* (2000) ADOS–G (Autism Diagnostic Observation Schedule (Generic)): a standard measure of social and communication deficits associated with the spectrum of autism. *Journal of Autism and Developmental Disorders*, **30**, 205–223.

Quinton, D. & Rutter, M. (1988) *Parenting Breakdown: The Making and Breaking of Intergenerational Links*. Aldershot: Avebury.

Robins, L. & Rutter, M. (eds) (1990) *Straight and Devious Pathways from Childhood to Adulthood*. New York: Cambridge University Press.

Rutter, M. (1966) *Children of Sick Parents: An Environmental and Psychiatric Study*. Maudsley Monograph No. 16. London: Institute of Psychiatry & Oxford University Press.

—— (1967) A & B scales, a children's behaviour questionnaire for completion by teachers: preliminary findings. *Journal of Child Psychology and Psychiatry*, **8**, 1–11.

—— (ed.) (1971) *Infantile Autism: Concepts, Characteristics and Treatment*. Edinburgh & London: Churchill Livingstone.

—— (1972) *Maternal Deprivation Re-assessed* (2nd edn 1981). Harmondsworth: Penguin Books.

—— (1975) *Helping Troubled Children*. Harmondsworth: Penguin Books.

—— (1990) Interface between research and clinical practice in child psychiatry – some personal reflection: discussion paper. *Journal of the Royal Society of Medicine*, **83**, 444–447.

—— & Giller, H. (1983) *Juvenile Delinquency: Trends and Perspectives*. Harmondsworth: Penguin Books.

—— & Graham, P. (1968) The reliability and validity of psychiatric assessment of the child. Interviewing the parents. *British Journal of Psychiatry*, **114**, 563–579.

—— & Hersov, L. (eds) (1977) *Child and Adolescent Psychiatry: Modern Approaches* (3rd edn 1994). Oxford: Blackwell Science.

—— & Quinton, D. (1984) Parental psychiatric disorder: effects on children. *Psychological Medicine*, **14**, 853–880.

—— & —— (1987) Parental mental illness as a risk factor for psychiatric disorders in childhood. In *Psychopathology: An Interactional Perspective* (eds. D. Magnusson & A. Ohman), pp. 199–219. Orlando, FL: Academic Press.

—— & Rutter, M. (1993) *Developing Minds: Challenge and Continuity Across the Life Span*. Harmondsworth & New York: Penguin Books & Basic Books.

——, Korn, S. & Birch, H. G. (1963) Genetic and environmental factors in the development of 'primary reaction patterns'. *British Journal of Social and Clinical Psychology*, **2**, 161–173.

——, Graham, P. & Yule, W. (1970*a*) *A Neuropsychiatric Study in Childhood*. Clinics in Developmental Medicine 35/36. London: Heineman/SIMP.

——, Tizard, J. & Whitmore, K. (eds) (1970*b*) *Education, Health and Behaviour*. Reprinted 1981. London: Longman. Reprinted 1981.

——, Schaffer, D. & Sturge, C. (1975*a*) *A Guide to a Multi-Axial Classification Scheme for Psychiatric Disorders in Childhood and Adolescence*. London: Institute of Psychiatry.

——, Cox, A., Tupling, C., *et al* (1975*b*) Attainment and adjustment in two geographical areas. I. The prevalence of psychiatric disorder. *British Journal of Psychiatry*, **126**, 493–509.

——, Yule, B., Quinton, D., *et al* (1975*c*) Attainment and adjustment in two geographical areas. III. Some factors accounting for area differences. *British Journal of Psychiatry*, **126**, 520–533.

——, Maughan, B., Mortimer, P., *et al* (1979) *15,000 hours: Secondary Schools and their Effects on Children*. London & Cambridge, MA: Open Books & Harvard University Press. Reprinted 1994, London: Paul Chapman Publishers.

Taylor, E. & Green, J. (eds) (2001) *Research and Innovation on the Road to Modern Child Psychiatry. Vol. 2. Classic Papers by Professor Sir Michael Rutter*, Appendix. London: Gaskell.

World Health Organization (1977) *Child Mental Health and Psychosocial Development: Report of a WHO Expert Committee*. Technical Report Series 613. Geneva: WHO.

—— (1992) *Manual of the International Statistical Classification of Diseases, Injuries and Causes of Death* (10th revision) (ICD–10). Geneva: WHO.

Index

Compiled by Caroline Sheard

accentuation effects 140
ADHD *see* attention-deficit hyperactivity disorder
ADI–R 96, 159
adoption studies 143–4
ADOS 59, 96, 159
adult attachment interview 139
Adult Personality Functioning Assessment 159
adult relationships, factors affecting 12–13
adulthood, transition to 10–13
adversity
    animal studies 132
    childhood, and adult functioning 5–6
    psychosocial, and child psychopathology 129–52
affective disorder
    genetic factors 23–5
    twin studies 24–5
Aitken, William 105–6
Angelmann syndrome 86
anorexia nervosa, genetic factors 23
antisocial behaviour
    and age at first partnership 10–11
    age at onset 8–9
    association with depressed mood in adult life 11–12
    cohort effect 118–19
    developmental trends 4
    genetic factors 27
    and psychosocial adversity 137–8
anxiety disorders
    comorbidity with depression 8
    developmental trends 4
APFD 159
Aristotle 38, 104
Asperger's syndrome 60, 67, 95, 97, 99
assortative mating 12
attachment security 134
attachment theory 12
attention-deficit hyperactivity disorder (ADHD)
    animal models 85
    and birth season 86

genetic factors 23, 25–7
    moderating and mediating factors 31–2
    neuroimaging 90
    transition to conduct disorder 86
    twin studies 25–6
autism
    aetiology
        1950s and 1960s 59
        1970s to mid-1980s 62–3
        late 1980s to early 1990s 64–7
        late 1990s 70–1
    animal models 98
    associations 65, 66, 67, 71, 96, 99–100
    behavioural research 100
    broader phenotype 65–6
    developmental trends 4
    diagnosis and delineation
        1950s and 1960s 56
        1970s to mid-1980s 59–60
        late 1980s to early 1990s 67–8
        late 1990s 71
        research 93–6
    first delineation of syndrome 55–6
    genetic factors 23, 25, 62–3, 64–6, 67, 70, 71, 96–7
    interplay between research and clinical practice 54–80
    interventions 98–100
        1950s and 1960s 58–9
        1970s to mid-1980s 63–4
        late 1980s to early 1990s 69–70
        late 1990s 72
    nature of the disorder
        1950s and 1960s 56–8
        1970s to mid-1980s 60–2
        late 1980s to early 1990s 68–9
        late 1990s 71
    neurobiology 96, 97–8
    neuroimaging 71, 98
    neuropathology 98
    post-mortem studies 70–1

research 93–103
Rutter's work 155, 157–8
standardised assessments 59, 96, 159
twin studies 25, 62, 64–5, 71, 96
Autism Diagnostic Interview – Revised 96, 159
Autism Diagnostic Observation Schedule 59, 96, 159

behavioural phenotypes 87–8
behavioural therapy in autism 58
behaviourism 131
Bellevue Hospital Nomenclature 107
Birch, Herb 153
birth trauma 89
'brain damage syndrome' 81
brain dysfunction 81–92
brain injury
at birth 89
postnatal 89

Camberwell interview 133, 154, 159
CAPA 159
CAPSAC 160
CARS 59
categorisation *see* classification
cerebellum in autism 98
change, mediation of 9
Chess, Stella 20, 153
Child and Adolescent Psychiatric Assessment 159
Child and Adolescent Psychiatry Specialist Accreditation
Committee 160
Child Psychiatry Research Society 159
child-rearing practices 131–2
Childhood Autism Rating Scale 59
childhood disintegrative disorders 95
classification
1700 to 1900 105–7
1900 to date 107–12
classical beginnings 104
the future 112
Rutter's work 156
cognitive tests in autism 57
cohort studies on psychosocial adversity 134
Colorado Family Reading study 28–9
comorbidity 112
conduct disorder and depression 7–8
competence, adolescent 12
conduct disorder 112
consequences 119–22
co-occurrence with depression 7–8
developmental trends 4
genetic factors 27–8
increasing prevalence 115–28
as predictor of early substance use 123–4
retrospective studies 117–18
sequelae 5
stable predictors and consequences 115–16
study design and cohort effects 116–19
and substance misuse 122–5
twin studies 27
and violence 119–21
congenital hypothyroidism 88–9
continuity of disorder, homotypic/heterotypic 4
Cullen, William 105
culture and developmental psychopathology 44
cumulative continuity processes 13

DAMP 96
Darwin, Erasmus 105
de Sauvages, B. 105
deficits in attention, motor control and
perception 96
depression
comorbidity with anxiety 8
comorbidity with conduct disorder 7–8
developmental trends 4
heterogeneity of category 7
development
distinction between normal and abnormal 40–2
diversity in process and outcome 42
developmental neurobiology 83–5
developmental neuropsychiatry 81–92, 155
developmental psychopathology 37–53
cultural and contextual influences 44
definitions 39–40
future directions 48–9
implications for practice 45–8
principles 40–4
research methods 45
developmental studies in psychosocial adversity 130
developmental trends in disorder 2–4, 7
deviant behaviour and peer relations 10
Diagnostic and Statistical Manual
conduct disorder 116, 117
DSM–I 108
DSM–II 108
DSM–III 109–10
autism 94
DSM–III–R 110, 111
autism 94, 95
DSM–IV 110–12
autism 93, 94–5
disintegrative psychosis 95
disorder
childhood prevalence 81, 82
developmental trends 2–4, 7
heterogeneity in categorisations 7–9
time trends 141
disruptive behavioural problems
age at onset 8–9
sequelae 4–5
dopamine receptors
and attention-deficit hyperactivity disorder 26
development 84
Dunedin Multidisciplinary Study of Health and
Development 2–3

ECA project 117–18, 118–19, 120, 121, 122, 123
echolalia 100
education 155, 157
emotional problems, sequelae 5
environment
correlation and interaction with genetic factors 143
mediation of risk by 143–4
models of influence 30–2
selection and shaping 9–13
shared/non-shared 20, 22, 140, 143, 144
Epidemiologic Catchment Area project 117–18, 118–19,
120, 121, 122, 123
epilepsy, association with autism 56, 57, 71
equifinality 42
evidence-based medicine 54

facilitated communication in autism 69–70
false belief test 62
families
    interview measures 133
    observational measures 133
Farr, William 106, 107
fenfluramine 64
follow-back analysis 4
fragile-X anomaly 60, 62, 67, 71, 86, 96

genetics
    affective disorder 23–5
    anorexia nervosa 23
    Asperger's syndrome 97
    attention-deficit hyperactivity disorder 23, 25–7
    autism 23, 25, 62–3, 64–6, 67, 70, 71, 96–7
    conduct disorder 27–8
    correlation and interaction with environment 143
    and developmental neuropsychiatry 83
    evidence for effects on behaviour 22–3
    investigation and theories in child psychiatry research 20–1
    models of influence 30–2
    obsessive–compulsive disorder 23
    and psychopathology 140–1, 144
    quantitative research 22–3
    reading disability 28–30
    Tourette's syndrome 23
geographical area and psychosocial adversity 135–6, 142–3
Good, J.M. 105, 106
Gouley, John 106–7

haloperidol in autism 99
head injury, postnatal 89
Heller's syndrome 95
hemiplegia 87
heritability estimates 22–3
hippocampus, developmental abnormalities 83–4
Hippocrates 104
hypoglycaemia, neonatal 89
hypothyroidism, congenital 88–9

idiot-savant 69
ILCD 107
indirect chain mechanisms 13
infantile psychosis see autism
Institute of Medicine, Research on Children and Adolescents with Mental, Behavioral and Developmental Disorders 37, 39
internal working models 138–9
International Classification of Diseases 107, 156
    ICD–8 108
    ICD–9 109
    ICD–10 111–12
        autism 93, 95
International List of Causes of Death 107
IQ tests in autism 60–1
    as predictors of outcome 57
    score patterns 56
Isle of Wight study 1, 20, 22, 116–17, 154

Jack Tizard Memorial Lecture 1, 9
juvenile delinquency 157
    and relations with behaviourally deviant peers 10

language
    deficit in autism 56, 57, 60

effect of brain lesions 87
lateralised syndromes 87
learning disability, differentiation from autism 57
Lesch–Nyhan syndrome 88
life events
    active processing 138
    and affective disorder 24
    and psychosocial adversity 136, 142
longitudinal studies 1–19
    prospective use 3, 4, 6
    on psychosocial adversity 130
    retrospective use 2–3, 4, 5–6

macrogyria in autism 98
marginalisation 13
marital status
    influence on offending 14
    and psychiatric morbidity 12
maternal deprivation 131, 134, 155–6
mental hygiene movement 129
metabolic disorders 88–9
minimal brain dysfunction 81–2, 86
mouse, hippocampus abnormalities 83–4
multifinality 42
multiple complex developmental disorder 96
multiplex disorder 96

National Autistic Society 58
National Comorbidity Study 117–18, 119
National Institute of Mental Health, National Plan for Research on Child and Adolescent Mental Disorders 37
NCS 117–18, 119
neonatal hypoglycaemia 89
neural plate 83
neural tube 83
neuroimaging 85, 90
    attention-deficit hyperactivity disorder 90
    autism 71, 98
neuronal development 83–5
New York State longitudinal study 8
Nomenclature of Diseases and Conditions 107
novelty-seeking behaviour 26

obsessive–compulsive disorder, genetic factors 23
offending
    influences of family characteristics and early behaviour 21–2
    influences on 14

parenting 157–8
parents
    effects of children on 133
    mental disorder 134, 155
Parr, B. 105
PDDs 94, 95–6, 97, 111
peer relationships
    and deviant behaviour 10
    and psychosocial adversity 135
    and resilience 132
perinatal abnormalities 85
personality disorder, childhood precursors 4
pervasive developmental disorders 94, 95–6, 97, 111
phenylketonuria (PKU) 88
'planning' tendency 138
Plato 38

■ 165

polymicrogyria in autism 98
Prader–Willi syndrome 86
psychoanalysis and psychosocial adversity 129–30
psychological phenotypes 87–8
psychopathology
    developmental *see* developmental psychopathology
    and psychosocial adversity 129–52
psychosocial adversity
    animal studies 132
    and child psychopathology 129–52
    testing causal hypotheses 139–40

RDC 109
reading disability
    genetic factors 28–30
    twin studies 28–9
research 54–5
    on autism 93–103
Research Diagnostic Criteria 109
residential care and psychosocial adversity 135
resilience 49, 142, 158
    and developmental psychopathology 43–4
    and peer relationships 132
retrospective recall, problems with 133
retrospective studies 2–3, 4, 5–6
    conduct disorder 117–18
Rett's syndrome 59–60, 62, 95
'right-hemisphere syndrome' 87
risk 158
    distal and proximal processes 137
    environmental mediation 143–4
    indicators and mechanisms 134
    and multi-factorial causation 142
    operational model of factors 31
    psychosocial 134, 134–5
risperidone in autism 99
ritualistic and compulsive phenomena in autism 56
Robbers' Cave experiments 132
Rutter, Michael
    biography 153–5
    clinical work 160
    contribution to training and standards in child and
        adolescent psychiatry 160
    publications 155–8
    research themes 158–60
    work on classification and categorisation in child
        psychiatry 108–9
    work on genetic factors in child pychiatric disorder 20–1

Schedule of Handicaps, Behaviors and Skills 59
schizophrenia
    developmental trends 4
    differentiation from autism 57–8, 94
schizophrenic syndrome of childhood *see* autism
schooling 155, 157
    and psychosocial adversity 135
self-organisation and developmental psychopathology 42–3
separation, parent–child 131, 134
sequelae of childhood disorder 4–5
serotonin in autism 64
sexual abuse, adverse adult outcomes 6
Smith–Magenis syndrome 88
social exclusion 13
social groups and psychosocial adversity 132
social relationships
    failure to develop in autism 56
    and psychosocial adversity 134–5
South London Urban Comparison study 154
stepping-stone effects 13
Stress, Coping and Development Group 154, 157
substance misuse
    age at first exposure as predictor 122, 123
    cohort effect 118–19
    and conduct disorder 122–5

TEACCH programme 63
theory of mind and autism 62, 68–9, 98
Thomas, Alex 20, 153
Tizard, Jack 154
Tourette's syndrome, genetic factors 23
transitions, early-adult 10–13
tuberose sclerosis and autism 67, 71, 96
turning-point effects 13–14, 140
twin studies 22–3
    affective disorder 24–5
    attention-deficit hyperactivity disorder 25–6
    autism 25, 62, 64–5, 71, 96
    conduct disorder 27
    psychosocial adversity 144
    reading disability 28–9

violence and conduct disorder 119–21
vitamin B6 in autism 64
vulnerability factors 137

Waltham Forest study 21
Williams' syndrome 88